EMERGING VIRUSES

EMERGING VIRUSES

Edited by

Stephen S. Morse
The Rockefeller University

New York   Oxford
OXFORD UNIVERSITY PRESS

Oxford University Press

Oxford   New York
Athens   Auckland   Bangkok   Bombay
Calcutta   Cape Town   Dar es Salaam   Delhi
Florence   Hong Kong   Istanbul   Karachi
Kuala Lumpur   Madras   Madrid   Melbourne
Mexico City   Nairobi   Paris   Singapore
Taipei   Tokyo   Toronto

and associated companies in
Berlin   Ibadan

Copyright © 1993 by Oxford University Press, Inc.

First published in 1993 by Oxford University Press, Inc.,
198 Madison Avenue, New York, New York 10016

First issued as an Oxford University Press paperback, 1996.

Oxford is a registered trademark of Oxford University Press

Library of Congress Cataloging-in-Publication Data
Emerging viruses / edited by Stephen S. Morse.
p.   cm.   Includes bibliographical references and index.
ISBN 0-19-507444-0
ISBN 0-19-510484-6 (Pbk.)
1. Virus diseases—Epidemiology.
[DNLM: 1.   Disease Outbreaks.   2. Virus Diseases
3. Viruses.   WC 500 E53]
RA644. V55E44   1993
616'.0194—dc20
DNLM/DLC   91-39612
for Library of Congress

9 8

Printed in the United States of America
on acid-free paper

Acknowledgments

First of all, my sincere thanks to the authors in this volume for all their generosity of spirit, hard work, and enthusiasm. I am grateful for the generous help of many colleagues and collaborators whose knowledge and insight are matched by their kindness and patience. Many of these exemplary souls appear as authors in this book, but I would like to mention some whose indispensable role might not otherwise be known.

I owe a special and great debt of gratitude to John R. La Montagne, Director, Division of Microbiology & Infectious Diseases of the National Institute of Allergy and Infectious Diseases, National Institutes of Health, my colleague in planning the Emerging Viruses conference, whose enthusiastic support, clear vision, and incisive suggestions during planning made this work possible in the first place, and without whose enthusiasm and interest none of this could have happened; to Ann Schluederberg, Chief, Virology Branch, Division of Microbiology & Infectious Diseases, whose intelligent good humor and clear prose are only two of the exemplary qualities that made her a pleasure to work with; and to Joshua Lederberg, an esteemed colleague and friend, who first got me interested in emerging viruses.

My own research is supported by the National Institutes of Health. For valuable discussions and special help on various aspects of emerging viruses, I am especially indebted (in alphabetical order, noting that these names are in addition to the authors in this volume, and apologizing to those I have inadvertently omitted) to Baruch Blumberg, Pravin Bhatt, S. Gaylen Bradley, Merrill W. Chase, Sheldon Cohen, Paul J. Edelson, Daniel M. Fox, Mirko Grmek, the late Edward H. Kass, Luc Montagnier, Walter Parham, Edward Tenner, and Emily Wilkinson. I thank Elizabeth Osborne at *The New Yorker* for locating a reference. Kirk Jensen, Senior Editor at Oxford University Press, offered valued encouragement and practical assistance. For design and typography, for the Index, and for the figure in Chapter 1, I am grateful to Margaret Ryon at The Rockefeller University Media Resources Department. My wife, Marilyn Gewirtz, deserves more than whatever thanks I can give her here. She has been a true collaborator, whose perceptive questions and suggestions have been invaluable at every step.

Preface

From AIDS and influenza to smallpox and zoster (shingles), many of the deadliest and most feared diseases—as well as some of the most common—have been viral. AIDS and influenza also typify an especially alarming aspect: the emergence of "new" diseases, often manifested explosively as epidemics. Throughout history and up to the present, such events seem to descend suddenly and unpredictably, appearing as vengeful and capricious natural disasters.

Despite the obvious importance of such events to our lives, the reasons for viral emergence have rarely, if ever, been systematically explored. There have been no books addressing this question for either the scientifically literate general reader or the specialist. This book is an attempt to fill that gap. The contributing authors to this volume are authorities in their areas who were selected both for their expert knowledge and for their ability to define and elucidate the fundamental issues (and sometimes to be provocative). They have aimed at an accurate and accessible brief review of some representative viruses and what is known about the factors responsible for their emergence, including mechanisms of evolution. The hope is thereby to encourage further thinking about this question, and to inform the reader (whether a scientist or social scientist in one of the fields represented here, a scientific generalist, or a general reader possessing a basic biomedical vocabulary), who may be daunted by the "new" diseases that now seem to appear in the news on a regular basis, and would like to know what lies behind them.

I believe that finding answers to the questions posed by emerging viruses requires attacking the problem from several different perspectives, often crossing disciplinary lines. Of course, some aspects are better understood or have been more thoroughly studied than others, but I feel it essential to represent the state of knowledge in each of these areas, even though some sections of the book may as a result seem to have a more tentative or descriptive quality than others. In science, stories are rarely complete, if ever, and an appreciation of the scientific process is valuable in itself. It is also useful in order to show where more information is needed.

This diversity of approaches also gives rise to a diversity of vocabulary, level of detail, and style in the various chapters. While many chapters presuppose some familiarity with biomedical terminology and basic concepts of molecular biology and immunology, an attempt has been made to accommodate those less fluent by briefly defining some of these terms in parentheses wherever feasible. While this will seem unnecessary and repetitive to technical readers, I hope it will encourage those who might otherwise find the subject matter intimidating. Many of the methods used for studying viruses, and associated terms, are also described in Richman's chapter.

In attacking the problem of emerging viruses, scientific knowledge of the agents is essential, and the recent flowering of molecular biology and molecular genetics has provided powerful tools for analyzing and tracking viruses, and is yielding fresh insights into viral evolution. But viruses are of necessity dependent on their hosts, requiring us to have an appreciation of the factors that may influence the interaction of a virus with a host. Although many of these factors are molecular or cellular, when the host is human, social factors can play a very significant role in both dissemination and expression of disease. On a larger scale, many epidemics can be understood only in their ecological context.

Despite our wish to anticipate emerging diseases, we cannot foretell the future. What we can do is to draw the best inferences possible from past experience; for this, history can be a valuable guide. The opening five chapters place emerging viruses within a framework of both history and natural history, from several different vantage points. Themes introduced in these chapters will recur throughout the book. Some readers may prefer to read the subsequent chapters in an order dictated by their own personal interests and background. For them, the book has been organized into sections and connecting material added where necessary to allow most chapters to be read independently.

At the outset, the problem of emerging viruses may seem too vast and too amorphous to tackle. That is probably why it has remained largely unexamined in the past. However, as I discuss in Chapter 2, there are often identifiable causes—such as the role of human activities in the environment—that underlie most episodes of viral emergence. A conceptual framework for infectious disease emergence is formulated, and evidence is presented for a unifying hypothesis of the origins of epidemics. William McNeill examines both what history teaches us about new diseases, and the limitations of the historical record. The remaining chapters of this section provide overviews of two types of diseases that often make the news: influenza, familiar but still dangerous, and viruses that cause hemorrhagic fevers, a mixed bag of disparate viruses with remarkable similarities in their natural history and pathogenesis.

Viruses are especially important to us because of their effects on us as their hosts. The unique dependence of viruses on living cells makes their relationship with the host an essential factor in their behavior. This theme is introduced in Chapter 1 by Lederberg, who states "the very essence of the virus is its fundamental entanglement with the genetic and metabolic machinery of the host." The three chapters by May, Fields, and Shenk expand upon the interrelationship between virus and host, moving in descending scale from ecosystem (May) to subcellular (Shenk). Interactions at the whole organism level, which include important constraints on viruses, are analyzed by Fields.

Because what we can study is necessarily determined by the tools available, methods for detecting viruses—for seeing the unseen—are of great importance. Many "new" viruses are only newly recognized. Recently developed techniques, such as PCR (the polymerase chain reaction) for amplifying DNA sequences, are making it possible to search for viruses that have been undetectable until now. Using HIV as the main example, Richman considers available methods, including PCR, while Ward discusses some developing technologies, such as confocal microscopy and new light-emitting compounds, that allow precise visualization of viral genetic sequences inside the cell, or more sensitive detection of viral components.

Armed with these tools to study viruses, we now turn to the very large question of what constitutes an emerging virus and where emerging viruses come from. Viruses have no locomotion, yet many of them have traveled around the world. Shope and Evans consider this essential process in viral emergence, giving several examples to illustrate their analysis. The subsequent chapters describe individual examples of emerging viruses. In general (as is discussed elsewhere in the book, and surveyed in Chapter 2), most epidemics are caused by existing viruses acquiring new hosts. The worldwide epidemic of HIV infection and the acquired immune deficiency syndrome (AIDS) is, of course, the major emerging viral threat. The origins of HIV have been the subject of considerable debate, and are still unresolved. The chapter by Myers and colleagues discusses current views of how HIV originated and evolved and illustrates how the tools of molecular biology can help to track the origins and spread of HIV. Other viruses may be introduced to humans in various ways, including by mosquitoes and other arthropods (described and analyzed in the chapter by Monath), or from contact with rodents (LeDuc and colleagues) or other vertebrates (Peters and colleagues); the chapter by Fenner on monkeypox is another specific example. Many "emerging viruses" have crossed species lines, only to appear suddenly in a new species (including man). However, as many of these instances are recognized only long after the fact, such interspecies transfers have been difficult to study and some key steps must usually be inferred. In a few instances, it has been possible to study this process as it was occurring or soon after it began. A selection from the most instructive recent examples, involving three different species, is presented here by Fenner, Mahy, and Parrish. Fenner describes human monkeypox, an interspecies transfer to humans which many feared would replace smallpox after that virus was eradicated, and discusses why monkeypox is not likely to become a threat to human health. Mahy and Parrish begin with the startling initial observations that brought these new diseases to notice (dead seals washing up on the British shore, puppies dying of a disease that "turns their hearts to sponges"), go on to describe how the responsible virus was identified, and then discuss how techniques of molecular biology were used to study the new virus and define its relationships to known viruses. Both are interesting glimpses into viruses that have emerged in populations of nonhuman species.

The last 10 chapters involve possible futures, first from the vantage point of the virus and then from our point of view as a species. The genetic plasticity and variability of many viruses has often been remarked on, and six chapters on mutation and evolution (by Holland, Temin, Palese, Murphy, and Strauss, and on evolutionary relationships between mosquitoes and viruses by Eldridge) explore molecular mechanisms responsible for viral variation and some possible implications for the evolution of "new" viruses. Holland demonstrates, and subsequent chapters emphasize, that viruses are not static and new variants often arise. This general tendency of genetic sequences to show variability is especially pronounced in many viruses. Largely because of HIV, retroviruses have received particular attention recently. Their great genetic plasticity, and issues raised by this variation, are considered by Temin. This discussion of retroviral variation and the earlier chapter by Myers and colleagues also complement each other. Palese examines influenza, another virus that typifies constant variation, and offers some comparisons of mutation rates for different RNA viruses. On the other hand, as Brian Murphy explores in the case of influenza, even at this level, the host imposes powerful constraints on viral evolution. (Other constraints imposed by the host are discussed by Fields earlier in the book.) Considering another mechanism of genetic plasticity, evidence for actual genetic rearrangements in RNA viruses is reviewed by Strauss. Finally, Eldridge considers how identifying the associations between particular mosquitoes and specific viruses can possibly shed light on the evolutionary origins of both.

If any of this knowledge is to be of value in preventing future tragedies, it must lead to appropriate action. Ultimately, human actions underlie many episodes of disease emergence, and our own influence and responsibility may therefore be greater than we usually suppose. The closing chapters (Lovejoy, Legters and colleagues, and Henderson) address the future from the ecological perspective (some possible scenarios of environmental change described by Lovejoy), and the practical. The chapter by Legters and colleagues is written in the form of a news story. (The episode, while fictitious, is loosely modeled on an actual—and devastating—1976 Ebola epidemic in Africa.) They question whether we have the resources to deal with a major foreign epidemic. Henderson, who directed the successful world program to eradicate smallpox (he is now Associate Director for Life Sciences in the White House Office of Science & Technology Policy), then analyzes existing warning systems and offers his suggestions for an international disease surveillance system that could make a significant difference—at a surprisingly modest cost. The final chapter, by Edwin Kilbourne, a pioneer in influenza vaccine development, is a short reprise of the opening chapters, readdressing and summarizing the major questions from his personal perspective.

This book does not attempt to be all-inclusive. Rather than aiming at an encyclopedic approach, the emphasis is on trying to elucidate some of the salient characteristics and underlying mechanisms of emerging diseases and how this might inform strategies for their control. To some extent, this involves comparative and "case study" approaches. It is hoped that this organization of the book will help to provide a framework for analyzing other examples, including other known viruses as well as viruses that may come to light in the future.

Although it has evolved considerably since then, this volume has its own origins in a conference, "Emerging Viruses: The Evolution of Viruses and Viral Diseases", sponsored by the Division of Microbiology & Infectious Diseases of the National Institute of Allergy and Infectious Diseases and the Fogarty International Center of the National Institutes of Health in cooperation with The Rockefeller University, and held in Washington, D.C., in May 1989 under the chairmanship of the Editor. As many of the authors in this volume were speakers at that meeting, the first to consider the question of emerging viruses, I hope that the book provides a useful record, but I also hope that this book goes beyond that. Chapters have been rewritten for this volume, some subjects not represented at the conference have been added, and the content has been revised (to 1991, and where possible updated while the book was in press in 1992). It is encouraging to see the exploration that led to this book also continuing on several fronts as this book was going to press, in the form of activities such as a Committee on Emerging Microbial Threats to Health convened in 1991 by the Institute of Medicine of the National Academy of Sciences in order to further address these questions at the policy level.

The subject of emerging infectious diseases and the origins of plagues is a vast one, spanning the biomedical sciences, molecular biology, medicine, history, and the social sciences, and its study is newly begun. It is hoped that this volume may help to answer some questions about emerging viruses, and to stimulate further exploration.

New York   S.S.M.
May 1992

Contents

HOW VIRUSES EVOLVE:
VARIATION AND EVOLUTION OF RNA VIRUSES

PROSPECTS FOR THE FUTURE

Foreword

"Science knows no country because it is the light that illuminates the world."
—Pasteur

Like science, emerging viruses know no country. There are no barriers to prevent their migration across international boundaries or around the 24 time zones.

The light of science must be focused on those forces that propel the emergence and migration of virus diseases. These events stem from attributes of microbes—either old ones that reemerge in new settings or new mutations that arise from the old. Numerous examples of epidemics that occurred as a consequence of these changes will be cited in the chapters that follow. There are, however, other forces at play: social and economic change, changes in human behavior such as sexual practices, and catastrophic events such as war and famine that result in mass migration of armies and refugees. Microbes thrive in these "undercurrents of opportunity" that arise through social and economic change, changes in human behavior, and catastrophic events such as war and famine. They may fan a minor outbreak into a widespread epidemic. One result of the turbulence of World War I, for example, was the spread of malaria in Europe as far north as Archangel above the Arctic Circle. The ancient Mediterraneans said that malaria flees before the plow. We might well add, it returns on the wings of war. The influence of factors such as these on the course of epidemics of viral diseases will also be discussed in the following chapters.

The microbial world is a boisterous place, and recent undercurrents of opportunity have occurred as this book goes to press. The current epidemic of cholera in South America was propelled by the consequences of progressive poverty and unsanitary dietary habits. And since Desert Storm and its aftermath, diarrheal diseases and respiratory infections in infants and children have reemerged with a vengeance in the Tigris-Euphrates Valley. The World Health Organization warns that the number of deaths will be in the thousands.

Can the chronicle of such events be foretold? Efforts to predict an epidemic and prepare to forestall it came to a head in 1975 with the occurrence of "swine flu" in a small number of soldiers at Fort Dix, New Jersey. Serologic evidence suggested that the virus isolated from these patients had the same antigenic components as the flu virus that caused the pandemic of 1918. One or two unexpected deaths among those infected heightened the anxiety.

To forestall the possible repetition of the 1918 catastrophe, within 9 months a specially formulated vaccine was mass produced and millions of Americans were immunized. For whatever reason, "swine flu" did not go global. The same can be said for Ebola virus infection. While deadly localized outbreaks occurred in Africa, it too failed to go global. But AIDS did do so. This poses the practical question: Do strategies exist to anticipate, detect, and then prevent future epidemics due to new viruses or the reemergence of old ones? Can we devise countermeasures to forestall the emergence of new plagues? These are among the issues to be addressed in this book.

All of these matters on emerging viruses are much more thoroughly reviewed here than I was able to do in a book published in 1981, *The Restless Tide: The Persistent Challenge of the Microbial World* (Washington, DC: National Foundation for Infectious Diseases). It was my purpose to inform the general public and the U.S. Government that the threat of epidemics was real and that it would persist. I warned that we had become complacent about such threats because of the success of antibiotics for the treatment of common pyogenic infections, and the success of vaccines for the prevention of common childhood virus infections such as polio, rubella, and measles. But this general optimism, I cautioned, overlooked the alarms offstage— the rising tide of antibiotic resistance among microbes; the undaunting genetic drift of microbes in the evolutionary stream; and modifications of life style, commerce, agriculture, and war.

My book was, at best, a small factor that led to public and scientific recognition in the last 10 years that infectious diseases are a persistent challenge. Rather, it was microbial mischief that attracted attention. They conspired with the changing circumstances of our times and fomented a succession of unexpected events— epidemics of genital herpes, Legionnaire's disease, toxic-shock syndrome, Lyme disease, and a surge in malaria that circled the globe. And then came AIDS. All of these events were widely reported in the popular press. "Has something new occurred?", asked Congressman Joseph Early during House Appropriation hearings for the National Institute of Allergy and Infectious Diseases in 1982. "Why do we have so many new infectious diseases?" "No", I said, "nothing new has happened. Plagues are as certain as death and taxes." They will arrive with the spread of insect vectors into new locales or as a consequence of migration of peoples. Plagues occur in the wake of social and economic changes in crowded urban centers, or as a consequence of new population patterns in rural areas where jungles and primeval forests collide with cropland.

Sophisticated surveillance with clinical, diagnostic, and epidemiological components on an international scale will be required to make a plausible prediction about future epidemics and to take corrective action before a disaster actually occurs. The effort must be broadly based: laboratory research on viruses and virus infections and the immune response to them using modern techniques of molecular biology and immunology; clinical research on pathogenesis; and field research on the etiology, epidemiology, and natural history of infections and the ecology of insect vectors. To be successful, an effort of this complexity must be dominated by a *central concern* to curtail the nationwide, indeed worldwide, proliferation of an epidemic from an unexpected origin. The work in this volume is an important step in that direction.

Richard M. Krause
National Institutes of Health

Contributors

Linda H. Brink
Countway Library of Medicine
Harvard Medical School
Boston, Massachusetts

J.E. Childs
Department of Immunology and
   Infectious Diseases
The Johns Hopkins University School
   of Hygiene and Public Health
Baltimore, Maryland

Bruce F. Eldridge
Professor and Director
Mosquito Research Program
Department of Entomology
University of California, Davis

Alfred S. Evans, M.D., M.P.H.
John Rodman Paul Professor of
   Epidemiology, Emeritus
Yale University School of Medicine
New Haven, Connecticut

Frank Fenner, M.D., F.R.S.
John Curtin School of Medical
   Research
The Australian National University
Canberra City, Australia

Bernard N. Fields, M.D.
Adele Lehman Professor and
   Chairman
Department of Microbiology &
   Molecular Genetics
Harvard Medical School
Boston, Massachusetts

G.E. Glass
Department of Immunology and
   Infectious Diseases
The Johns Hopkins University School
   of Hygiene and Public Health
Baltimore, Maryland

W. Hall
Pathology Division
U.S. Army Medical Research
   Institute of Infectious Diseases
Fort Detrick, Frederick, Maryland

Hon. D.A. Henderson, M.D., M.P.H.
Associate Director for Life Sciences
Office of Science and Technology
   Policy
Executive Office of the President
Washington, D.C.

John J. Holland
Professor, Institute for Molecular
   Genetics, and Department of
   Biology
University of California, San Diego

N. Jaax
Pathology Division
U.S. Army Medical Research
   Institute of Infectious Diseases
Fort Detrick, Frederick, Maryland

P.B. Jahrling
Disease Assessment Division
U.S. Army Medical Research
   Institute of Infectious Diseases
Fort Detrick, Frederick, Maryland

E.D. Johnson
Disease Assessment Division
U.S. Army Medical Research
   Institute of Infectious Diseases
Fort Detrick, Frederick, Maryland

Karl M. Johnson, M.D.
Rockville, Maryland

Edwin D. Kilbourne, M.D.
Distinguished Service Professor
   of Microbiology
Mt. Sinai School of Medicine
New York, New York

Richard M. Krause, M.D.
Senior Scientific Adviser
Fogarty International Center
National Institutes of Health
Bethesda, Maryland

T.G. Ksiazek
Special Pathogens Branch, Division of
    Viral & Rickettsial Diseases
National Center for Infectious
    Diseases
Centers for Disease Control
Atlanta, Georgia

Joshua Lederberg
President Emeritus and
    University Professor
The Rockefeller University
New York, New York

James W. LeDuc
World Health Organization
Geneva

Llewellyn J. Legters, M.D., M.P.H.
Professor and Chair, Department
    of Preventive Medicine and
    Biometrics
Uniformed Services University of
    the Health Sciences
Bethesda, Maryland

Thomas E. Lovejoy
Assistant Secretary for External
    Affairs
The Smithsonian Institution
Washington, D.C.

Kersti MacInnes
HIV Sequence Database and
    Analysis Unit
Theoretical Division, Los Alamos
    National Laboratory
Los Alamos, New Mexico

William H. McNeill
Professor of History Emeritus
University of Chicago

Brian W.F. Mahy
Director, Division of Viral &
    Rickettsial Diseases
National Center for Infectious
    Diseases
Centers for Disease Control
Atlanta, Georgia

Robert M. May, F.R.S.
Royal Society Professor
Department of Zoology
Oxford University

Thomas P. Monath, M.D.
Ora Vax, Inc.
Cambridge, Massachusetts

Stephen S. Morse
Assistant Professor
The Rockefeller University
New York, New York

Brian R. Murphy
Chief, Respiratory Viruses
    Section
Laboratory of Infectious Diseases
National Institute of Allergy and
    Infectious Diseases
National Institutes of Health
Bethesda, Maryland

Gerald Myers
Director, HIV Sequence Database
    and Analysis Unit
Theoretical Division, Los Alamos
    National Laboratory
Los Alamos, New Mexico

Lynda Myers
St. Johns College
Santa Fe, New Mexico

Peter M. Palese
Professor and Chairman
Department of Microbiology
Mt. Sinai School of Medicine
New York

Colin R. Parrish
Assistant Professor, James A.
   Baker Institute for Animal Health
New York State College of Veterinary
   Medicine
Cornell University
Ithaca, New York

C.J. Peters, M.D.
Special Pathogens Branch, Division of
   Viral & Rickettsial Diseases
National Center for Infectious
   Diseases
Centers for Disease Control
Atlanta, Georgia

Douglas D. Richman, M.D.
Professor, Departments of Pathology
   and Medicine
University of California, San Diego;
   and Division of Infectious Diseases,
VA Medical Center, San Diego

P.E. Rollin
Institut Pasteur, Paris
(When this chapter was written:
National Research Council
Postdoctoral Associate, Disease
Assessment Division, U.S. Army
Medical Research Institute of Infec-
tious Diseases, Fort Detrick, Frederick,
Maryland)

Thomas E. Shenk
Professor, Department of Molecular
   Biology
Princeton University
Princeton, New Jersey

Robert E. Shope, M.D.
Professor of Epidemiology and
   Director, Yale Arbovirus Research
   Unit
Department of Epidemiology
   and Public Health
Yale University School of Medicine
New Haven, Connecticut

James H. Strauss
Professor, Division of Biology
California Institute of Technology
Pasadena

Ernest T. Takafuji, COL MC USA
Office of the Surgeon General
Department of the Army
Falls Church, Virginia

Howard M. Temin
American Cancer Society Research
      Professor, McArdle Laboratory
University of Wisconsin, Madison

R. Trotter
Pathology Division
U.S. Army Medical Research
      Institute of Infectious Diseases
Fort Detrick, Frederick, Maryland

David Ward
Professor, Department of Human
   Genetics
Yale University School of Medicine
New Haven, Connecticut

A.J. Watson
Division of Nephrology
The Johns Hopkins University School
   of Medicine
Baltimore, Maryland

Robert G. Webster
Chairman, Department of Virology
   & Molecular Biology
St. Jude Children's Research Hospital
Memphis, Tennessee

J. White
Pathology Division
U.S. Army Medical Research
      Institute of Infectious Diseases
Fort Detrick, Frederick, Maryland

EMERGING VIRUSES

1

Viruses and Humankind: Intracellular Symbiosis and Evolutionary Competition

JOSHUA LEDERBERG

Some may say that AIDS has made us ever vigilant for new viruses. I wish that were true. Others have said that we could do little better than to sit back and wait for the avalanche. I am afraid that this point of view is much closer to the reaction of public policy and the major health establishments of the world, even to this day, to the prospects of emergent disease.

A relatively small number of investigators have been preoccupied with the biology of viruses and have a very personal and intimate acquaintanceship with how they tick; these scientists are therefore much more sensitive to the viruses' potentialities for evolutionary change in the evolution of their symbiotic relations with their hosts. Never has there been a more concentrated collection of intellect devoted to that kind of question than is represented in this book.

However deeply gratifying this is, I do marvel that the present examination is virtually without precedent. Of course, many books and symposia on viruses cover every aspect of their biology and epidemiology. For the most part, these have been sharply focused on particular categories, whether of the host, the vectors, or the taxonomic location of the virus itself. But the historiography of epidemic disease is one of the last refuges of the concept of special creationism, with scant attention to dynamic change on the part of the agents of disease.

It is not hard to imagine the sources of resistance to these evolutionary concepts. It is scary to imagine the emergence of new infectious agents as threats to human existence, especially threatening to view pandemic as a recurrent, natural phenomenon. In reaction to the daunting pace of technological change and the sudden alteration of balance, the natural has been extolled. In 50 years, the earth has become so small on the scale of technological alterations of the environment; the atmosphere, the oceans, our aquifers are no longer infinite sinks. Many people find it difficult to accommodate to the reality that Nature is far from benign; at least it has no special sentiment for the welfare of the human versus other species. Those who are horrified at any tinge of our "tampering with natural evolution" need to be reminded that this has been intrinsic to human culture since Prometheus: the invention of fire, of agriculture, of language, of human settlements, of an overall peopling of the planet perhaps a thousand-fold denser than we had been evolved for—not to mention a sudden doubling of life span in our century that leaves the latter half of it beyond the scope of what had ever been shaped by natural selection. So contemporary man is a manmade species. In a biological sense, we may achieve new genomic equilibria with these radically altered environments; but the price of natural selection is so high that I doubt we would find it ethically acceptable: it conflicts violently with the nominally infinite worth that we place on every individual. So we have drastically tampered with human evolution, in large measure by suspending that process in favor of artifice.

That artifice has of course been the greatest threat to every other plant and animal species, as we crowd them out in our own quest for *Lebensraum*. A few vermin aside, *Homo sapiens* has undisputed dominion—and we could, where we choose, even eradicate rodent and insect pests in confined areas we chose to make oligoxenic at the expense of some of the birds and the bees and some marginal chemical poisoning of ourselves, and an irrevocable loss of evolutionary diversity among the species, an eventual narrowing of the options for our own survival.

Bacterial and protozoan parasites linger a bit longer; but they do have distinctive metabolism, and our ingenuity in devising antibiotics can be expected to outpace theirs in evolving resistance (albeit not without some struggle) provided only that we apply the needed technological resources. And for the most part, still more appropriate technologies of hygiene and vaccination will do most of the job. Our only real competitors remain the viruses; for it is by no means clear that antiviral antibiosis can generally be achieved in principle: the very essence of the virus is its fundamental entanglement with the genetic and metabolic machinery of the host.

Our main recourse has been prophylactic vaccination; and for a number of viruses this will surely work, though very few share the idiosyncrasies of variola (smallpox) that made it the most rational target for our initial effort at global eradication, at an evolutionary victory of the first order. But as we find in abundance, many viruses are more adroit than variola in antigenic evolution, and we shall have to be very nimble indeed to keep up with the diversification of influenza, particularly when we get recurrence of more lethal strains, such as neurotropism already well known in bird strains.

Other viruses will adapt by changes of range of host or of vector—the more threatening as we know so little of the biochemical bases of that specificity. And some vector-borne agents will surely learn the tricks of direct aerosol transmission, as has been claimed for pneumonic transmission of bacterial plagues. Why not? For the few antiviral drugs now available, we are, of course, already seeing the emergence of resistant viral strains, just as with bacteria. The viruses I know best, the bacteriophages, are of course no threat to public health. They may occasionally be pests in the fermentation industry; D'Herelle (and Martin Arrowsmith, the hero of Sinclair Lewis' novel) once thought they might have some merit in therapeutics. They have conveyed to me dramatic images of the wipeout of large populations, sometimes as the result of host range mutations. They have also taught us a great deal about the basic biology of viruses, lessons that can be extrapolated first hand—for example, the transduction of host genes by viruses, and the integration of viral genomes into the host chromosomes. The intrinsic hypervariability of certain categories of viruses is often mentioned; and we know this will be aggravated further in maladjusted genetic complexes. It is after all genetic stability that has had to be meticulously evolved; we will see mutation rates as high as are compatible with generational viability when the regulatory controls are disrupted. The vertebrate immune system illustrates how the hypermutability of immunoglobulin genes is a trick relearned in evolution—and matched by the trypanosome's versatility in varying its surface antigens.

Our view of virus as a parasite is complicated by that of a virus as a genetic element, a two-way channel. The viruses are routinely subject to phenotypic modification by the host cells and, from time to time, the viruses incorporate host genes in their standard genomes and vice versa.

This view still looks at host and parasite as independent and autonomous genetic systems. Let us examine their relationship still more broadly.

When we try to classify the genetic elements within cells we find a continuum, with the nucleus and its macrochromosomes at one pole, a range of other particles in between, and the frank extraneous cytocidal and cytolytic viruses at the other. Even among the chromosomes, especially in plants, we find micro- or B chromosomal elements that share every attribute of a parasite except that they show vertical transmission rather than routine lateral mobility; they also differ in their highly attenuated pathogenicity.

Other particles occupy the cytoplasm. We know most of all today about the mitochondria and the chloroplasts. The eukaryotic cell is now recognized as a symbiosis, those elements very likely having been evolved from what were once free living microbes. Indeed, it is not difficult to cure yeast of their mitochondria with acriflavine, and *Chlamydomonas* and other green plant cells of their chloroplasts with streptomycin.

Conversely, we know of many "viruses" in plants and animals that display vertical transmission. These include the rodent leukemogenic viruses and, close by, the mouse mammary tumor milk factor (now called mouse mammary tumor virus), and abundant examples in plants. It will be astounding if we were not to find still other viruses that have become routinized as cytoplasm organelles in parallel with the mitochondrial and chloroplast systems, like some of the endosymbiotic bacteria of insects that have become indispensable to the normal economy of their specific host.

At one time much polemical energy was spent arguing whether some of these entities were viruses, on the one hand, or cytogenes on the other, as if these were disjunctive concepts. The word plasmid was invented in 1952 to help moot a logically empty controversy (Lederberg, 1952). The expression has come to be used mainly in the narrower sense of the small circular DNAs that abound in bacteria (it is hard to find bacteria that don't have them). However, it was intended to apply as well to mitochondria and to temperate viruses. We are going to discover many, many more entities like that in the cytoplasm of eukaryotic cells as well (Gaubatz, 1990).

To look still more broadly, we discovered that terrestrial life is a dense web of genetic interactions. The plant cell is an intracellular symbiosis, the photosynthetic chloroplast fixing solar energy for the benefit of the host. And I will not take time to articulate how the tree repays that debt. Then, when I eat a green plant and sow its seeds, our genetic systems are also interacting to mutual benefit. The lichen is not much different: that the cell boundaries are likewise still intact between algae and fungus. One can find intermediate interactions, even across broad species lines, of hyperparasitism, the nuclei of one fungus parasitizing the cytoplasm of another. This blends into heterokaryosis within a species, with the regular dikaryons (cells with two nuclei) of the Basidiomycetes, the mushrooms. In the laboratory there is an easy and elegant demonstration of nutritional symbiosis of complementary auxotrophic mutants in heterokaryons. Each mutant separately is unable to grow because each requires a nutrient that it cannot make; together, each of the two nuclei placed into one cell provides the genetic information needed by the other, and the hybrid cell can grow. In streptomycetes it is difficult to distinguish these internuclear interactions from chromosomal ones.

We can thus see the continuum of interaction of genetic systems we have coevolved (Fig. 1.1). There is a synecology at the very top level that is absolutely undeniable, the exchange of what are ultimately gene products, the metabolites, the energy that is fixed in green plants. Syncytia—fused cells—form more abundantly than most people realize where these interactions become possible at a more intimate level, and one can see polymers, enzymes, RNA messages, and so on as the units. And then synkaryosis, the primitive step in sexual recombination, is a further step in that continuum. Consider further the interrelationships of still smaller autonomous

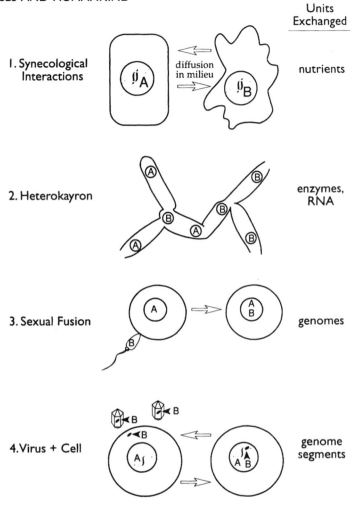

Figure 1.1 Interactions of genetic systems: a lesson in continuity.

Arranged in order of descending size. For each level of interaction, representative examples are indicated. A, B are genetic segments (complementary or antagonistic).

1. **Synecological interactions:** E.g., bird eats plant cell. *Interchange of nutrients (ultimate gene products);*
2. **Heterokaryon:** Anastomosis of hyphae, or cell fusion. *Interaction of metabolic systems, transfer RNA, messenger RNA, etc. (proximate gene products);*
3. **Sexual fusion.** *Interaction (and recombination) of genomes;*
4. **Virus and cell:** Integration of infecting virus into cell nucleus; conversely, induction of latent virus. *Interaction of genome segments.* (Transition: Virus free in environment, virus in cytoplasm, or virus integrated into chromosome.)

genetic elements like viruses and plasmids, and mitochondria, as falling at different points on this spectrum with no sharp line between them (Margulis and Fester, 1991).

This pattern of mutualism must have prevailed from the very earliest stages of biosynthetic evolution, perhaps even prior to the organization of the cell as we now know it. The recombination of self-replicating molecules to facilitate biosynthetic complementation would have accelerated primitive chemical evolution from the earliest times.

Refocusing on the pathogenic interactions, we recall that since Frank Macfarlane Burnet (Burnet and White, 1972), Theobald Smith (1939), and others, we have understood that evolutionary equilibrium favors mutualistic rather than parasitic or unilaterally destructive interactions. Natural selection, in the long run, favors host resistance, on the one hand, and temperate virulence and immunogenic masking on the parasite's part on the other. But I garner limited assurance from those precedents. Yes, demographic obliteration is not the most likely outcome of a novel introduction or the emergence of a major new virus. Most likely, the outcome of those exigencies will not be worse than what happened to the rabbits in Australia after the introduction of myxoma virus.

But apart from the personal human catastrophe that such a pandemic would entail (short of prompt species obliteration), I would also question whether human society could survive left on the beach with only a few percent of survivors. Could they function at any level of culture higher than that of the rabbits? And, if reduced to that, would we compete very well with kangaroos?

Let me summarize: the units of natural selection are DNA, sometimes RNA elements, by no means neatly packaged in discrete organisms. They all share the entire biosphere. The survival of the human species is not a preordained evolutionary program. Abundant sources of genetic variation exist for viruses to learn new tricks, not necessarily confined to what happens routinely or even frequently.

The first inklings that genetic recombination could occur at all in bacteria, in F$^+$ E. coli, were at a rate of 10^{-7}, or one in ten million, and one had to look very hard to have any evidence that they existed at all. And some bamboo plants flower only once per century and the careless observer might think that they never recombine. Some generalizations to the limits of genetic change in viruses are equally hasty.

REFERENCES

Burnet, F.M., and D.O. White (1972). *Natural History of Infectious Disease,* fourth ed. Cambridge: Cambridge University Press.

Gaubatz, J.W. (1990). Extrachromosomal circular DNAs and genomic sequence plasticity in eukaryotic cells. Mutat. Res. **237**:271-292.

Lederberg, J. (1952). Cell genetics and hereditary symbiosis. Physiol. Rev. **32**:403-430.

Margulis, L., and R. Fester (eds.) (1991). *Symbiosis as a Source of Evolutionary Innovation: Speciation and Morphogenesis.* Cambridge, Mass.: MIT Press.

Smith, T. (1939). *Parasitism and Disease.* Princeton: Princeton University Press.

2

Examining the Origins of Emerging Viruses

STEPHEN S. MORSE

The sudden appearance of the AIDS epidemic in our midst demonstrates once again that infectious diseases can still be important causes of illness and death. HIV (human immunodeficiency virus, the AIDS virus) has been front-page news for so long that it is hard to remember that it first came to our notice just over a decade ago. Influenza, one of our most familiar viruses, still periodically causes massive epidemics (the most massive are called pandemics because the entire world is usually affected), and another influenza pandemic is virtually inevitable. There have been several influenza pandemics in this century alone, the most severe being the notorious pandemic of 1918-1919 that resulted in over 25 million deaths worldwide. Lyme disease, although bacterial rather than viral, is another infectious disease recently emerged to prominence in the United States. From such regular experiences, it is easy to get the justifiable impression that we are being inundated by infectious diseases.

These manifestations reinforce a general feeling that sudden disease outbreaks will emerge in capricious ways as "acts of God." The factors responsible for sudden manifestations of viral diseases such as AIDS or epidemics of influenza have been poorly understood and therefore have always seemed inexplicable. However, critical comparative examination indicates that there are factors common to most, perhaps almost all, known examples of viral emergence. In this chapter, I will summarize my own views as to what these factors are, and formulate a conceptual framework for disease emergence. Where it seems appropriate, I have included a few examples involving bacterial diseases, as I believe many of the underlying mechanisms are similar.

WHAT ARE THE ORIGINS OF EMERGING VIRUSES?

We may use the term "emerging viruses" to refer to viruses that either have newly appeared in the population or are rapidly expanding their range, with a corresponding increase in cases of disease (Morse and Schluederberg,

1990). Table 2.1 lists some examples, including many of the human viruses discussed in this book, with their conventional taxonomic classification. (Some of the examples in this chapter are drawn from other chapters of this volume, where additional information and references may be found. Detailed information on the biology of many of the viruses discussed here can be found in Fields, Knipe et al., 1990. Brief capsule descriptions of many viruses can be found in Porterfield, 1989; arthropod-borne viruses are catalogued in Karabatsos, 1985. Benenson, 1990, gives capsule summaries of both viral and nonviral infections, emphasizing epidemiologic and public health aspects.)

The Newly Recognized

Before considering these viruses, I wish first to mention another group of potentially emergent viruses: those viruses that are already widespread but, while not new in the human population, are newly recognized. (Human viruses that are not yet widespread fall into another category, discussed below.) A recent example is human herpesvirus 6 (HHV-6). Although identified only a few years ago (Salahuddin et al., 1986), HHV-6 appears to be extremely widespread (Lopez et al., 1988), and has recently been implicated as the cause of roseola (exanthem subitum), a very common childhood disease (Yamanishi et al., 1988). Since roseola has been known since at least 1910 (Zahorsky, 1910), HHV-6 is likely to have been common for at least decades, and probably much longer.

A related category is the association of some infectious agents with chronic diseases, such as the long established association of chronic hepatitis B infection and hepatocellular carcinoma. The most surprising recent example is infection with the bacterium *Helicobacter pylori* as a probable cause of gastric ulcers (Peterson, 1991) and possibly gastric cancer (Nomura et al., 1991; Parsonnet et al., 1991). As with roseola, the disease (in this case, gastric ulcers) was known for a long time but the identification of the putative cause is quite recent.

Conceivably, on occasion, a change in the microbe or (more frequently) in host nutritional or immune status might result in a new or more serious disease. But usually, although these diseases (especially the chronic diseases) can be important causes of illness, these newly recognized but common agents are not likely to emerge suddenly or threateningly because they are already widespread and are likely to have reached an equilibrium in the population: we have lived with these diseases for a long time, although without knowing their cause. Recognition of the agent may even be advantageous, offering new promise of controlling a previously intractable disease. If *Helicobacter* is a major cause of ulcers, a new and potentially promising avenue of treatment, specific antimicrobial therapy, is now opened up.

The Roles of Viral Evolution

Setting aside the newly recognized but ubiquitous, we might begin an examination of emerging viruses by asking how a new virus might originate. It must be noted that "newly evolved" viruses will usually descend from a parent that already exists in nature. This is a consequence of Darwinian evolution. Even HIV, the most novel of recently described viruses infecting humans, has its relatives in nature. Given these constraints of organic evolution, then, there are fundamentally three sources (which are not necessarily mutually exclusive): [1] evolution *de novo* of a new virus (more precisely, usually the evolution of a new viral variant); [2] introduction of an existing virus from another species; [3] dissemination of a virus from a smaller population in which the virus might have arisen or originally been introduced.

It is often assumed that "new"diseases must be the result of the evolution of new viruses. It would therefore seem useful to evaluate the relative importance of viral evolution versus transfer and dissemination of viruses to new host populations (the latter being the process I have called "viral traffic"; Morse, 1991) in the emergence of "new" viral diseases. Both processes need to be better understood; both surely are important, but perhaps in different ways. Many viruses show a high mutation rate and have great evolutionary potential. This continuing process has probably been important in producing the great diversity of viruses recognized today. While many viral variants can be identified both in nature and in the laboratory, their significance as a source of new viral diseases is hard to determine, and there appear to be relatively few documented examples in nature. Undoubtedly more examples will be found as further efforts are made using the more sensitive detection methods now available. However, most variants that have been identified in nature (e.g., Western equine encephalomyelitis, discussed by Strauss, and the possible example of Rocio encephalitis, discussed by Monath) often resemble the parental virus in the kind of disease caused, although host range may differ. Canine parvovirus, for example, discussed by Colin Parrish, represents a different host range. Some exceptions are known, in which a new viral variant shows greatly increased virulence or causes a different type of disease. Influenza, which I will discuss again later in another context, provides some of the most notable examples, including an H5 influenza variant in chickens, discussed in Chapter 4 by Webster. It was also recently suggested that a mutation in a viral gene is responsible for a fulminant form of hepatitis B infection (Carman et al., 1989, 1991; Liang et al., 1991; Omata et al., 1991). The conclusion from these data is that viral variation per se undoubtedly plays a role in some situations, and may be of greater importance over long time periods, but so far has

TABLE 2.1. Some Examples of "Emerging" Viruses

Virus	Signs/Symptoms	Distribution	Natural host
Family: Orthomyxoviridae (RNA, 8 segments)			
Influenza	Respiratory	Worldwide (often from China)	Fowl (and pigs)
Family: Bunyaviridae (RNA, 3 segments)			
Hantaan, Seoul, etc.	Hemorrhagic fever with renal syndrome	Asia, Europe, U.S.	Rodent (e.g., *Apodemus*)
Rift Valley Fever*	Fever, ± hemorrhage	Africa	Mosquito; ungulates
Oropouche*	Fever	Brazil, Trinidad, Panama	Midge
Family: Togaviridae (Alphavirus genus) (RNA)			
O´nyong-nyong*	Arthritis, rash	Africa	Mosquito
Sindbis*	Arthritis, rash	Africa, Europe, Asia, Australia	Mosquito; birds
Family: Flaviviridae (RNA)			
Yellow Fever*	Fever, jaundice	Africa, S. America	Mosquito; monkey
Dengue*	Fever, ± hemorrhage	Asia, Africa, S. America, Caribbean	Mosquito; human/monkey
Rocio*	Encephalitis	Brazil	Mosquito; birds
Kyasanur Forest*	Encephalitis	India	Tick; rodent
Family: Arenaviridae (RNA, 2 segments)			
Junin (Argentine HF)†	Fever, hemorrhage	S. America	*Calomys musculinus*
Machupo (Bolivian HF)	Fever, hemorrhage	S. America	*Calomys callosus*
Lassa fever	Fever, hemorrhage	W. Africa	*Mastomys natalensis*
Family: Filoviridae (RNA)			
Marburg, Ebola	Fever, hemorrhage	Africa	Unknown
Family: Retroviridae (RNA + reverse transcriptase)			
HIV§	AIDS	Worldwide	Human virus (? originally from primate)
HTLV‡	Often asymptomatic; adult T-cell leukemia, neurological diseases (e.g., tropical spastic paraparesis)	Worldwide, with endemic foci	Human virus (? originally primate virus)
Family: Poxviridae (DNA)			
Monkeypox	Smallpox-like	Africa (rainforest)	Rodent (squirrel)

[From S. S. Morse and A. Schluederberg (1990). Emerging viruses: The evolution of viruses and viral diseases. J. Infect. Dis. 162:1-7. ©1990 by The University of Chicago Press.]
*Transmitted by arthropod vector
† HF: Hemorrhagic fever
§ HIV: Human immunodeficiency virus
‡ HTLV: Human T cell leukemia/lymphoma virus (human T-lymphotropic virus) I, II (types I and II)
Bold: Viruses with greatest apparent potential for emergence in near future

not proved to be the major engine driving viral emergence. Examples of specific viral variants produced within different individuals during infection (Ahmed et al., 1991; Kilbourne et al., 1988; Salvato et al., 1991), and the relative rarity of observing progressive accumulation of mutations within an infected host over time (Rocha et al., 1991) suggest stabilizing effects of natural selection on viruses. Viral evolution is likely to be more important for increasing adaptedness in a new host immediately after a virus is introduced

TABLE 2.2.

Some Emerging Viruses and Probable Factors in Their Emergence

Virus Family, Virus	Probable Factors in Emergence
Arenaviridae	
Junin (Argentine HF)	Changes in agriculture (maize; changed conditions favoring *Calomys musculinus*, rodent host for virus)
Machupo (Bolivian HF)	Changes in agriculture (changed conditions favoring *Calomys callosus*, rodent host for virus)
Bunyaviridae	
Hantaan	Agriculture (contact with mouse *Apodemus agrarius* during rice harvest)
Seoul	?Increasing population density of urban rats in contact with humans; spread of rat hosts
Rift Valley Fever	Dams, irrigation
Oropouche	Agriculture (cacao hulls encourage breeding of *Culicoides* vector)
Filoviridae	
Marburg, Ebola	Unknown; in Europe and U.S., importation of monkeys
Flaviviridae	
Dengue	Increasing population density in cities, and other factors (e.g., open water storage) favoring increased population of mosquito vectors
Orthomyxoviridae	
Influenza	?Integrated pig-duck agriculture
Retroviridae	
Human immunodeficiency virus (HIV)	Medical technology (transfusion); sexual transmission; contaminated hypodermic equipment; other social factors*
HTLV	Medical technology (transfusion); contaminated hypodermic equipment; other social factors (virus is already naturally widespread in some populations)

* Hepatitis B and Hepatitis C, in different viral families, have similar causes of emergence

into a new species or population, as demonstrated by the coevolution of virus and host that followed the introduction of myxoma virus in Australia (discussed by May in Chapter 6).

Human Viruses and the Zoonotic Pool

At least over the period of recorded history, then, "emerging viruses" have usually not been newly evolved viruses. Rather, they are existing viruses conquering new territory (Table 2.2). The overwhelming majority are viruses already existing in nature that simply gain access to new host populations. The most novel of these emerging viruses are zoonotic (naturally occurring viruses of other animal species); rodents are among the particularly important natural reservoirs. This seems logical, considering that the total number and variety of viruses in animal species is probably very large, and hence offers a large pool of potential "new" virus introductions. In such cases, introduction of viruses into the human population is often the result of human activities, such as agriculture, that cause changes in natural environments. Often, these changes place humans in contact with previously inaccessible viruses. The success of a new virus then depends on its ability to spread within the human population after introduction. A similar situation would apply to viruses already present in a limited or isolated human population. After all, the viruses best adapted to human transmission are likely to be those that already infect people. Here, too, human intervention is providing increasing opportunities for dissemination of previously localized viruses. The example of HIV demonstrates that human activities can be especially important in disseminating newly introduced viruses that may not yet be well adapted to the human host and that do not spread efficiently from person to person.

Human pathogens, which may include agents currently in an isolated human population, are often best positioned to cause future epidemics, and bear careful scrutiny. But the numerous examples of zoonotic diseases suggest that the "zoonotic pool"—introductions of viruses from other species—is also an important and potentially rich source of emerging diseases. Even if the odds of a randomly chosen organism being a successful human pathogen are low, the great variety of microorganisms in nature offers many chances. As one example, field sampling and disease surveillance efforts over the years have resulted in the identification to date of more than 520 arthropod-borne viruses (arboviruses) (Karabatsos, 1985). Most of these are of unknown disease potential; Monath estimates in Chapter 13 that about 100 of the known arboviruses cause human disease. As shown by examples cited throughout this chapter, and throughout the book, chance will also affect which zoonotic agents will make contact with humans. But historical examples of zoonoses that have caused major outbreaks or epidemics, or become established as human diseases, such as Hantaan (Korean hemorrhagic fever), yellow fever, Rift Valley fever, pandemic influenza (usually reassortant viruses containing genes derived from avian influenza viruses), and others, indicate that a large number of potential introductions exist in nature and that some of them might become successful as emerging diseases given the right conditions.

Periodic discoveries of "new" zoonoses also suggest that the known agents are only a fraction of the total number that exist in nature. One example of an animal virus discovered only recently is Guanarito, the cause of Venezuelan hemorrhagic fever (Salas et al., 1991). The virus is rodent-borne and appears similar to other arenaviruses such as Junin.

The zoonotic pool can also include organisms in environments that have been little studied. In Chapter 17, Mahy discusses seal plague, a virus that may well be a common infection in marine mammals. Marine viruses may occasionally come ashore to cause disease in terrestrial mammals or humans. Several diseases are caused by members of the calicivirus family. It has been suggested that vesicular exanthema of swine, a serious viral disease caused by a calicivirus, was a virus of marine origin introduced into pigs by feed containing material from sea lions, and that many caliciviruses of terrestrial mammals may have been introductions from marine sources (Smith and Boyt, 1990). Caliciviruses have been described in humans; most recently, hepatitis E virus (the enterically transmitted non-A non-B hepatitis that is usually water-borne and is widespread in tropical areas including parts of South America) has been classified as a calicivirus (Reyes and Baroudy, 1991; Reyes et al., 1990).

Our knowledge of viral and microbial host range determinants is too rudimentary to allow us to predict which agents are most likely to emerge from the zoonotic pool as human diseases. Chance and environmental factors will also play a part in that process. The evidence indicates, however, that microbial pathogens of other species have been an important source of new diseases in the past, and this is likely to continue.

EMERGENCE AS A TWO-STEP PROCESS, AND THE IMPORTANCE OF VIRAL TRAFFIC

Given this complexity, our approach to understanding emerging infectious diseases should emphasize understanding the mechanisms underlying emergence. Consideration of the above shows that viral emergence is essentially a two-step process: [1] introduction of the virus (whatever its origin) into a new host, followed by

[2] dissemination within that new host population. The two events could occur almost simultaneously, or, more usually, be separated by considerable periods of time. The second step might not occur at all, for example if a virus is not able to transmit well within a new host species or does not have sufficient opportunity to disseminate. However, changing conditions might increase the chances of this second step occurring.

I coined the term "viral traffic" for these movements of viruses to new species or new individuals. To rephrase the conclusions stated above, we can say that, with rare exceptions, most outbreaks of "new" viruses appear to be caused by changes in viral traffic (Table 2.2; see also Chapter 11). Changing environmental conditions are often responsible for viral traffic. Because people are major agents of ecological change, often these changes are brought about by human activities, so interspecies transfers of infectious organisms are not nearly as random as they seem.

A variety of human activities can precipitate emergence, but some types of activities appear especially likely to do so. Some of these are listed in Table 2.2, and include specific types of agricultural practices, or changes in agricultural practices. Hantaan virus, the cause of Korean hemorrhagic fever, first came to Western attention when troops in Korea succumbed to the disease, but it causes over 100,000 cases a year in China, and has been known in Asia for centuries. The virus is a natural infection of the field mouse *Apodemus agrarius*. The rodent flourishes in rice fields; people usually contract the disease during the rice harvest, from contact with infected rodents. Closely related viruses, Seoul virus and Seoul-like viruses, are found in urban rats worldwide; James LeDuc and colleagues (Chapter 14) have found infection to be quite common among rats in inner-city Baltimore. Junin virus, the cause of Argentine hemorrhagic fever, is an unrelated virus with a remarkably similar history to Hantaan. Conversion of grassland to maize cultivation favored a rodent that was the natural host for this virus, and human cases increased in proportion with expansion of maize agriculture. Other viruses with similar life histories are likely to appear as new areas are placed under cultivation.

The most startling example is pandemic influenza, which also appears, at least in some instances, to have an agricultural origin, integrated pig-duck farming in China. This is startling because influenza has always been the classic example of viral evolution at work, and scientists have long believed that new epidemics are caused by mutations in the virus. Although this appears to be true of the smaller annual or biennial epidemics we frequently experience, influenza viruses that cause pandemics do not generally arise by this process. Instead, genes from two influenza strains reassort to produce a new virus that can infect humans. Pandemic influenza viruses have always come from China, but the reason has been obscure. Evidence amassed by Robert G. Webster, Christoph Scholtissek, and others, and discussed in this volume by Webster, indicates that waterfowl, such as ducks, are major reservoirs of influenza and that pigs can serve as "mixing vessels" for new mammalian influenza

strains. Scholtissek and Naylor have suggested that integrated pig-duck
agriculture, an extremely efficient food production system traditionally
practiced in certain parts of China for several centuries, puts these two
species in contact and provides a natural laboratory for making new
influenza reassortants (Scholtissek and Naylor, 1988).

In the industrialized world, bovine spongiform encephalopathy
(BSE), known colloquially as "mad cow disease ", appeared in Britain
within the last few years. BSE is an impressive recent example of an
apparent interspecies transfer of an infectious agent, in this case the
apparent transfer of scrapie from sheep to cattle. The cattle probably
became infected after eating byproducts from scrapie infected sheep.
It has been suggested that changes in rendering processes, allowing
incomplete inactivation of scrapie agent, may have been responsible
(Wilesmith et al., 1991). The example is instructive, although fortunately BSE is not likely to be a major threat to human health; the
human equivalent, Creutzfeldt-Jakob disease, is rare even though
scrapie has been known in sheep for at least two centuries and there
have presumably been many possibilities for human exposure comparable to the acquisition of BSE by cattle (Morse, 1990).

Viruses transmitted by arthropods, which include some of the most
notorious diseases such as dengue and yellow fever, are often stimulated by expansion of stored water supplies, because many of the
arthropods (especially mosquitoes) that transmit these viruses breed in
water. There are many examples, most involving water for irrigation or
stored drinking water in cities. Japanese encephalitis in Asia is more
frequent around rice fields, which are flooded for cultivation. Outbreaks of Rift Valley fever in some parts of Africa have been associated with dam building, as well as with periods of heavy rainfall. Thomas
Lovejoy mentions the example of Lake Bayano in Panama, whose creation as part of a hydroelectric project caused a local increase in cases
of Venezuelan equine encephalomyelitis, another serious mosquito borne
viral disease with potential for reestablishment in the United States.

Dengue virus deserves special mention because it is also lapping
at our shores. A 1981 outbreak in Cuba involved over 300,000 cases,
and much of the Caribbean regularly experiences dengue outbreaks.
There are four known dengue viruses, or serotypes (Chapter 13). A
particular concern is the more severe form known as dengue hemorrhagic fever, which occurs in many areas where dengue is
hyperendemic, and has been postulated to result from sequential
infection with different dengue viruses that now overlap geographi-
cally in many tropical areas (Halstead, 1989). The frequency of
dengue hemorrhagic fever is increasing as several types of dengue
virus, extending their range, now overlap. Dengue virus is very
common in Asia, where the high prevalence of infection is attributed
to the proliferation of open containers needed for water storage as
the population size exceeds the infrastructure. In urban environ-

ments, rain-filled tires or plastic bottles are also often breeding grounds of choice for mosquito vectors. The resulting mosquito population boom is complemented by the high human population density in such situations, increasing the chances of transmission between infected and uninfected individuals.

These problems can be exacerbated by many types of human activities that may disseminate vectors as well as viruses. Both yellow fever virus and its principal vector, the *Aedes aegypti* mosquito, are believed to have been spread from Africa via the slave trade. The mosquitoes were stowaways in the ships, possibly in containers that were kept to provide water for the slavers' human cargo. In a repetition of history, although in a more benign pursuit, another vector of dengue virus, *Aedes albopictus* (the Asian tiger mosquito), was recently introduced into the United States in shipments of used tires imported from Asia. From its entry in Houston, Texas, in 1982, the mosquito has established itself in at least 18 states. A previously unknown Bunyavirus, probably a virus native to North America that was acquired by the mosquito after its arrival here, was recently isolated from *Aedes albopictus* in Missouri (Francy et al., 1990). This virus does not appear to be a cause of human disease, but more recently, Eastern equine encephalomyelitis virus, which can cause serious disease in both humans and horses, was found in *Aedes albopictus* from Florida (Centers for Disease Control, 1992). The *Aedes albopictus* mosquito has also been introduced into Brazil and parts of Africa through the same trade in used tires that brought it to the United States (Centers for Disease Control, 1991), and the mosquito appears on its way to becoming worldwide.

I will give only one more example of this sort of transport, raccoon rabies in the United States. In the last few years, rabies in raccoons has moved from the southeast, where it has been localized for some time, to the northeast, and raccoons now seem well on their way to becoming a major wildlife source of rabies. For the first third of 1990 alone, New Jersey found 37 rabid raccoons, after identifying its first rabid raccoon only in October 1989. The Centers for Disease Control implicated sport hunting as the main factor in this explosive spread of raccoon rabies. In order to ensure an adequate supply of raccoons, hunters from Virginia imported Florida raccoons to the north.

Another factor in viral traffic is human traffic itself (some medical technologies, such as organ transplants and blood, could also be considered as a surrogate, but this is now usually carefully controlled in Western countries). Highways and human migration to cities, especially in tropical areas, can introduce remote viruses to a larger population. HIV, discussed in Chapter 12, is the most notorious recent example, but it is not alone. There is evidence that mosquitoes carrying dengue viruses in Thailand were spread along railroads, a vehicle also previously suggested by McDonald from studies in Malaysia (Wellmer, 1983). On a global scale, similar opportunities are offered by rapid air travel. The Public Health Service reported 124 suspected cases of imported dengue in the United States in 1988, of which 27 (in 17 states) were definite and another 25 were uncertain. Lassa fever, a virus endemic to west Africa, caused an unexpected death in Illinois just over 3 years ago: a man who contracted the virus while visiting Nigeria for a funeral became sick after returning to the United States.

FAILED PUBLIC HEALTH MEASURES

In 1991, epidemics around the world included dengue in Brazil and yellow fever in Nigeria (some 600 deaths were reported in an outbreak lasting from April through July 1991). A classic bacterial disease, cholera, has been raging in South America (for the first time this century) and Africa. According to a report from the Pan American Health Organization, the rapid spread of cholera in South America may have been favored by recent reductions in chlorine levels used to treat water supplies (Anderson, 1991). Incidentally, the mystery of why cholera suddenly appeared in South America after a lapse of almost a century may also have been solved; the Pan American Health Organization suggested that cholera was probably introduced into South America when a freighter from China released contaminated bilge water into a Peruvian harbor, from whence it spread into local shellfish and later disseminated through contaminated water supplies (Anderson, 1991).

Yellow fever and cholera are not new diseases, and the reasons for these outbreaks are similar to those we have already discussed. However, many diseases gain a foothold because of inadequate preventive measures, sanitation, or nutrition. Better water supplies would have lessened the magnitude of the cholera outbreaks. Adding yellow fever immunization to the worldwide Expanded Program on Immunization of the World Health Organization (WHO), which has been proposed by Monath, might well prevent further epidemics like the one in Nigeria.

Several United States cities have experienced epidemics of childhood measles in 1990 and 1991. A recent government report attributes much of the increase in measles cases to cutbacks in childhood vaccination programs, with the result that some children were inadequately immunized or immunized too late.

These examples emphasize the point that some effective weapons already exist and are in use, but even the most powerful weapons are useful only if properly deployed (this point is also made forcefully by Karl Johnson in Chapter 5.) Much disease could be prevented simply by consistent and universal application of traditional public health and sanitation measures. Conversely, as shown by examples such as the resurgence of cholera, many disease outbreaks follow the breakdown of such measures.

PRACTICAL ACTION: SURVEILLANCE AND RESPONSE CAPABILITIES

I conclude that viral traffic, often abetted by human actions, is the major factor in viral emergence. Because human activities are often involved in emergence, anticipating and limiting viral emergence is more feasible than previously believed. Basically, people are creating much of the viral traffic, even if we are doing it inadvertently. We need to recognize this and learn how to be better traffic engineers.

Knowledge of viral traffic can help identify where to look and what to look for, as I will briefly discuss later. At a practical level, there must be mechanisms in place for recognizing disease emergence and for initiating action, and I shall therefore discuss these specific organizational aspects first.

Global disease surveillance is an essential first step. Weaknesses in vaccine development, production, and deployment also need to be addressed. For surveillance, a promising start is the plan described in Chapter 27 by D.A. Henderson, who spearheaded the highly successful international smallpox eradication program and therefore has both experience and insight into the realities of disease surveillance and control. His proposal would establish a network of international centers for disease surveillance and human health. Centers would be located in tropical areas, especially near cities; each center would include clinical facilities, diagnostic and research laboratories, an epidemiological unit that could include disease investigation and local response capability, and a professional training unit. Each center would be part of an international network, which would also include academic and government laboratories, to coordinate data collection and evaluation, conduct relevant research, provide backup support, and activate an international rapid response system when warranted.

There is no fully developed network for human health. The closest parallels in human health are the polio surveillance network of the Pan American Health Organization, and, with a more specific focus but wider global reach, the WHO influenza surveillance system. Henderson modeled his center concept on the network of laboratories in the Consultative Group on International Agricultural Research (CGIAR). The network proposed by Henderson could even be interfaced with the CGIAR, which includes the International Laboratory for Research on Animal Diseases (ILRAD) in Kenya. A joint network of animal and human health research centers, operating internationally and combining efforts when appropriate, would make great sense both scientifically and economically. Although specific details need to be worked out, a proposal like Henderson's is realistic and deserves enthusiastic support.

Surveillance must be linked to a proactive worldwide rapid response system. There is at present no international system for rapid response. The WHO provides an admirable vehicle for targeted programs, and the smallpox eradication program and Expanded Program on Immunization, among others, have been notable successes. The WHO is also a superb forum for international communication, but WHO's present limitations in budget and research capabilities severely circumscribe its ability to respond quickly to new diseases or to rapidly identify new priorities. However, any network should function in connection with WHO as an umbrella to establish international cooperation.

Henderson discusses the available agencies for response, and concludes that the best current model for rapid response is the well respected Epidemic Intelligence Service (EIS) of the U.S. Centers for Disease Control (CDC), which uses mobile epidemiologic teams that are sent to the site of a disease outbreak. CDC has at times offered this assistance internationally, through a Division of Global EIS, and many feel the most efficient measure would be to expand CDC into an international resource, at least pending further development of multinational response teams or of additional nationally based capabilities in other countries. The international system of Pasteur Institute affiliates has also been effective.

In the United States, federal responsibilities for disease surveillance and international health programs are fragmented and diffuse, without clearly defined lines of cooperation or responsibility. While the responsible agencies often cooperate well, this is not built into the structure, and many things can fall through the cracks. There may also be duplication of efforts. Therefore it would make sense to coordinate federal efforts.

It is sobering to realize that good models for worldwide surveillance and research networks have been tested, but promising first attempts have not been further refined or expanded. The Rockefeller Foundation program provides an effective model of how international laboratory capabilities can be developed. In the 1950s and 1960s, the Rockefeller Foundation established a number of laboratories worldwide, especially in the Third World. American experts helped to set up each laboratory and to train local personnel. Other professionals in the host country were sent to the United States and Europe to be trained and were encouraged to return home afterwards to direct the laboratories. Each laboratory was seen as a collaboration between Western and Third World colleagues, with an emphasis on developing local capabilities, local autonomy, and national pride. Cooperation with host governments was actively encouraged, and the program was designed to make the host country feel an equal partner in an important mutual enterprise. At the same time, there were specialized laboratories in the United States for training and support, such as what is now the Yale Arbovirus Research Unit. Much of our present knowledge of viral ecology was acquired as a result of this effort, and most of the over 500 known arthropod borne ("arbo") viruses were discovered as a result of this program despite the comparatively primitive technology that was then available.

VIRAL TRAFFIC CONTROL

What would all these programs be looking for? Traditionally, surveillance means identifying any unexplained disease outbreak in the geographic area of the surveillance center or laboratory. In Henderson's proposal, clinicians and diagnostic facilities would be available to identify, treat, and follow up on all such outbreaks. Improved local health would be a beneficial side product.

This is valuable in and of itself, but, in addition, our burgeoning knowledge of viral traffic also makes more focused approaches possible. Especially in tropical areas, ecological or demographic changes including deforestation, dam building, changes in agricultural products or in land use, and major demographic changes such as population migrations, often precipitate viral emergence. These are "traffic signals" for viral traffic: we should see them as warning signals. Knowing these viral traffic signals makes the surveillance task more manageable. We can emphasize watching for the traffic signals, and concentrate attention and resources where indicated by these traffic signals.

There is a need to recognize that the types of environmental change I have mentioned and categorized as viral traffic signals have often caused unanticipated health effects. The traffic signals should alert people to the possibility of emergence, and therefore viral traffic planning should be an adjunct to development plans. Development agencies should automatically include these health considerations in evaluating major land use or development decisions.

If one wished to formalize this, one could develop regular "viral (or microbial) impact assessments", analogous to environmental impact assessments, for all projects or events likely to involve such changes. This could include evaluations of viral "fauna" in key local vertebrate, biting arthropod, and human populations. I am not sure such detailed assessments are necessary except as a reminder to make us aware of the microbial traffic being created, but these studies would yield considerable information on viral ecology, a study presently in its infancy. Biotechnology actually makes this sort of study technically possible now. Powerful detection technologies such as the polymerase chain reaction (PCR) can be adapted to detect

undiscovered members of given viral families rapidly and effectively, so that even unknown viruses may be detected relatively
easily and selected for later detailed study. Additional basic research would undoubtedly develop still easier methods.

For the future, in addition to paying attention to viral traffic signals, we
can begin developing a more systematic understanding of viral traffic. I
have sketched above in outline the state of the art of viral traffic. At present,
a major limitation of the approach suggested in the preceding paragraph is
that methodology for assessing the likelihood that a given animal virus
will emerge as a human pathogen is still rudimentary, even putting
aside the role of chance in this process, so that it is not yet possible
to know how best to make inferences, let alone use the information
for prediction. There are some obvious factors that potentially limit
the geographic range of a virus. For arthropod-borne or zoonotic
viruses, one of the best understood is the requirement for a suitable
vector or natural host. Hantaan virus, by and large, is limited by the
range of its major natural host, *Apodemus agrarius*. A similar requirement applies to an arthropod-borne virus.

Further research could greatly advance knowledge, leading to
more precise viral traffic analysis, a sort of "driver's manual" for
viral traffic. Because people are so important in traffic, close collaboration between biomedical and social scientists will be indispensable, and interdisciplinary approaches should be encouraged. It
could be stimulated by additional funding for traffic research to the
National Institutes of Health and to interdisciplinary sources.

More immediately, we need better viral traffic engineering. Like
the famous gentleman who had spoken prose all his life without
knowing it, we are major engineers of biological traffic, but are
unaware of it. Mostly because we do not realize how important a
force people are in this respect, we do the job of traffic engineering
very poorly. There are many improvements possible, such as more
careful surveillance of viruses and vectors transported in commerce.
We can make more effective use of control measures we now have at
our disposal. Many control programs have failed because they were
scrapped after they alleviated the crisis they were designed to combat.
Mosquito control programs are notorious victims of their own success.

In this respect, local action is also valuable. We tend to think of
massive projects, but education and locally applied precautions,
such as mosquito or rodent control, can make a difference. With
economic assistance, it may be possible to move towards reducing
open water sources and improving water supplies on a large scale.
This can have a major impact on water-borne diseases, such as
cholera, and on mosquito populations, decreasing not only viruses
but also other major tropical killers such as malaria.

Many of these problems may begin in the tropical Third World,
but they are not localized to these areas. Most viruses that today are

worldwide were once localized or "exotic". Yellow fever and dengue are two examples, but, again, AIDS is the most striking. If HIV had been discovered in nature before it emerged to spread round the world as a human disease, it would probably have seemed as "exotic" to us as Ebola does now (the same observation is also made by C.J. Peters). In fact, from all available data, it may well have had much the same origin as Ebola.

In addition, not all emerging diseases are exotic. Consider Lyme disease, which emerged in the northeastern United States. Even though Lyme disease is bacterial rather than viral, its emergence is another example of microbial traffic, and was very likely due to the same sorts of environmental changes, such as increases in deer populations and in amounts of forested land in proximity to human dwellings, that we have been considering. This simply emphasizes that emerging disease is a worldwide problem, with similar mechanisms responsible all over the world.

AIDS was once an emerging viral disease. Like the other diseases discussed here, it too could have been stopped at the precrisis stage. It is therefore not surprising that the AIDS problem and the emerging virus problem should be closely related.

It is a great irony that our efforts against AIDS are still weakened by the same problems as those I have discussed here. Criticizing the fragmentation of federal efforts, the National Commission on AIDS recently concluded that federal AIDS policy was like "an orchestra without a conductor" and that "coordination of these efforts is the missing link to an effective national strategy." (The Commission expands on these themes in National Commission on AIDS, 1991.)

What are the resources needed for anticipating and controlling emerging diseases? Most of all, we will need trained people, and active laboratory facilities and research programs in which training can take place. Each year, there are fewer people available and trained to do field virology and epidemiology. Physical resources for studying these problems, and for identifying and controlling them in the field, are now extremely limited. As pointed out by several of the other contributors to this book, there are very few laboratories anywhere in the world that are either funded or equipped to do research on newly emerging or very hazardous viruses.

It is essential to strengthen research in relevant areas. These areas include viral ecology, viral traffic analysis, driving forces and constraints in viral evolution, technologies for detection, and increased understanding of how viruses cause disease and how they interact with their hosts and with host cells (viral pathogenesis and immunology).

The precipitating causes of viral traffic are often environmental changes, with emerging viruses yet another consequence of damage to the environment. Emerging disease is another strong argument for sensitivity to our environment. It is therefore a common ground

uniting otherwise diverse environmental, agricultural, human resources, economic development, and health interests. Only together
can a consensus for survival be developed. The environmentalists'
motto, "Think globally, act locally", also applies to strategies for
disease prevention.

I personally believe that science is now providing powerful tools and
approaches that can appropriately be used for better anticipating and
controlling emerging diseases. Despite our experiences with AIDS and
other recent epidemics, we are poorly prepared for viral emergence, and the
gap between science and practice continues to widen.

We now have the scientific information to design appropriate
programs. The more serious lag is therefore in mobilizing ourselves
to attack the problem with all the tools available and in organizing
effective systems for action. Experience with the AIDS crisis, and
major outbreaks of viral disease in the Caribbean and Central and
South America, should force the realization that new crises will
always be imminent, and, sadly, in the absence of effective action,
tragedies like the AIDS epidemic will be repeated. History has borne
this out too many times. The problem of emerging viruses is not
likely to disappear. If anything, it will increase; episodes of disease
emergence are likely to become more frequent as environmental
change accelerates. At the same time, rapid transportation and
increasing urban density will continue to enhance the dissemination
of previously localized viruses.

Constructive action has been paralyzed in the past by a combination of apathy and uncertainty. The AIDS epidemic is a powerful
reminder of the price of apathy. It is also a demonstration that
infectious diseases can still be a major threat to human life. Although we cannot yet predict specific disease outbreaks, and may
never be able to, we now understand many of the factors leading to
emergence. More important, because we better understand their
origins, we should be in a position to circumvent emerging diseases
at fairly early stages. The major consequence of this knowledge is
that solutions are now within human ability to implement. In fact,
as I hope this essay has shown, human actions are themselves one
major factor in emergence. Part of the question therefore becomes
whether people will continue unwittingly to precipitate emerging
diseases and suffer the consequences, as has happened throughout
history, or will begin to take responsibility for these human actions.

ACKNOWLEDGMENTS

A number of the examples in this chapter are drawn from the work of the other
contributors to this volume, with my thanks. My research is supported by NIH
grants RR 03121 and RR 01180, U.S. Department of Health and Human Services.

REFERENCES

Ahmed, R., C.S. Hahn, T. Somasundaram, L. Villarete, M. Matloubian, and J.H. Strauss (1991). Molecular basis of organ-specific selection of viral variants during chronic infection. J. Virol. 65:4242-4247.
Anderson, C. (1991). Cholera epidemic traced to risk miscalculation [News]. Nature 354:255.
Benenson, A.S. (ed.) (1990). Control of Communicable Diseases in Man, fifteenth ed. Washington, D.C.: American Public Health Association.
Carman, W.F., M.R. Jacyna, S. Hadziyannis, P. Karayiannis, M. McGarvey, A. Makris, and H.C. Thomas (1989). Mutation preventing formation of e antigen in patients with chronic HBV infection. Lancet ii:588-591.
Carman, W.F., E.A. Fagan, S. Hadziyannis, P. Karayiannis, N.C. Tassopoulos, R. Williams, and H.C. Thomas (1991). Association of a precore genomic variant of hepatitis B virus with fulminant hepatitis. Hepatology 14:219-222.
Centers for Disease Control (1991). Aedes albopictus introduction into continental Africa, 1991. Morbidity and Mortality Weekly Reports 40:836-838.
Centers for Disease Control (1992). Eastern equine encephalitis virus associated with Aedes albopictus—Florida, 1991. Morbidity and Mortality Weekly Reports 41:115, 121.
Fields, B.N., D.M. Knipe, et al. (eds.) (1990). Virology, second ed. New York: Raven Press.
Francy, D.B., N. Karabatsos, D.M. Wesson, C.G. Moore Jr., J.S. Lazuick, M.L. Niebylski, T.F. Tsai, and G.B. Craig Jr. (1990). A new arbovirus from Aedes albopictus, an Asian mosquito established in the United States. Science 250:1738-1740.
Halstead, S.B. (1989). Antibody, macrophages, dengue virus infection, shock, and hemorrhage: A pathogenic cascade. Rev. Infect. Dis. 11: Suppl. 4, S830-S839.
Karabatsos, N. (ed.) (1985). International Catalogue of Arboviruses Including Certain Other Viruses of Vertebrates, third ed. San Antonio, Tex.: American Society of Tropical Medicine and Hygiene.
Kilbourne, E.D., B.C. Easterday, and S. McGregor (1988). Evolution to predominance of swine influenza virus hemagglutinin mutants of predictable phenotype during single infections of the natural host. Proc. Natl. Acad. Sci. USA 85:8098-8101.
Liang, T.J., K. Hasegawa, N. Rimon, J.R. Wands, and E. Ben-Porath (1991). A hepatitis B virus mutant associated with an epidemic of fulminant hepatitis. N. Engl. J. Med. 324:1705-1709.
Lopez, C., P. Pellett, J. Stewart, C. Goldsmith, K. Sanderlin, J. Black, D. Warfield, and P. Feorino (1988). Characteristics of human herpesvirus-6. J. Infect. Dis. 157:1271-1273.
Morse, S.S. (1990). Looking for a link. Nature 344:297.
Morse, S.S., and A. Schluederberg (1990). Emerging viruses: The evolution of viruses and viral diseases. J. Infect. Dis. 162:1-7.
Morse, S.S. (1991). Emerging viruses: Defining the rules for viral traffic. Perspect. Biol. Med. 34:387-409.
National Commission on AIDS (1991). America Living With AIDS. Washington, D.C.: U.S. Government Printing Office.

Nomura, A., G.N. Stemmermann, P.-H. Chyou, I. Kato, G.I. Perez-Perez, and M.J. Blaser (1991). *Helicobacter pylori* infection and gastric carcinoma among Japanese Americans in Hawaii. N. Engl. J. Med. **325**:1132-1136.

Omata, M., T. Ehata, O. Yokosuka, K. Hosoda, and M. Ohto (1991). Mutations in the precore region of hepatitis B virus DNA in patients with fulminant and severe hepatitis. N. Engl. J. Med. **324**:1699-1704.

Parsonnet, J., G.D. Friedman, D.P. Vandersteen, Y. Chang, J.H. Vogelman, N. Orentreich, and R.K. Sibley (1991). *Helicobacter pylori* infection and the risk of gastric carcinoma. N. Engl. J. Med. **325**:1127-1131.

Peterson, W.L. (1991). *Helicobacter pylori* and peptic ulcer disease. N. Engl. J. Med. **324**:1043-1048.

Porterfield, J.S. (ed.) (1989). *Andrewes' Viruses of Vertebrates*, fifth ed. London: Baillière Tindall.

Reyes, G.R., M.A. Purdy, J.P. Kim, K.-C. Luk, L.M. Young, K.E. Fry, and D.W. Bradley (1990). Isolation of a cDNA from the virus responsible for enterically transmitted non-A, non-B hepatitis. Science **247**:1335-1339.

Reyes, G.R., and B. M. Baroudy (1991). Molecular biology of non-A, non-B hepatitis agents: Hepatitis C and Hepatitis E viruses. In *Advances in Virus Research* (K. Maramorosch, F.A. Murphy, and A.J. Shatkin, eds.), vol. 40, pp. 57-102. San Diego: Academic Press.

Rocha, E., N.J. Cox, R.A. Black, M.W. Harmon, C.J. Harrison, and A.J. Kendall (1991). Antigenic and genetic variation in influenza A (H1N1) virus isolates recovered from a persistently infected immunodeficient child. J. Virol. **65**:2340-2350.

Salahuddin, S.Z., D.V. Ablashi, P.D. Markham, S.F. Josephs, S. Sturzenegger, M. Kaplan G. Halligan, P. Biberfeld, F. Wong-Staal, B. Kramarsky, and R.C. Gallo (1986). Isolation of a new virus, HBLV, in patients with lymphoproliferative disorders. Science **234**:596-600.

Salas, R., N. de Manzione, R.B. Tesh, R. Rico-Hesse, R.E. Shope, A. Betancourt, O.Godoy, R. Bruzual, M.E. Pacheco, B. Ramos, M.E. Taibo, J.G. Tamayo, E.Jaimes, C. Vasquez, F. Araoz, and J. Querales (1991). Venezuelan haemorrhagic fever. Lancet **338**:1033-1036.

Salvato, M., P. Borrow, E. Shimomaye, and M.B.A. Oldstone (1991). Molecular basis of viral persistence: a single amino acid change in the glycoprotein of lymphocytic choriomeningitis virus is associated with suppression of the antiviral cytotoxic T-lymphocyte response and establishment of persistence. J. Virol. **65**:1863-1869.

Scholtissek, C., and E. Naylor (1988). Fish farming and influenza pandemics. Nature **331**:215.

Smith, A.W., and P.M. Boyt (1990). Caliciviruses of ocean origin: A review. J. Zoo Wildl. Med. **21**:3-23.

Wellmer, H. (1983). Some reflections on the ecology of dengue hemorrhagic fever in Thailand. In *Geographical Aspects of Health* (N.D. McGlashan and J.R. Blunden, eds.), pp. 273-284. London: Academic Press.

Wilesmith, J.W., J.B.M. Ryan, and M.J. Atkinson (1991). Bovine spongiform encephalopathy: epidemiological studies on the origin. Vet. Rec. **128**:199-203.

Yamanishi, K., T. Okuno, K. Shiraki, M. Takahashi, T. Kondo, Y. Asano, and T. Kurata (1988). Identification of human herpesvirus-6 as a causal agent for exanthem subitum. Lancet **i**:1065-1067.

Zahorsky, J. (1913). Roseola infantum. JAMA **61**:1446-1450.

3

Patterns of Disease Emergence in History

WILLIAM H. McNEILL

The sudden appearance of new infections, or at least of locally new infections, previously unrecognized, has been very frequent in human history and sometimes of very great importance in affecting the course of public affairs—that which we commonly think of as history. Among instances that can be reconstructed with a certain degree of confidence, the really striking examples all come from some new pattern of human movement, initiating new contacts across what had previously been disease boundaries. This meant that infections new to one partner in the encounter moved into what the epidemiologists call a virgin population, sometimes with very dramatic consequences indeed.

What got me started on writing my book *Plagues and Peoples* (McNeill, 1976) was reading about Cortez and what happened to him and his men after they had been attacked by the Aztecs and were driven from Tenochtitlan in 1520. By all rights, they should have been pursued the next day and had their hearts cut out on top of the temple in the center of the city. Instead, there was almost no pursuit, and in the weeks after the Spaniards had been defeated, the former subjects of the Aztecs joined Cortez. Together they then besieged the capital city of Tenochtitlan until Cortez marched in and destroyed the temple instead of being destroyed on its top, as surely should have happened. After all, there were only about 400 Spaniards left after the retreat from Tenochtitlan and they were exposed in a big open plain and absolutely vulnerable. But nothing happened, or rather, the wrong thing happened.

When I read this story, I felt that it violated all ordinary canons of human behavior. What went wrong? While puzzling over this, I read an account of the *noche trista*, as the Spaniards called their defeat, which mentioned the fact that smallpox had broken out in Tenochtitlan on that same *noche trista*. The nephew of Montezuma, who had organized the attack upon Cortez, died, and the historian mentioned this death and its cause to explain why the pursuit was so half hearted.

I had enough general understanding of what an infection such as smallpox let loose on a virgin population might do to be able to imagine what was going on in Tenochtitlan that night. It wasn't just the nephew of Montezuma who died. Aztec civilization died too. Think of the confrontation. On the one hand were the Spaniards, who grew up in a world in which smallpox was an endemic childhood disease, so that it would hardly be possible to become an adult without having had smallpox in youth. Opposed to them, the Aztecs were completely inexperienced. Then when they attacked the Spaniards, the disease broke out and one side—the Spanish side—was untouched while the other side died like flies.

After that, why do you think the Indian subject allies joined Cortez? They had witnessed a divine demonstration. Something up there said: "Don't attack Spaniards. Join Spaniards. We are showing which side we are on in this contest." The consequence was victory for Cortez, and persisting epidemiological disequilibrium assured continuing victories of Europeans in encounters with the Indians for the next three centuries. Indeed, the whole history of our country, and of the Americas at large, centering as it does around the repopulation of the land by immigrants from Europe and Africa, is a function of the disease disequilibrium that existed after 1500 between the Old and the New World.

In contrast, consider what happened in Africa where the disease balance went quite the other way. Europeans who went to Africa died of fevers to which the African peoples were already acclimated. So Africa remained African, except for the very southernmost parts of the continent, because of the formidability of its diseases as compared to other parts of the world. Incidentally, the variety of human infections in tropical Africa is a powerful reason for thinking that human evolution occurred in these lands, where the disease elaboration is the greatest anywhere on the face of the earth.

Having realized how powerful and important disease inequalities of this sort could be in human history, I began looking through the whole recorded past. From these researches, I suggest to you that the human encounters with disease may be schematized in the very simplest fashion as follows: Our remoter ancestors evolved in Africa where they established an ecological equilibrium with very numerous infections and infestations. Then sometime not so very long ago, by which I mean 50,000 to 100,000 years before our time, some ingenious character decided that he could put a bear skin on his bare back and then carry a tropical microenvironment with him into temperate zones where it froze in winter. This allowed escape from a whole host of tropical infections. After this extraordinary emancipation, human beings expanded around the earth at a very rapid pace. In terms of biological evolution, the time involved was like the twinkling of an eye. Within a few thousand years, humans reached

every habitable land except for a few small islands of the remoter
oceans. Humanity thereby launched itself upon its global career as
a predator upon other forms of life. In the process, humanity left
behind all but a few infections. It was probably the healthiest time
that human beings have ever experienced. The resulting ecological
disequilibrium assured population growth, which in turn impelled human
hunting bands to expand very rapidly around the whole earth.

Now the history of civilized times is the gradual rectification of
this initial disequilibrium. Bit by bit, disease organisms moved into
this temperate world–the world that human beings, tropical animals
outside their natural niche, had created for themselves. There
appear to be certain horizon points in this process. For example,
when human populations become large enough, they can sustain
viral infections that provoke lasting immunity among survivors.
These are the classic childhood diseases, such as measles, smallpox,
mumps, and two or three others. The point at which local human
populations become large enough to sustain such infections is a
distinct threshold. When it was crossed, exposed populations acquired a very powerful epidemiological weapon in any contact with
smaller societies, that did not have such endemic infections. That in
fact is why there are so few civilizations in Eurasia, because a society
with that kind of epidemiological advantage, when encountering a
previously isolated population, almost but not quite destroys it. It
is rather like the process of digestion. The expanding endemically
diseased society breaks down the political and cultural structure of
peripheral, disease inexperienced populations, allowing survivors
to enter into the civilized body politic. What happened to the Aztecs,
when Cortez encountered them, is a case in point, for the resistance
to Christianity, along with resistance to wholesale incorporation
into the Spanish imperial system, was also destroyed by the discred-
iting that came to the political leadership and to the religious ideas
that had structured Amerindian life before smallpox hit.

The history of civilized disease is one of step-by-step intensifica-
tion of infection, perhaps approaching a stabilization analogous to the sort
of ecological stability, or near stability, that presumably had once existed in
tropical Africa. Then modern medicine came along and renewed ecological
disequilibrium all over again. It is rather like a reprise of the escape
from the burden of infectious disease that occurred when human
beings first left their tropical cradle land. For, demographically
speaking, medical intervention was scarcely significant before the 1880s
but then achieved a series of triumphs to 1968. The extinction of smallpox
in that year may turn out to be the apex of this process, allowing human
populations to experience again a situation analogous to the situation that our ancestors had known when they first left the tropics.

Disease organisms are now finding new avenues of ingress into the
mass of human bodies that has multiplied so extraordinarily in the

recent past. AIDS is what we have principally on our minds at the
moment, but I must say that it is a poor country cousin in terms of the
slowness of its propagation and the obviousness of behavioral adjustments that would check its spread. Other kinds of infections go
much more rapidly and will be much more difficult to control by
behavioral adaptation. The historical parallel to AIDS is clearly
syphilis, which appeared abruptly in Europe in 1494 and had no
perceptible demographic impact anywhere in the world, presumably because those who died of syphilis would have died from
something else at almost the same age. I also imagine that the
historical career of AIDS will be very similar in its demographic
impact; it is always worth reminding oneself that more people die in
automobile accidents each year than (I think it is still correct to say)
have yet died of AIDS in the United States. Demographically, in
terms of its effect on population, it is not yet a major phenomenon.
It may be in the future but it hasn't yet become so.

For syphilis, as far as I can understand from the historic record,
its major impact was a change in sexual manners, and the propagation of puritanism in the Christian churches. I have not been able to
find out whether there were comparable adjustments of sexual
practices in the Asian world because records of sexual behavior in
Asia have not been carefully studied. A similar sort of sexual
adjustment may well turn out to be the major impact of AIDS on the
human population as a whole.

Earlier, I mentioned the importance an infection may have when
it breaks across older geographical boundaries and hits a new population with catastrophic consequences. This doesn't say anything
about the emergence of really new diseases–those not merely new to
a particular human population, but new to the world. Obviously
new diseases do arise, but I think I am on very firm ground in saying
that they are historically untraceable.

Ancient descriptions of an outbreak of some lethal epidemic are
completely inadequate to allow one to say,"Aha, this is the point at
which a really new disease first hit the human population." Decid-
ing the exact nature of recorded infections is usually impossible.
Even the famous plague of Athens in 430 B.C. described by Thucydides
with apparent precision, and with an elegant succession of symptoms, cannot be confidently identified with any modern infection.
There are almost as many diagnoses of that plague as there are
doctors who have addressed themselves to the page and a half of the
Greek text that describes it.

In addition, it is, I suppose, self-evident that no contemporary
observer, Thucydides or anybody else, could know that a particular
infection, hitting a particular population, was absolutely new, as
against something that came in from somewhere else. Thucydides
actually says that the plague probably came from Egypt. Given the

limitations of human communications, no contemporary observer can be in a position to say that any particular outbreak is in fact the first time that a given disease ever affected a human population. This is still the case. I doubt that the moment of mutation or transfer when a disease organism first finds a new species of host is ever going to be observed. Perhaps we now know enough to confine such an event within certain geographical and time limits, say a decade or so, in a region of Africa, as is now believed about AIDS. But I don't think anyone is ever going to get much more precise than that. There are significant delays before a new infection is recognized. One has to wait until cases of the new disease come to relatively highly developed diagnostic centers, of which there is not an infinite number in the world. Even then, there are likely to be further delays in recognizing it as due to some new, previously unrecognized form of infection.

The case of AIDS here is quite instructive. It was first recognized, I think, about 1978. But reconstructed cases suggest that it had been around for maybe a couple of decades in the United States before that time, and probably even longer in other parts of the world, Haiti, or Africa. But who knows how far back into the human past it goes, and behind that, very likely although this is not certain either, to some kind of monkey population. Such history is terribly vague, even though it happened, so to speak, under our eyes.

In most disease partnerships, a very rapid adaptation between hosts and parasites occurs, and presumably this involves genetic change, both on the part of the host and on the part of the infectious agents. Perhaps adaptation may only select from an initial range of variability, but sometimes an apparently new mutation is fixed or alters its population frequencies drastically. Unfortunately, clinical reports are likely to be more revealing here than the historical record. Historical records are no help because the people who made the records with which historians work did not move in a universe of discourse that allowed for biological evolution through mutual adaptation and mutation. I am not perfectly sure that test tubes will take knowledge very much further because scientists are not going to be able to replicate in their laboratories the ecological networks and balances within which real disease changes occur.

Setting these theoretical questions aside, the possibility of really drastic epidemiological disaster bringing a halt to the modern surge of human population seems to me something we all should take very seriously. To paraphrase Piers Plowman, What a fair field full of folk waiting to be fed upon! If you look at the world from the point of view of a hungry virus (speaking metaphorically of course)—or even a bacterium—we offer a magnificent feeding ground with all our billions of human bodies, where, in the very recent past, there were only half as many people. In some 25 or 27 years, we have doubled in number. A marvelous target for any organism that can adapt itself to invading us.

A question I thought about when I wrote my book *Plagues and Peoples* is what is the expected frequency for a successful disease transfer from one species to another? I have no light to cast, aside from one simple observation. The appearance of viral diseases— diseases I called diseases of civilization, and which we know as standard childhood diseases—perhaps lagged not more than 1,000 years behind the emergence of human populations large enough, and in sufficiently dense communication, one with another, to sustain them. The horizon at which infections ancestral to the viral childhood infections of historic times seem to be present is about 2000 B.C. in Mesopotamia. Now, the earliest emergence in Sumeria of a dense population with a total number of perhaps half a million came about 3000 B.C. By that time, there were about a dozen cities of about 30,000-50,000 inhabitants in Sumer, and they were in communication with one another. And for about 1,000 years, between approximately 3000 B.C. and 2000 B.C., we have no record of epidemics that might signify the incorporation into that society of one or another of these viral infections. Even after 2000 B.C., the best evidence is merely an inscription that refers to epidemics and the Goddess of Epidemic as an established and recognized phenomenon. The epidemics referred to might not necessarily be viral, and they might have been enteric infections carried by water rather than by droplet infection. One can't identify the infection clearly as one of the later recognized childhood diseases. So I am jumping to a conclusion in saying that 1,000 years separate the emergence of the demographic possibility and the appearance of such diseases. Yet it is the best estimate I can make of what may have happened.

It is ironical to suppose, as I do, that the brilliantly successful elimination of most human infections in the last 100 years or so–it all happened between 1884, when Koch discovered the bacterium of cholera, through the 1960s when smallpox was eliminated–actually set up the possibility of some new disease invasion.

The fate of the rabbits of Australia seems to me perhaps the worst case one can imagine. When (deliberately, under Dr. Fenner's jurisdiction) myxomatosis was introduced to Australia to control the rabbits, Fenner and colleagues studied what happened with all the sophistication of modern science (Fenner, 1983). Initially the lethality rate was 99.8 percent. But the rates of lethality diminished very rapidly. Adaptation between the new virus and the rabbit population of Australia occurred with a speed which, in a sense, is reassuring. After 7 years the lethality rate was down to around 25 percent and the number of rabbits in Australia had stabilized at about 20 percent of what it had been before myxomatosis was introduced.

Now this seems to me a very exact model of what might happen to human populations exposed to a new and very lethal virus in the world today. The idea that the medical profession would constitute an effective obstacle to the propagation of such an infection seems optimistic, to say the least. Doctors would simply be the first to go with 99.8 percent lethality! Just think about it.

In general, let me leave you with the thought that perhaps what we face as human beings is a conservation of catastrophe. I wrote an essay about this, which was published in Daedalus recently (McNeill, 1989). It is sort of musing upon the limits of medical and other dimensions of our human capacity to make things the way we want them, and, by skill, organization and knowledge, to insulate ourselves from local and frequent disasters. Every time we do this we change natural ecological relationships, at the cost of creating a new vulnerability to some larger disaster, which happens less frequently, but is sure to happen sooner or later when that artificial system, for whatever reason, breaks down.

An example that is most immediately obvious is what the Army Corps of Engineers is doing with the Mississippi, and has been doing since I was a child. When I was young, spring floods occurred regularly on the Mississippi and there would be stories about how much of Louisiana and Arkansas was under water each year. The Corps of Engineers, beginning in the 1920s sporadically, and then more systematically in the 1930s, began building dikes to hold the Mississippi within fixed limits. The result of this is that the Mississippi now deposits silt in its bottom every year. The dikes then have to go higher, and the river goes higher, in response to which the dikes go still higher, and the river goes higher, and so on. In Louisiana, even at slack water the river is now flowing several feet above the level of the ground. The Chinese did the same in the Yellow River Valley beginning about 800 B.C. As a result, they have had a series of vast catastrophes when the river broke its dikes and took a new course to the sea. The same thing will happen with the Mississippi. It has, in fact, chosen its new course to the sea, as was explained in a very interesting article in the New Yorker several years ago (McPhee, 1987). It very nearly made it in 1973, during high water season, when despite the most modern technology, the river came close to breaking through. Well, the dikes can go still higher, but everybody knows that eventually the system will topple over. One can't have the Mississippi 800 feet above ground level. So some day there is going to be a very big flood in the lower Mississippi, wreaking much greater damages than annual floods ever did before the dikes were built.

This is an easily graspable physical model of what human intervention in the natural ecosystem does. We create new situations that become unstable. Medical intervention, which has been so dramatically successful in the last 100 years, is another example. It makes the situation unstable. And from what others have said, clearly viruses are what is most likely to break those dikes and create some kind of vast new catastrophe for humankind.

This is not a reason for holding back and not trying to understand and remake natural balances; quite the contrary. But we should also realize the limits of our powers. It is worth keeping in mind that the more we drive infections to the margins of human experience, the wider we open a door for a new catastrophic infection. We will never escape the ecosystem and the limits of the ecosystem. Whether we like it or not, we are caught in the food chain, eating and being eaten. It is one of the conditions of life.

REFERENCES

Fenner, F. (1983). Biological control, as exemplified by smallpox eradication and myxomatosis [The Florey Lecture, 1983]. Proc. R. Soc. (Lond.) B **218**:259-285.

McNeill, W.H. (1976). *Plagues and Peoples.* Garden City, N.Y.: Anchor Press/Doubleday.

McNeill, W.H. (1989). Control and catastrophe in human affairs. Daedalus **118**(1):1-12.

McPhee, J. (1987). The control of nature (Atchafalaya). The New Yorker, Feb. 23, pp. 39-100. [Reprinted: McPhee, J. (1989). Atchafalaya. In *The Control of Nature*, pp. 3-92. New York: Farrar, Strauss and Giroux.]

4

Influenza

ROBERT G. WEBSTER

Influenza is probably one of the oldest emerging viruses. It is still emerging. Still the sixth most important cause of death in the United States, it goes far back into ancient Greece and Rome, although the ancient descriptions of influenza were so imprecise that we cannot be sure that they were specifically influenza rather than some other respiratory infection. However, we have reasonably clear records beginning from the middle ages. Hirsch, in the last century, identified and tabulated reports of influenza outbreaks from the fifteenth century onward, using as his criteria a respiratory infection with sudden onset in the context of an epidemic lasting 2 to 3 weeks and then disappearing, exactly like the pattern of modern influenza epidemics (Hirsch, 1883).

There are three features of influenza that make us think that the disease in all of the records collected by Hirsch really was influenza. First, the epidemics occurred periodically. There was no set pattern and, from time to time, they disappeared. The second point was that some epidemics were much more severe than others and usually, as now, affected the elderly people. Third, fairly frequently these epidemics came from the east, spreading to Europe from Asia, across Russia. These are still the hallmarks of influenza epidemics today.

For those not in the influenza field, a brief description of influenza virus is in order (Murphy and Webster, 1990). The virus contains RNA, in eight segments, each segment corresponding to a gene of the virus. The segmented genome of the virus facilitates genetic reassortment, or reshuffling, when different strains may infect the same host. As with almost all viruses, the packaging of the virus consists of various proteins. There are three major varieties of the influenza virus, called A, B, and C. They look identical, but influenza A is by far the most mutable, as Palese and Murphy will describe in other chapters, and is responsible for almost all major epidemics. For this reason, this chapter will deal with influenza A exclusively. Two proteins on the surface of the virus particle, the hemagglutinin, or H protein, and the neuraminidase, or N protein, are of special importance. Seen as "spikes" in electron micrographs, they are involved in the interaction between the virus and host cells.

Each hemagglutinin molecule consists of three chains, like three ropes coiled together, and is a glycoprotein, with sugar molecules attached at specific places. The H and N proteins are major antigens of the virus, which is to say that the immune system of infected individuals actively responds to these proteins and makes antibodies against them. In influenza A, there are numerous varieties, called subtypes, of both the H and N proteins. Some 13 subtypes of the H protein are known, designated by arbitrary numbers (we recently described a fourteenth one; Kawaoka et al., 1990). Because of the importance of the H and N proteins, influenza strains are often designated by their subtype of each protein. When we speak of an "H2N8" influenza, we mean a virus strain that possesses, as its surface proteins, hemagglutinin of subtype number 2 (H2) and neuraminidase of subtype 8 (N8). It is a kind of formula identifying the virus strain. All of these are H and N subtypes of influenza A virus.

If we use sero-epidemiology, that is, test for antibodies in the blood in different populations, to look back at influenza strains that have infected in the past, we can go back as far as 1890 by testing sera of elderly people still living. We find an influenza epidemic about 1890 caused by an H2N8 virus, followed in 1900 by an epidemic caused by an H3N8 influenza virus. Then in 1918 we had the virus that we all know about, the so-called Spanish flu (H1N1 to virologists). The greatest natural disaster since the beginning of the century, it probably influenced the ending of the First World War, at least according to German historians, who attributed to it a vast effect. It wasn't the Americans coming to Europe, it was the virus they brought with them that actually did the job.

In recent times, after Richard Shope (the father of the Robert Shope whose chapter appears elsewhere in this book) discovered swine influenza, we had the human series of influenza pandemics. Wilson Smith and his colleagues discovered and described the influenza virus in 1933, making more accurate studies possible. After that, we had the first change, H2N2, in 1957. This was the first major change in human influenza since 1919. Then in 1968 H3N2 appeared; more recently, in 1977, an H1N1 influenza virus reappeared. A couple of points can be made from these facts. All human influenza epidemics involved viruses with H subtypes 1, 2, or 3. We saw them back at the end of the last century; we are seeing them again. Are all human epidemics confined to H1, H2, H3? We still don't know.

Let us stop for a moment and consider the sorts of variation that occur in influenza viruses. The first kind of variation occurs as a result of accumulation of point mutations in those two spike proteins, the hemagglutinin and neuraminidase, which we call antigenic drift. After the appearance of the Hong Kong flu in 1968, for example, almost every other year we have another epidemic of influenza right up to 1992. This is due to accumulation of point mutations driven by the immune response (Fitch et al., 1991). Point mutations, substitutions in one or a few of the individual amino acids making up the H protein, occur randomly as the virus is copied in infected cells. The immune response takes care of some variants in the hemagglutinin, but variants emerge that are not neutralized by the antibodies that individuals have made in response to the original infection and so the system goes on with an accumulation of point mutations. From structural studies of the H protein, we know that this accumulation of point mutations is in the top of the globular head of the H protein molecule surrounding the region of the molecule that binds to the virus receptor on the cell surface. While receptor binding is essential to allow the virus to infect host cells, the head of the H molecule can accommodate a large number of changes without affecting functions like receptor binding, which is hidden in the center of the threefold molecule. Because there is a lot of plasticity in this molecule, it can accumulate many changes to avoid the immune response.

But there is another kind of change that represents the other method of evolution of influenza. This is the so-called antigenic shift, which has led to all the major pandemic strains, including the 1918 "Spanish flu", the Asian flu (1957), Hong Kong flu (1968), and Russian flu (1977), which is really a misnomer because it occurred in Anshan Province in northern China. The point to be made from this is that they occur in China, just as I mentioned above for the epidemics of previous centuries.

I am going to deal in some detail with the 1968 epidemic, because this was when I joined the influenza community after leaving Canberra, where I received my basic training in immunology and biology.

When the 1968 pandemic appeared, it swept around the world as these pandemics always do. Martin Kaplan at the World Health Organization in Geneva, workers at the National Institutes of Health in the United States, and Edwin Kilbourne, along with many other people, wondered where this virus came from. Very quickly, studies by Walter Dowdle (at the U.S. Centers for Disease Control) and others established that this virus had a hemagglutinin that was related to viruses in ducks, and related to viruses in horses, and the concept emerged that perhaps this virus, or at least part of it, came from the lower orders, that is from animals.

At that stage, the National Institutes of Health decided it was time to understand the reservoirs of influenza in nature, and we were given this mission. A certain amount of information was already known. Richard Shope had established influenza in swine in the United States. Classical swine influenza is endemic to all hog farms in the United States; the pigs get sick only in the fall but the virus is always there. In 1968, it had become apparent that, in addition to this classical swine flu, the viruses from humans, such as Victoria or Hong Kong, also spread back into the pig. Thus the pig apparently plays an important role. Other animals were also known to harbor influenza viruses. From 1968, for the next 10 years or so, Virginia Hinshaw and I studied influenza in many exciting places in the world. We looked at quite a number of possibilities. For example, we considered the horse, although we eventually found that it is not a major source of new influenza strains in humans. However, it is an interesting situation. It was already known by 1968 that the horse has two subtypes of influenza, an H3 and an H7. It is surprising to realize that one of these subtypes is now apparently disappearing. So influenza is not only evolving; on the other hand it is disappearing. H7 influenza viruses haven't been seen clinically in the world for the last 10 years. We did a survey and we can find some evidence in Outer Mongolia and Poland, but otherwise this particular strain of flu has dissappeared from horses. The H3 subtype of influenza in horses, on the other hand, is evolving (Webster and Guo, 1991). It was recently spread by airplane. In 1987, two American horses brought into South Africa infected local horses. Instead of being a mild endemic disease, as it is in the United States, when it got into a totally virgin population this virus killed 50 foals, and so on. The severity therefore depends a great deal on the immune status of the host population.

What we eventually did find as a result of all these animal studies surprised us. After studying all these other species, we then made the mistake of studying the wild duck, and we found that all subtypes of influenza, H1 through H13, are present in the wild duck population. The ultimate reservoir of influenza is in the aquatic birds of the world.

In the wild duck, these influenza viruses cause no disease. They probably ultimately are adapted to the duck because the virus replicates a little in the respiratory tract, mainly in the intestinal tract, and the birds spread their virus through the water systems. Every August you can go to Canada and take samples from all of the local lakes in the Canadian shield and you can isolate your own kind of influenza virus, causing no disease at all in these species.

More recently, we have found that there is another reservoir of influenza, the little shore birds that migrate north in the spring time from South America, particularly the ruddy ternstone and red knot. We believe that populations of these shore birds maintain the virus in the spring and the ducks maintain the virus in the fall. Some of these viruses are shared; some are not. Types H3, H4, and H6 predominate in ducks; types H1, H2, and H9-13 in shore birds. An interesting point, also verified by more recent studies, is that the avian reservoir in nature can be divided into two pathways, the New World and the Old World, in which the influenza viruses belong to different lineages. That is probably because the migration of birds is north and south, and there is only a limited amount of mixing across the Alaskan Straits, so Old World and New World migratory birds rarely cross paths.

In many ways the discovery of the avian reservoirs of influenza was a big non-event because here we have all of these influenza viruses and they are causing no disease. And in many senses the scientific community considered this a bit irrelevant. But nature has taken care to show us the potential. In 1980, Graham Laver, another noted influenza virologist, sent me a cutting from the *Canberra Times*. One hundred young seals had died in the Boston region, and the cause was called seal flu. We followed this and indeed the disease was caused by influenza, in current terminology an H7N7 influenza, isolated not only from the lungs but also from the brains of the seals. Using the molecular genetic technology then current, RNA-RNA hybridization to compare the genetic information of this virus with that of other influenza strains, we found that the closest relatives to this virus were viruses from ducks, gulls, turkeys and so on. We concluded that the eight individual gene segments probably came from viruses circulating in that aquatic bird reservoir. Incidentally, laboratory workers who came in contact with the virus while taking samples from infected seals got conjunctivitis, an eye inflammation due to the virus (Webster et al., 1981). Although this was a very mild consequence of infection, it indicates how easily an influenza virus can spread. So, again, while these avian viruses are not serious in their aquatic bird reservoir, when they spread into a susceptible species, in this case the seal, they can be disastrous and could kill a third of the population. Other viruses could be similar. More recently we have looked at another virus that has spread into the seal population, an H4 virus, and sequenced the hemagglutinins of influenza viruses isolated from seals, turkeys, ducks, and chickens. To define the evolutionary pathways, we mapped the sequence changes in the hemagglutinin. From this analysis, we saw that this seal virus hemagglutinin also belongs to a virus of the avian reservoir.

Another incident, that occurred in 1983, further proves that the influenza viruses in the aquatic reservoir are not so benign. An influenza virus was identified in chicken houses in Pennsylvania in April 1983. We were very fortunate that an astute veterinarian isolated an H5N2 virus from a very mild respiratory infection. Then, suddenly, in October, the virus became virulent. Every chicken in the houses was killed. How do we cope with such an epidemic? The Agriculture Department used the standard methods of eradication, killing the infected chickens and exposed neighboring birds and burying the carcasses. But we can't help asking ourselves what we would have done if this virus had occurred in humans. We can't dig holes and bury all the people in the world. It is a very serious situation. One antiviral drug that shows real promise in influenza epidemics is an agent called amantadine. The U.S. Department of Agriculture wouldn't let us use amantadine on the chickens, but we tried it in the laboratory on the virus strain isolated from the outbreak. Strains of virus resistant to the drug developed within a week. So we have to think of alternative strategies to cope with such an emerging situation.

Where did this virus come from, and how did it get to be so severe? When we looked at the various genes by nucleic acid hybridization techniques, just as we did earlier for the seal virus, we found that the eight genes of the chicken virus came from this aquatic reservoir which we thought was rather benign: the genes came from gulls, ducks, turkeys, and so on. The genetic information suggested that it was just a mutation in the hemagglutinin gene that was required for the change in virulence between April and October. We confirmed this in the laboratory by making reassortants, in which we introduced the new hemagglutinin gene with the other seven genes all from the mild virus. When this reassortant virus was tested in eggs, it killed all the embryos and was totally virulent, just like the severe virus we isolated from the dying chickens. So the last step in the development of that virus was something to do with the hemagglutinin. That is not to say that the other genes are not involved; they certainly are. But it was the replacement of the hemagglutinin gene that made the difference. By mixing through the aquatic reservoir, the formerly mild virus had picked up the necessary genes, the last changes. The pivotal changes occurred in the hemagglutinin. A single point mutation in that hemagglutinin gene, indeed, was sufficient to change that benign virus into one that was completely lethal (Webster et al., 1986). In fact, what happened was surprising. There are two potential glycosylation sites (places where sugars can be attached to the protein) in this region of the hemagglutinin molecule. In the original H protein, only one of these sites had sugar attached. In the H protein from the virulent virus, this sugar was lost. This is because there was a point mutation that caused the amino acid lysine to be substituted for the amino acid threonine in that position. As a result, the site for attaching the carbohydrate was lost. For virulence, the H protein needs to be cut—cleaved—in that position, and the carbohydrate side chain in the original virus shielded the hemagglutinin from cleavage. The change allowed the new virus to spread through the tissues and kill (Kawaoka and Webster, 1988). In summary, a virus evolved from this benign reservoir, passaged and multiplied in the chicken population.

These two cases, the seal and the chicken, are very similar and also relevant to human health. Historically, the chicken population in Pennsylvania is like the world as it is at the moment. There are hundreds of thousands, even millions of chickens just waiting to be infected. In fact, human agency introduced the virus into those houses and it was disastrous. A single point mutation in a virus was enough to make this evolutionary pattern take place.

Returning briefly to the pig and its role in the evolution of influenza viruses, we now believe that the pig probably plays a very important role. Back in 1968, when the Hong Kong virus appeared, Kundin and others in Asia isolated the H3N2 viruses in pigs as well (Kundin, 1970). Many countries in the world had them. Since then, every few years, we find these H3N2 viruses in the pig population, particularly in Asia (Kida et al., 1988). Are they coming from humans or are they coming from the aquatic reservoirs? The answer is that they are coming from both sources. Viruses are moving from the aquatic bird population into pigs, and viruses from humans are moving into pigs. Conversely, viruses in pigs are moving into humans. Just a few years ago we had another "swine flu" incident that went almost unnoticed. Investigators at the Centers for Disease Control reported recently that a pregnant woman died in Wisconsin in 1988 (Wells et al., 1991). The virus isolated was a swine virus, and all the genes in that virus came from a pig. The indication is that, periodically, these viruses do get transmitted to humans. Luckily, they lack the gene composition that will allow virus to spread from human to human. This lack is what also limited the spread of the 1976 Fort Dix swine flu isolate. We know very little about this process. One piece of evidence comes from looking at the receptor binding properties of the viruses that were in pigs. This property of the H protein is required for infecting cells. The classical human binding properties, at positions 226-228 of the H protein, are the amino acids Leucine-Serine-Serine. We find that these swine viruses we have tested that are circulating in Southeast Asia have the sequence Glutamine-Serine-Glycine, which is also more typical of a duck virus rather than of the human type. Thus, we find in the pig population viruses with receptor binding properties typical of those in duck; they also appear somewhat as though they are on the way to becoming human viruses. The concept is emerging that the pig is the mixing vessel.

To return to the human situation, it is now apparent that the Asian strain that occurred in 1957 acquired not one gene from pigs. The virus probably emerged by reassortment between the viruses in humans at that time, and the virus from some aquatic reservoir. And the human viruses acquired three genes, PB1, H and N, from this avian reservoir. This was a pandemic strain that caused high mortality around the world.

In 1968 the Hong Kong virus did the same thing. It acquired the hemagglutinin and the PB1 gene. The PB1 gene didn't come from the Asian strain then circulating. Again, based on sequence analysis, we think that the PB1 came in from the avian reservoir. So the transfer of information resulting in the last two pandemic strains has come directly from the avian reservoir (Kawaoka et al., 1989).

The conclusion can be stated simply: All the genes of the influenza viruses of the world are being maintained in the aquatic bird population, in gulls and ducks, and periodically they are transmitted to other species, including humans, usually after reassorting (Webster et al., 1992).

In closing, I would just like to return to the 1918 catastrophe. The influenza pandemic of 1918-1919 caused a greater number of mortalities than any other single event, including the Civil War, World War I, World War II, or any war. The same influenza viruses are still maintained in the aquatic bird reservoir. Even though influenza is very ancient, it still has the capacity to evolve, to acquire new genes, new hosts. The potential is still there for a pandemic like 1918-1919 to happen again.

REFERENCES

Fitch, W.M., J.M.E. Leiter, X. Li, and P. Palese (1991). Positive Darwinian evolution in human influenza A viruses. Proc. Natl. Acad. Sci. USA **88**:4270-4274.

Hirsch, A. (1883). *Handbook of Geographical and Historical Pathology* (C. Creighton, trans.), vol. I, pp. 7-54. London: The New Sydenham Society.

Kawaoka, Y., and R.G. Webster (1988). Molecular mechanism of acquisition of virulence in influenza virus in nature. Microb. Pathog. **5**:311-318.

Kawaoka, Y., S. Krauss, and R.G. Webster (1989). Avian-to-human transmission of the PB1 gene of influenza A viruses in the 1957 and 1968 pandemics. J. Virol. **63**:4603-4608.

Kawaoka, Y., S. Yamnikova, T.M. Chambers, D.K. Lvov, and R.G. Webster (1990). Molecular characterization of a new hemagglutinin, subtype H14, of influenza A virus. Virology **179**:759-767.

Kida, H., K.F. Shortridge, and R.G. Webster (1988). Origin of the hemagglutinin gene of H3N2 influenza viruses from pigs in China. Virology **162**:160-166.

Kundin, W.D. (1970). Hong Kong A-2 influenza virus infection among swine during a human epidemic in Taiwan. Nature **228**:857.

Murphy, B.R., and R.G. Webster (1990). Orthomyxoviruses. In *Virology* (B.N. Fields, D.M. Knipe, et al., eds.), second ed., Chap. 40 (pp. 1091-1152). New York: Raven Press.

Scholtissek, C., and E. Naylor (1988). Fish farming and influenza pandemics. Nature **331**:215.

Webster, R.G., J. Geraci, G. Petursson, and K. Skirnisson (1981). Conjunctivitis in human beings caused by influenza A virus of seals. N. Engl. J. Med. **304**:911.

Webster, R.G., Y. Kawaoka, and W.J. Bean Jr. (1986). Molecular changes in

A/chicken/Pennsylvania/83 (H5N2) influenza virus associated with virulence. Virology **149**:165-173.

Webster, R.G., W.J. Bean, O.T. Gorman, T.M. Chambers, and Y. Kawaoka
(1992). Evolution and ecology of influenza A viruses. Microbiol. Rev.
56:152-179.

Webster, R.G., and R. Rott (1987). Influenza virus A pathogenicity: The
pivotal role of hemagglutinin. Cell **50**:665-666.

Webster, R.G., and Y. Guo (1991). New influenza virus in horses. Nature
351:527.

Wells, D.L., D.J. Hopfensperger, N.A. Arden, M.W. Harmon, J.P. Davis,
M.A. Tipple, and L.B. Schonberger (1991). Swine influenza virus infections. JAMA **265**:478-481.

5

Emerging Viruses in Context: An Overview of Viral Hemorrhagic Fevers

KARL M. JOHNSON

Viral hemorrhagic fever is itself an emergent concept: a product of events of the twentieth century, albeit some of the diseases we recognize as such today were clearly known to man many centuries ago (Gajdusek, 1962). They were all zoonotic infections and this fact, together with the violent ongoing ecological change that has occurred on this planet since the end of World War II and the emergence of modern virological science, has led to a perception that these are "emerging" diseases. If this is true in one sense, it is important to realize that from the viewpoint of the agents themselves, it is plainly not so. The viruses almost surely antedate our species.

I confess to some difficulty in understanding what was meant by "emerging". Webster's *Unabridged Dictionary*, as usual, came to the rescue. The word is from the Latin *emergere*. Definitions cited include "to reveal itself to notice so as to call for immediate attention", "to issue from an inferior or obscure condition." On the same page I found another word, a deletion mutant, if you will, *emerere*, whence emeritus, "To serve out one's term." Thus, you confront here emergent viruses surveyed by an emeritus virologist.

Still searching for a way to present the subject of emerging hemorrhagic fever viruses, I noted that the first dictionary definition for emerge was "to rise from, or as from, an enveloping fluid." For a Montana trout fisherman the simile was irresistible. Compare these diseases to the life cycle of the mayfly. Mayflies spend most of their lives underwater as egg and molting nymphs. One to three years may be required. Finally, there comes a magic moment when the nymph comes to the surface, sheds its skin and becomes an emerger. Rapidly, it unfurls its wings to dry and the insect, now called a dun, drifts with the current. Shortly the dun flies off to the shrubs or trees lining the river and molts a final time to become the imago or spinner. Hours to a few days later, after mating, the spinner deposits eggs in the water and dies. Even in Montana, fishermen find that it is much easier to work with emergers, duns, and spinners if they want to catch a trout than to try to do it with the nymph. To become a nymph expert is considered by some to be the highest art in trout fishing.

Can we, with all of our history, ever recognize "new diseases" while they are still in the nymphal stage before they have emerged to become duns and go through their life cycle? Viral hemorrhagic fevers have surely spent most of their life cycles "underwater". They are zoonotic diseases, that is, are naturally occurring viruses of other animal species. In the historical sense man has come to know them only as emergers, duns or, in rare instances, as spinners. I have selected several of these viruses as examples to illustrate when, how, and why these diseases emerged, where they stand today, and where they are going. This discussion is designed to allow us finally to ask whether there are other metaphorical mayflies yet to rise to the surface and how we might seek and identify them as nymphs.

What we know today about the viral hemorrhagic fevers is only a tiny drop compared to what we have learned about many other viral infections. For example, we have not had available for these viruses the kind of resources that it took to identify CD4 as the receptor for the AIDS virus, HIV, and there are very few places where any work is going on with these viruses. There are several reasons for this. First of all, these diseases generally occur or originate in parts of the world where technology is usually not available to study them in great detail. Secondly, although most of these viruses have not frequently been transmitted from person to person by aerosol, they do have the capacity to infect man that way, as we have learned to our sorrow through a number of instances of hospital- and laboratory-acquired infections that resulted in serious disease and even death. This means that for serious microbiological work one has to have maximum containment facilities, so-called P4 or BL (Biosafety Level) 4 laboratories, which are expensive to equip and maintain. To my knowledge, there is no university in the world that has such a laboratory. In the United States and in a few other countries, suitable facilities can be found only at a handful of special national laboratories. Therefore, if research programs with these viruses continue at all, which is unfortunately itself questionable in these days of budgetary constraints, they will continue to be fundamentally organized at a national level.

GENERAL CLINICAL FEATURES OF HEMORRHAGIC FEVER AGENTS

With this prologue, let us consider the viruses and their diseases. Although caused by many different RNA viruses, with corresponding variations in the specific manifestations of disease, the pathogenesis of viral hemorrhagic fevers appears to have certain common threads. One key theme, at least in man, is the importance of cells of the monocyte-macrophage lineage in these infections. The circulating monocyte and the tissue macrophage serve as essential first line of defense in many infections. The ability of a virus to replicate in these cell types, with a variety of possible consequences, is intimately linked to host resistance and to expression of disease. Certain manifestations of hemorrhagic disease are probably induced by the response of the macrophage to infection. In contrast, when it comes to parenchymal disease (liver, kidneys, etc.), these agents tend to sort out in different subsets. The reasons for this, for example in terms of virus-receptor interaction, are virtually unknown.

In general, infection in humans with any one of these agents frequently causes serious disease and, in many instances, a tremendous lethality. There are exceptions. One of the most interesting is Lassa virus, the cause of Lassa fever in West Africa. It now appears that in terms of infection rates, probably less than 1 percent of all infections of Africans with Lassa virus will eventually result in serious and fatal disease. In contrast, fatality rates appear to be far higher in people of non-African stock.

"CLASSIC" HEMORRHAGIC FEVERS: YELLOW FEVER, DENGUE, AND HANTAAN

To go from the general to the specific, let us examine three "classic" hemorrhagic fevers, in terms of their emergence. These diseases were recognized, in varying degree, long before their causative agents were identified, before the advent even of the science of virology. These "classic" diseases are yellow fever, dengue, and hemorrhagic fever with renal syndrome.

The prototype is yellow fever. It has been said, rightly I think, that the history of yellow fever is, in many important ways, the history of the New World. In its natural state, in Africa, the yellow fever virus is propagated in a sylvan cycle involving monkey–mosquito–monkey. We now know that the critical event in the emergence and maturation of this disease was most likely the accidental, selection by humans of a variant of *Aedes aegypti*, an African rain forest mosquito that breeds in tree holes. The selected variant was one that bred in horizontal tree holes, and was therefore able to thrive in a rather similar structure, the water containers of ships used to bring slaves from Africa to the Americas.

Thus domesticated, *Aedes aegypti* and yellow fever wrought havoc in the New World for more than 2 centuries wherever humans gathered, whether in cities or in the armies attacking the gates of those cities.

After the recognition of the essential mosquito–human–mosquito virus cycle, yellow fever was rendered a sterile spinner in our cities within 20 years, not by virologists but by sanitarians who implemented vigorous and successful mosquito control programs.

A vaccine was shortly developed to deal with the original sylvan cycle, which man had robbed for its unknowing destiny. Unfortunately, having a vaccine is one thing and using it is quite another. The current trend of the smoldering "spinner" in South America, and especially in Africa, is not auspicious for man (World Health Organization, 1987).

Dengue hemorrhagic fever, the second classic disease, is the hemorrhagic form of dengue fever. Dengue hemorrhagic fever effectively became an "emerger" in 1949 although, in retrospect, it probably occurred at least 100 years ago and clinical dengue fever, in its nonhemorrhagic form, was described long before that. Dengue virus, like its viral relative, yellow fever, is usually transmitted by the mosquito *Aedes aegypti*. Dengue hemorrhagic fever is a tropical urban disease of childhood. After several decades of work and considerable controversy, it now seems clear that the odds for developing dengue hemorrhagic fever increase manyfold in secondary, as compared to primary, dengue virus infection (Burke et al., 1988). The macrophage appears to be the only human cell type capable of supporting dengue virus replication and there is convincing experimental evidence that virus-antibody complexes actually enhance such replication by promoting cell infection via macrophage receptors for the Fc portion of the antibody molecule (Brandt et al., 1983).

There are four recognized dengue virus immunotypes (varieties that are recognized as distinct by the immune system), and two of these were first isolated during a hemorrhagic fever epidemic. Were they recent mutants? Unlikely, in my opinion. Elegant retrospective detective work has produced serological evidence that volunteers infected with dengue virus in Army sponsored studies in the Philippines, more than 60 years ago, had received a type 4 dengue virus as the infecting agent. Type 4 is one of two that were "new" viruses at the time of the recognition of the hemorrhagic syndrome.

What then was the basis for the explosive emergence of dengue hemorrhagic fever shortly after the end of World War II in the Philippines, in Thailand, and elsewhere in Southeast Asia? We cannot be sure, but I share the belief of many who, much closer to the problem, cite a number of recent changes in distribution of human, virus, and mosquito populations that allow people to come in contact with successive immunotypes of dengue virus. These factors include radical change in infant mortality due to the advent of antimalarial and antibiotic drugs; rapid inward migration to cities without access to closed water systems, which led to large populations of *Aedes aegypti*; and the endemic presence, finally, of three or four dengue immunotypes.

This mayfly is an expanding "dun", not likely to be rendered a "spinner" until effective vaccines are available. I wonder if it will happen even then. Dengue hemorrhagic fever has begun to appear in tropical America and the ecological parameters involved are disturbingly similar to those in Asia: an expanding, degrading, urban environment. Today, dengue hemorrhagic fever is the leading viral hemorrhagic fever in the world.

Hemorrhagic fever with renal syndrome (HFRS), the third classic disease, is a clinically distinctive syndrome now known to have worldwide distribution. The prototype is Korean hemorrhagic fever, caused by the virus now called Hantaan. Modern description of the disease dates to about 1913 in what is now Siberia, but there is Chinese literature to suggest that it was recognized at least a millennium earlier. This is not unlikely in view of the Asiatic source of the causative Hantaan virus.

The aptly named striped field mouse, *Apodemus agrarius*, is both reservoir and primary vector of this agent in eastern Asia. Chronic infection of the mouse with persistent viruria represents the core of virus maintenance and transmission to humans. In other words, many of the mice are chronically infected, usually without overt illness, and chronically shed virus in their urine. People become infected through contact with virus that is shed in the urine or other secretions of infected mice. Unlike yellow fever and dengue, but similar to several of the examples I will provide later, arthropods–insects or ticks–are not involved in transmission.

Korean hemorrhagic fever has undoubtedly impacted agricultural man in Eurasia for many centuries. Rice culture in this part of the world is still done by the same methods that have been used for centuries. Planting is in the spring, harvesting in the fall, and much manual labor is involved. Most cases of the disease occur in the fall of the year, when people go into the rice fields to harvest. At that time, both the *Apodemus* population and the prevalence of chronic infection in the mice reach annual peaks.

The long sought agent, now called Hantaan virus, was identified in rodents by applying convalescent human sera to rodent tissue sections and then identifying infected cells with fluorescent antihuman conjugate to show where the patients' antibodies bound to the infected cells (Lee et al., 1978). This finding led to "emerger" status of at least three related viruses, and the recognition of a unique genus in the family Bunyaviridae, the Hantaviruses. The Hantaviruses are vigorous "duns". More than 100,000 cases of HFRS occur in China annually, and the incidence of the seasonal and harvest disease will surely increase with that of rural human populations either until agriculture is mechanized, in which case something else will probably happen, or until a vaccine is available.

"NEW" HEMORRHAGIC FEVER AGENTS: ARENAVIRUSES AND OTHERS

As distinct from these classic diseases, there have been a variety of newly recognized hemorrhagic fevers. Omsk, Kyasanur Forest, and Crimean-Congo hemorrhagic fevers are examples I will mention only in passing. Each of these diseases was recognized during or since World War II. These three are tick borne diseases, and Crimean-Congo in particular is notorious for causing lethal hospital-acquired outbreaks, by aerosol transmission, in regions as far flung as Pakistan and South Africa (Burney et al., 1980).

The "new" viruses I will focus on for the rest of this chapter are three members of the arenavirus family, namely Junin, Machupo, and Lassa; Marburg and Ebola viruses, the members of a unique family, the Filoviridae; and Rift Valley fever. The names of the viruses, in general, match the disease names except in the case of Junin and Machupo viruses, which are respectively the causative agents of Argentine and Bolivian hemorrhagic fever.

The syndromes caused by arenaviruses illuminate many of the factors which have contributed to the emergence of "new" zoonotic viral diseases in the past 50 years. Rather like the unrelated Hantaviruses, each of these is caused by an agent that is host-specific for a rodent species that has recently come into close contact with large numbers of humans. Chronic viruric infection of the rodent, that is, chronic shedding of virus in the urine of infected animals, provides the means for transmission to man, resulting in a variably immunosuppressive and hemorrhagic illness with about a 20 percent mortality.

Intraspecies virus maintenance in the rodent involves interaction between the agent and the rodent reproductive system. The biology of these viruses served as a model for the strategy used to eventually recover Hantaan virus, which is totally unrelated but biologically similar in its ability to chronically infect specific rodent species. Two of these diseases, Argentine hemorrhagic fever (Junin) and Lassa fever, are stable or enlarging "duns"; one, Bolivian hemorrhagic fever (Machupo), is a relic "spinner", at least for the present, for reasons I will explain shortly.

The emergence of each of these diseases was the direct result of major manmade ecologic perturbation. For millennia, the Argentine pampa was a fertile temperate grassland populated in more recent times by cattle and a rich wild fauna. The dominant rodent was *Akodon azarae*. Between the great wars of this century, however, plowing of the land for production of maize began. The pace of this process rapidly accelerated during World War II as Argentina became bread basket for both sides in the conflict. The pampa did not give in easily, however. Yields of maize were often low because prolific annual grasses and weeds had to be battled by hand. At the end of the war, however, herbicides were introduced and agriculture was immediately, and I mean immediately, transformed on the

pampa. Now the grasses were controlled until the maize plants
reached nearly full height. An understory of shade tolerant, rather
than solarphilic, grasses was also selected for. The altered ecology
produced a new dominant mouse, *Calomys musculinus*. This small
cricetine rodent had always been there, but only in small numbers.
Now this species was selected to become the dominant animal
because a mainstay of its diet is seeds of shade tolerant grasses. In a
given year, *Calomys* populations in maize fields may average more
than 20 times those in adjacent cultivars of alfalfa or soy beans (de
Villefañe et al., 1977). It transpired that *Calomys musculinus* is (and
surely long has been) the natural reservoir and vector of Junin virus.
By 1953 Argentine hemorrhagic fever, the disease caused by Junin
virus, was clinically described and the virus was isolated about 5
years later. The disease is still increasing its geographic range.

Farther to the north, on the tropical plains of eastern Bolivia, a
different story unfolded at almost exactly the same time. Beni
province of Bolivia was frontier country, reminiscent of our own dry
west 150 years ago. Sparsely populated and unfenced, it contained
thousands of stringy beef cattle. Everything was owned by a Brazilian family called Casa Suárez, the House of Suarez. This company
had German meat processing facilities and a fleet of ships that took
beef down the Amazon river system and then to Europe and the
Americas. These ships brought back the rice, maize, beans, and fruit
to feed the cowboys of the Beni. The Casa Suárez suddenly disappeared, however, when a major social revolution in Bolivia resulted
in the return of the land to the citizens in 1952. No more rice boats
arrived, so the people had to resort to subsistence agriculture. The
sites that the people selected to grow their food were small forested
outcrops in the prairie where the soil was much better than on the
leached and alternately flooded sun baked grasslands. Phosphorus
content, for example, was fiftyfold higher in the ground of these
"alturas" than in the adjacent lateritic flats. At the forest-grassland
edge lived a small mouse called *Calomys callosus*, a relative of the
Argentine *Calomys*. Although we don't know how or why, this
mouse was somehow quite well adapted for living in the houses and
gardens of man. Much as with its Argentine cousin, it therefore
flourished and shared its virus, in this case Machupo virus, with its
new human hosts. As a consequence, beginning in 1960 outbreaks
occurred of a type of hemorrhagic fever never before seen in the
region. This story ends a little more happily, perhaps, than the
others. Recall that this one is a "spinner". By 1964 the virus was
isolated, its epidemiology was elucidated, and the disease was effectively controlled (Johnson et al., 1967). Let this be a lesson for all
who desire to build a research program on a single new disease! Less
than 100 cases of Bolivian hemorrhagic fever have been recognized
in the past 20 years in that region. The reason is that highly viruric

Calomys also experience virus-induced hemolytic anemia and have grossly and chronically enlarged spleens. Teams on horseback make the rounds of the towns and ranches, trap a few mice, open them up, and where large spleens are found, carry out an intensive trapping campaign. Thus, this disease has become a mayfly "spinner". Whether that will hold forever remains to be seen. The virus is not gone, by any means, from the region.

Lassa fever and the virus of the same name emerged suddenly in 1969 as the result of a chain of nosocomial infection in nursing staff at a mission hospital in Nigeria. A clinical description of this disease in Sierra Leone had been published more than a decade earlier, but went completely unnoticed. This disease involves another rodent. One genotype of the rodent *Mastomys natalensis*, notable for its proclivity to invade and reside in houses, proved to be the major Lassa reservoir vector.

Lassa fever is distributed focally over much of West Africa (World Health Organization, 1975). A hyperendemic focus of Lassa fever now exists in eastern Sierra Leone and is directly related to discovery and rather chaotic development of surface diamond mine deposits in that area. The diamond fields produced mass human invasion and the kind of ecology where money is used, leading to boom towns with plentiful food scattered around, at least from the rodents' point of view, instead of the traditional ecology of the area, in which food is scarce and *Mastomys* makes little headway, which has been the classical rural pattern of man in West Africa for a very long time. In contrast to the Bolivian *Calomys*, this mouse is expert at avoiding traps. So rodent control is not an effective solution for disease control. Antiviral therapy is effective where available (McCormick et al., 1986), and a Lassa vaccine is now struggling to emerge.

Marburg and Ebola viruses were recently elevated to family status as the Filoviridae. The name, "thread viruses", is based on their morphology. These viruses made their appearance in the 1960s and 1970s in the form of frightening nosocomial and occupational outbreaks, initially among polio vaccine production workers in Germany in contact with Ugandan green monkeys and their kidney tissues, then in independent hospital epidemics of devastating proportions during 1976 in the Sudan and Zaire (Pattyn, 1978). Mortality from these infections can range to nearly 90%, and that is 90% of infections, not just clinical illnesses. I can report, from personal experience, that in Zaire in 1976 an international team of investigators spent approximately 3 weeks collectively holding its breath. The reason was that the hospital in question that had been the epicenter of this epidemic had been wiped out. Thirteen out of 17 of the doctors and nurses there were dead. A real question was: Had we finally run into the Andromeda strain, like the deadly virus in the novel?

It turned out not to be the case. In general, this virus is not transmitted by aerosol from man to man. But it certainly has that potential and one wonders what might happen if and when the day comes that an agent of this degree of lethality obtains the right kind of receptors, or whatever is needed, to replicate in the respiratory tract and be transmitted. This would be, I think, the most lethal of influenzas. Is there an uneasy, even if unlikely, parallel here to the still unclear emergence of the human immunodeficiency lentivirus?

These diseases, therefore, are true "emergers", still waiting to rise from the enveloping fluid. The reason is that even today we do not yet know anything regarding their "nymphal" stages, namely their zoonotic reservoirs and possible vectors. Man has truly stumbled onto these agents. We know they are in Africa; we don't know where. I am personally not happy to report that there is hardly anybody trying to find out.

Finally, a few words about Rift Valley fever. This agent has a unique history of emergence as a hemorrhagic disease. The virus was first recovered in 1931 in East Africa during major epizootics of lethal or teratogenic disease in sheep and cattle of European origin. So the recipe, 50 years ago, was foreign animals, local virus, new disease. For several decades associated human disease, principally noted among veterinarians and slaughterhouse workers, was described as brief and influenza-like with occasional occurrence of sight-threatening retinitis. In 1977, however, shortly after a nosocomial outbreak of Marburg disease that made physicians and virologists in South Africa more aware of new hemorrhagic fevers, several cases of fatal hepatitis and hemorrhage were recorded during an epizootic of Rift Valley fever on the plateaus surrounding Johannesburg. During the next year the virus somehow reached, by uncertain means although almost definitely not directly from South Africa, immunologically virginal domestic animal and human populations in the lower Nile delta of Egypt. Several million human infections and thousands of hemorrhagic deaths ensued. The exact mode of virus entry into this region is still unclear, but changes in patterns of human and animal intercourse between Saharan and sub-Saharan Africa, which were significantly altered by construction of the Aswan Dam, were almost certainly responsible. In the meantime, the virus lies patiently for years in drought resistant mosquito eggs over much of the continent, waiting for rain and new opportunity.

PROSPECTS FOR THE FUTURE

What do these experiences offer in the context of considering disease emergence? In the first place, I think it is clear that in each case, medical and scientific energy was reactive, not proactive. Modern communications, the intercontinental airplane, liquid nitrogen, and now largely post modern technology were responsible for the rapid recognition and partial elucidation of these diseases. That energy, in turn, was fueled by the intellectual and economic hegemony enjoyed by our country during a 40-odd year period after the end of World War II. Those days are over.

Second, but perhaps of primary significance, most of the "new" hemorrhagic fevers emerged only because of large and often still accelerating ecologic changes made by a burgeoning *Homo sapiens*. After nearly 3 decades of personal experience in field and laboratory, I find it difficult not to adopt the burden of René Dubos who more than 25 years ago described himself as a "despairing optimist". Long before the greenhouse effect became an "emerger", these hemorrhagic fevers foretold that our earth is, in fact, a progressively immunocompromised ecosystem.

Are there any more hemorrhagic "nymphs" out there waiting to emerge? Can we grab them before they become airborne? I personally doubt that there are many left. We have hacked and slashed our way into just about all of the unique ecologic niches on the globe. Perhaps ironically, the year 1976, taken by some as the emergence year of modern biotechnology, is also the year that marks the emergence of the last new hemorrhagic fever.

This is not to say that we now know the names of all potentially virulent zoonotic viruses on earth. There may well be more trouble ahead as progressive stages in manmade ecologic degradation select infected wild vertebrates and invertebrates for population growth and proximity to the primary human instrument of change. We might anticipate such events by paying attention to details of this evolutionary cataclysm in a macro-sense, and use new micro-sense tools, such as the polymerase chain reaction. We should not forget that the viral hemorrhagic fevers have given us two new families, the Filoviridae and the Arenaviridae and a biologically unique genus, Hantavirus, which belongs to the largest animal virus family of all, the Bunyaviridae. Genetic materials of these virus taxons are progressively available. Furthermore, the latter two families have multipartite genomes and are perhaps likely to be more busily engaged in natural recombinant evolution than agents with nonsegmented nucleic acid.

Hantaviruses, in particular, intrigue me. Does the divorce of these agents from requirement for a biologically functional arthropod host signify recent evolution? If so, might we not search our own species and other primates for Hantaviruses? I think here of agents that have nothing to do with hemorrhagic fever, but which may cause subtle chronic, noninflammatory infection of the sort we observe in rodents in the models of similar phenomena elucidated for arenaviruses. Such speculative viruses might be nonzoonotic new human pathogens, new in the sense of previously unrecognized. We have many new tools. Do we have the creativity and courage to know where to fish?

Finally, a word about we. Who is going to be working on zoonotic viruses, the diseases they cause, and their possible human counterparts in the next century? A past generation of leaders of the National Institute of Allergy and Infectious Diseases (NIAID) closed NIAID's own laboratory of tropical virology 25 years ago, and its principal field station a few years later. The Centers for Disease Control program, long squeezed into a semiportable module to provide maximum or BL4 containment required for work with many of these agents, now has a greatly expanded facility, but not the fiscal support to staff it. Finally, the U.S. Army program, clearly the last and best funded operation of its kind in the entire world, has recently come under increasing and misguided fire, in my opinion, over the largely dead horse issue of biological warfare. Surely, a better consortium of national effort and communication is needed or we shall soon add zoonotic medical virology to the growing list of earth's extinct species. I hope that this book will stimulate a growing awareness of this danger. Please know, in any case, that as an emerging yet evanescent historian, I am deeply concerned.

REFERENCES

Brandt, W.E., J.M. McCown, M.K. Gentry, and P.K. Russell (1982). Infection enhancement of dengue type 2 virus in the U937 human monocyte cell line by antibodies to flavivirus cross-reactive determinants. Infect. Immun. 36:1036-1041.

Burke, D.S., A. Nisalak, D.E. Johnson, and R.McN. Scott (1988). A prospective study of dengue infections in Bangkok. Amer. J. Trop. Med Hyg. 38:172-180.

Burney, M.I., A. Ghafoor, M. Saleen, P.A. Webb, and J. Casals (1980). Nosocomial outbreak of viral hemorrhagic fever caused by Crimean hemorrhagic fever-Congo virus in Pakistan, January 1976. Am. J. Trop. Med. Hyg. 29:941-947.

Gajdusek, D.C. (1962). Virus hemorrhagic fevers. J. Pediatr. 60:841-857.

Johnson, K.M., S.B. Halstead, and S.N. Cohen (1967). Hemorrhagic fevers of Southeast Asia and South America: A comparative appraisal. Progr. Med. Virol. 9:105-158.

Lee, H.W., P.W. Lee, and K.M. Johnson (1978). Isolation of the etiologic agent of Korean hemorrhagic fever. J. Infect. Dis. 137:298-308.

McCormick, J.B., I.J. King, P.A. Webb, C.L. Scribner, R.B. Craven, K.M. Johnson, L.H. Elliott, and R. Belmont-Williams (1986). Lassa fever: Effective therapy with ribavirin. N. Engl. J. Med. 314:20-26.

Pattyn, S.R. (ed.) (1978). *Ebola Virus Haemorrhagic Fever.* Amsterdam: Elsevier/North-Holland.

de Villafañe, G., F.O. Kravetz, O. Donadio, R. Percich, L. Knecher, M.P. Torres, and N. Fernandez (1977). Dinámica de las comunidades de roedores en agro-ecosistemas pampásicos. Medicina (B. Aires) 37: Suppl. 3, 128-140.

World Health Organization (1975). International symposium on arenaviral
    infections of public health importance. Bull. WHO **52**:318-766.
World Health Organization (1987). Yellow fever epidemic, Nigeria. WHO
    Weekly Epidemiol. Rep. **62**:155.

6
Ecology and Evolution of Host-Virus Associations

ROBERT M. MAY

The first question that ecologists ask of a virus, as they would ask of any other organism, is what is its basic reproductive rate, what is its fitness? What, on average, are the number of offspring, as it were, that each infected case produces?

Viral, bacterial, and protozoan infections—microparasites—can be grouped together as infections in which it is usually necessary just to distinguish uninfected, infected, and immune people (Anderson and May, 1979), as opposed to what might be called macroparasites, such as most helminth infections, where one really has to deal with the number of worms in a given individual. For microparasites, which include most viruses, the basic reproductive rate (R_0 in the mathematical notation I shall use) is essentially the average number of secondary infections produced when you put one infected host into a wholly susceptible population. It is important to know the basic reproductive rate, R_0, because if R_0 is greater than 1, then if you put a handful of infected people into a population, there will be an exponentiating chain of infection, until eventually it will be brought to a halt when some of the secondary candidates for infection have already experienced infection.

In short, if R_0 is bigger than 1, the situation exists where the virus can invade, persist, maintain its population, and, as it were, emerge. Whereas, if R_0 is less than 1, then though you may introduce the entity, and though it may produce secondary infections, it will not be self-sustaining.

HIV is one example that we have examined. For HIV, in some rough intuitive sense that can be made precise, the basic reproductive rate (R_0, the number of secondary infections produced early in the epidemic by each infected individual in a particular risk category), is clearly proportional to the average probability (β) that a susceptible partner will be infected over the duration of the relationship, multiplied by the average number of partners acquired over the course of infectiousness which, in turn, will be the average rate of acquiring new partners (c) times the average duration of infectiousness (D).

Translating these terms into an equation (May and Anderson, 1988):

$$R_0 = \beta cD \qquad \text{(Eqn. 6.1)}$$

where β is the average probability that a susceptible partner will be infected over the duration of the relationship, c is the average rate of acquiring new partners, and D is the average duration of infectiousness.

Clearly, there are, of course, a lot of sins and complexities smuggled into this blithe use of average. Some of these things, the duration of infectiousness D for example, primarily depend on the biology of the virus. Some are a mixture of biological and social variables, such as the probability β of infecting a partner, which clearly depends, to some extent, on such biological factors as the number of viral particles needed to infect, and possibly the genotypes of the transmitter and transmittee. But it also depends on social variables such as, for example, the use of condoms and the type of sexual act. Finally, the average number of partners per unit of time, c, is essentially wholly a behavioral variable that can change markedly from time to time or group to group. There are many uncertainties surrounding the estimation of the average number of partners, but I wish only to make the point that if we look at the kind of inadequate and woefully slowly mounted surveys of sexual behavior in developed, much less developing countries, there are many differences between groups. Not the least of these is that in a British survey of some 1,000 homosexual and heterosexual men in 1986, if you ask how many sexual partners each man had last year, there is a wide distribution but the average for homosexual men is somewhere in the neighborhood of 10 partners per person. For heterosexual men, there is also a wide distribution, but the average is about an order of magnitude less, which means that the quantity c will also be about an order of magnitude less, at least insofar as the other variables remain roughly the same for the two groups, with a resulting reduction in R_0 by a factor of about 10 (Anderson and May, 1988).

There has been a good deal of confusion about this. It is important to distinguish clearly between β (average probability that a susceptible partner will acquire the infection from his or her infected partner) being bigger than 0, meaning that the overall transmission is probable or possible, and R_0 being >1, which is the actual criterion for, as it were, emergence in sustainable epidemic form. A sustainable epidemic requires not merely that transmission be possible (β>0), but that the entire combination of characters that go into characterizing the reproductive rate of the virus (R_0) be effectively greater than 1.

In passing, for the mathematically inclined, I will add to my earlier remark that a lot of sins are swept under the rug when I talk about averages. For example, the average rate of acquiring partners isn't simply the arithmetic mean of the distributions, but rather is a more complicated moment of the distribution involving both the mean and the variance-to-mean ratio. There are many other complexities that require one to go beyond intuitive ways of thinking, which are a helpful guide in order to get things started, onto more precise analytic models. This point will be reiterated throughout this chapter.

THRESHOLDS AND THE DYNAMICS OF HOST-PARASITE ASSOCIATIONS

Many others have considered threshold phenomena, such as minimum population sizes required before a disease becomes self-sustaining, and the way threshold phenomena can depend upon host density as well as behavior. For example, Bartlett (1957) and others have shown, I think fairly well, that to maintain measles endemically you need something like a population of 300,000 or so. It is a disease that wasn't with us in hunter-gatherer days, and many of the other directly transmissible viral infections—with their high threshold host densities—were probably also absent.

There is the flip side to that, thinking about the disemergence, as it were, of viruses. When we try to eradicate an infection by vaccinating, we don't have to vaccinate everybody. We simply have to vaccinate a sufficiently large fraction to drive the remaining susceptible population, the candidates for spreading infection, below the critical threshold (or, mathematically, reduce R_0 to <1). For smallpox, this threshold may correspond roughly to vaccinating something like 80 percent of many populations, rather than 100 percent. It is a story that has been documented in beautiful detail in a review article by Arita et al. (1986) relatively recently. For a more detailed discussion of these questions, see Anderson and May (1985; 1991).

After these general remarks, I wish to focus, admittedly in a slightly abstract way, on more analytic ways of thinking about this. For this purpose I want to go from the complex world of humans to a much simpler world. In fact, I will begin with an imaginary world of an insect population that has discreet, non-overlapping generations and whose population is regulated by a lethal pathogen that spreads in an epidemic fashion through each generation before reproduction. So the number of adults in the next generation (N_{t+1}) is the number in the present generation (N_t), multiplied by their intrinsic capacity for increase in the absence of infection (we usually label this rate λ), but then discounted because that fraction that are infected in generation t die and do not reproduce.

I can calculate what the fraction is, as a function of the host density in generation t, from the simple Kermack-McKendrick epidemic relationship, or more complex realistic variants of it, which say essentially if N is below a certain threshold the epidemic doesn't take off, corresponding to R_0 below 1. If N (that is, N_t) is above threshold the epidemic does sweep through the population, the fraction affected increasing as the population density increases.

The resulting map that carries me from the number of creatures this generation to the number next generation shows a simple propensity to increase at the normal reproductive rate, λ, when the population number is below the threshold needed for the virus to emerge in those generations; once the population size goes above the threshold, the virus emerges and kills a larger and larger fraction.

The reason I bring this up is partly to emphasize, yet again, this threshold concept but partly, also, to say something about the complexity of the dynamics of the host-virus association. You may think that with a relationship like this (increase at low density, decrease at high density), the population would settle to the point where this density dependent relationship intersects the nirvana of zero population growth, upon which the population of each generation is unchanging, equal in number to that of the last. But, in fact, if I iterate that simple deterministic relationship, that simple difference equation with its one constant parameter (the reproductive rate λ), setting a fixed value for λ and plotting the values of population density in successive generations, I don't get things settling to a point, or even to a simple cycle, but rather to some fuzzy probabilistic looking distribution. For low values of λ, the graph tends to oscillate somewhat above and below the threshold, depleting susceptibles and then bouncing back above threshold. At higher densities, or at higher values of λ, but not very high values, we see wider oscillations, a more boom-and-busty population. That simple deterministic relationship gives me something that looks, for all of the world, like random noise. This phenomenon of deterministic chaos, of simple trivial Newtonian clockwork models that generate unexpectedly the illusion of randomness is, of itself, fascinating. But I also believe that one cannot really conduct a good analytic discussion of the population biology and population genetics of host-viral associations without this awareness, because it is intrinsic in the nature of most host-parasite relations that one is easily swept into this domain of nonsteady cyclic or chaotic behavior. For a more detailed discussion of this example, see May (1985).

This, to me, seems relevant to the 2-year interepidemic cycles of measles before the advent of vaccination, and the more raggedy cycles of many childhood diseases that one saw in both Britain and the United States in the days before vaccination. These are beginning to be understood better as transmogrified versions of the dynamical complexities that I have just discussed in a deliberately oversimplified example.

The emergent moral is that the threshold relationships that govern the ability of viruses, as any other organism, to invade and persist, themselves change from time to time and from place to place in response to changing environmental settings as host density and host behavior change. If we do not conduct our understanding and discussion of these phenomena within an analytic framework of the kind I have sketchily outlined, we are reduced to the kind of vague waffle of ecological niches and so on, of which I believe we already have too much.

I am afraid, and I say this constructively, there is a sad tendency to feel, when it comes to evolutionary questions, that the kind of rigor one brings to the laboratory bench, or to many other enterprises, is somehow not necessary and one can read two graceful essays by Stephen Jay Gould and one elegant book by Dawkins, and then everybody can be an evolutionary biologist. My point is that the dynamics of these things are complex, and these discussions, if not conducted within an appropriate, carefully thought through analytic framework, are likely to be vacuous.

COEVOLUTION OF HOSTS AND PATHOGENS

Once a virus has emerged, as it were, in the sense that it has become established or is spreading in epidemic fashion, how do the relations between host and pathogen tend to coevolve? Is it true, as so widely asserted, particularly in medical texts, that there is a tendency to evolve toward avirulence?

Again, I want to begin with a deliberately oversimplified mathematical model which, for all of its simplicity, might look a bit complicated. We will use this to consider the real-life situation with many strains of a pathogen co-occurring rather than the simpler single-pathogen model we used before.

Levin and Pimentel (1981) at Cornell University developed a very simple model for this. In their model, there is a host susceptible to two strains of pathogens. The number of susceptible hosts is replenished by births; the number is depleted as susceptible hosts are infected either by strain 1 or strain 2 of the pathogen, or by hosts simply being run over by a bus and killed. Hosts infected by strain 1 move into the infected Class 1; they can move out as a result of natural deaths (at a rate designated by b) or of disease induced deaths (at a rate designated by the symbol α_1). Similarly for those infected in Class 2, at a disease-induced death rate α_2. The final kink is that strain 1 is nastier: it kills hosts at a faster rate. Therefore, α_1 is bigger than α_2: the virulence of strain 1 is greater. But strain 1 is also more transmissible, in the sense that all hosts infected with both strains manifest the pathogenicity of strain 1. That is to say, strain 1 takes over infections with strain 2. So strain 1 is both more transmissible and more virulent.

The question is: How does this system move? Does it move towards selecting the avirulent strain, the nicer strain 2, or does it move towards selecting the more transmissible strain 1? And the answer is, there is no general answer. It depends on the ratio of virulence in relation to the transmission advantage. If strain 1 is much nastier, and kills much faster in relation to a modest transmission advantage, then strain 2 emerges victorious. Conversely, if the transmission advantage of strain 1 is large in relation to the virulence difference, strain 1 wins. There is also a narrow window of co-occurrence.

More generally, we can define, as before, R_0 as the basic reproductive rate or Darwinian fitness of the pathogen or parasite strain, but in these kinds of simple models R_0 is essentially the rate at which new infections are produced, which often will depend on host density, multiplied by the length of time over which infections are being produced. This latter factor is the reciprocal of the rate at which infected hosts move out of the infected classes; recall that they can do this either by dying as a result of the infection (at a rate α), by dying of other causes such as being run over by a bus at a rate b (assuming that the probability of this occurrence is not enhanced by being sick, as it may well be in the real world), or simply and more cheerfully, by recovering (at a rate υ). One can find the total rate at which infected hosts move out of the infected classes by taking the sum of the rates of these separate events. Hence we have

$$R_0 = \frac{\lambda(N)}{(\alpha+b+\upsilon)} \qquad \text{(Eqn. 6.2)}$$

Here $\lambda(N)$ represents the transmission rate, or rate at which an infected individual produces new infections, and α, b, and υ are respectively rates of death (α, b) or recovery (υ).

Since R_0 is basically the measure of Darwinian fitness of the pathogen, it should be no surprise that, in general, the strain with the largest value of R_0 will tend to win.

Now, if virulence were completely unconnected with transmission or recovery, then indeed, one would maximize R_0 in Equation 2 by having $\alpha=0$, and one would get the most avirulent strain. But, of course, most of the nasty things that pathogens do, most of the causes of virulence and disease-induced death, are associated with the production of transmission stages and are entwined with recovery rates, and there are various constraints that vary with different viruses and hosts. These complexities mean that there is no general statement that can be made. What we need to do, and what so rarely has been done, is to evaluate the relations among virulence, recovery rates and transmissibility; that is, to evaluate the interdependencies of α, λ and υ.

Frank Fenner is the real hero of this part of my essay. His classic studies on the introduction of myxoma (rabbitpox) virus into Aus-

tralian rabbit populations could give us data to begin to approach
the task defined above. With typical Australian percipience, reference strains of the rabbits were kept in the laboratory and used
continually to evaluate field strains of the virus. From the initial
very nasty strain of myxoma virus, highly virulent with essentially
no recovery in infected rabbits, one found in the field progressively
less and less virulent grades of virus, with faster and faster recovery
rates of infected rabbits. One can plot that relationship between
virulence and recovery rate (between α and υ), and then whack it
into the sort of deliberately oversimplified formula I discussed
earlier (Equation 6.2). Unfortunately, it is much harder to get a
handle on another parameter, the way transmission depends on
virulence (λ as a function of α), because the nastier grades tend, on
the one hand, to be more transmissible, with larger lesions, but on
the other hand, they also drive rabbit populations to lower density,
which is a complicating factor. Just as an approximation, ignoring
such complications for which decent data are lacking anyway, one
can calculate the dependence of R_0 on virulence grade using only the
empirical relation between recovery and virulence. The result is that
R_0 has a peak. The really nasty strains kill the rabbits too fast to do
well, but the really avirulent strains allow rabbits to recover too fast
to permit effective transmission, and one has the suggestion from
this model of settling to an intermediate grade of virulence. Simple
statements in introductory texts to the contrary, this also appears to
be roughly what fairly quickly happened in the field. The same
fairly fast shift to an intermediate grade of virulence also occurred
with myxoma virus in Britain, a very different ecological setting
with a different vector, fleas, rather than mosquitoes as in Australia.
A more detailed discussion both of the basic issues, and of the rabbit-
myxoma example, is in May and Anderson (1983).

The moral is that the coevolutionary trajectories pursued by
virus-host associations, and more generally by most pathogen-host
associations, involve complicated tradeoffs between virulence, transmissibility, and host resistance (this last including a factor I haven't
discussed, the cost of resistance on the part of the host). Those
tradeoffs will be constrained in different ways by the natural history
of particular associations and may obey complex or chaotic dynamics. Let me just emphasize once more that an analytic framework
must be used to discuss these things. In the absence of it, one tends,
even in excellent books touching on evolutionary virology, to get
naive group selection statements that say parasites evolve to
avirulence because that is for the good of the group, as if they were
some marvelous, ideally communistic society that had subjugated
all Darwinian notions of selection acting on the individual, just for
the good of the group.

GENETIC DIVERSITY AND THE INTERACTION BETWEEN HOSTS AND PATHOGENS

Which brings me to part three of this chapter. If I were a more disciplined individual there would be no part three, because it is very much to my own enthusiasms. I want to go a bit more widely and come back to this theme of the complexity of the dynamics of the associations between host and parasite. If we really want to understand host and parasites, we have got to put the genetics in, as I have not yet done.

As a very simple caricature of the problem, we could imagine one locus, two allele models, with two genotypes, A and a. The gene frequency of A in generation t+1 will be its frequency in the previous generation, t, times its relative success (the fitness of genotype A divided by the sum of that same fitness plus the frequency of the other genotype times its success). For those fitnesses, instead of doing what population geneticists usually do and just calling them constants or making something up, we can actually go further. In case you were wondering why there was all that stuff earlier about insects, note that that model calculated the fitness of something with a pathogen specific to each genotype sweeping through it. The model shows how useful even a simple analytic framework can be. Now, if the genotype A is rare, the pathogen of this particular strain doesn't propagate, but as A becomes more common the pathogen starts killing the host off and the fitness falls, depending on what fraction the pathogen actually kills.

Conversely, for the genotype a, which is rare when A is common, up to a certain point a is more fit than A and its frequency increases. Above this, a is less fit than A, and the frequency decreases. A purely static analysis would suggest a nice balanced polymorphism here. But, as you know by now from our earlier experience with this model, this relation actually gives a very kinky map. It won't surprise you, on the basis of what I said earlier, that that map, for quite modest values of the reproductive rate of a pathogen, can give us cycles or chaos. If I let the pathogen regulate the population, not merely determine gene frequency, I get completely chaotic fluctuations in gene frequency (May and Anderson, 1983).

I want to conclude with something that is on the boundary between this notion of the complex dynamics of host-parasite systems and purely aesthetic considerations. It is a bit of a swindle.

A fully coevolutionary genetical host and pathogen model has dynamics very similar to those of a forced pendulum, substituting more appropriate host-pathogen parameters, such as initial gene frequency of the host and the parasite, for pendulum parameters such as initial angular position and the initial angular speed. I think one gets rather similar conclusions from both situations, except that, unlike me, people who work on pendulums have the patience and money to plot the results, which takes an entire night on a Cray supercomputer. Such plots show various paths to several alternative possible orbits, including a sort of overhead clockwise orbit, and an overhead counterclockwise orbit, as well as two other defined final states that are not overhead orbits, and a number of places in between where the pendulum is never settled. The different initial conditions that carry us to these different end states are interwoven, with more and more detail and more and more fine structure the closer we look at it. Indeed, the regions of initial conditions that lead to different end states are interwoven in such a way as to exhibit fractal geometries.

So too with the host–parasite interaction. There are various alternative states. The essential point is not merely that they are complicated, but that the broad boundaries of initial conditions that attract to one state rather than the other completely defy our intuition about simple deterministic clockwork systems. There is not just one broad band of initial conditions, with one specific outcome leading to another, but rather, as we look at this on finer and finer scales, we find that the initial conditions that give us the different final states are interdigitated, woven together like fine layers of pastry on ever finer scales, finer and finer. Even if we knew all of the parameters, and even if we could trust a simple model, prediction is essentially impossible because of the sensitivity to initial conditions.

CONCLUSIONS

I conclude by summarizing this essay in essentially three categories of morals. Cardinal Newman once said, "No souls are saved after the first 20 minutes", but he was talking about a more trivial topic. You will be saved if you understand the following:

All viral host associations have thresholds that govern the possibility of the virus invading or persisting, and thus, in whatever sense we mean this, emerging in the population. These thresholds depend on host density and behavior, and they will change from time to time and from place to place as the ecological setting, host behavior, and host density change.

If we ask, can we foresee patterns of future emergence, the answer will necessarily be that any such foresight must be embedded in an analytic discussion that recognizes the way changing threshold parameters will depend on the "lifestyle" of the virus in relation to its changing setting.

Second, coevolution of virus and host, like other such associations, can exhibit many patterns. There is no generalization. The virus may become less virulent, more virulent, or exhibit unchanging virulence; the virus may become less transmissible, more transmissible, or show unchanging transmissibility. All of this depends on the tradeoffs among virulence, transmissibility, and the cost of resistance, which are also constrained by the nature of the host-pathogen association. If transmission of a virus is enhanced by modifying behavior, as in rabbits and many other things, then the virus might not have the option of becoming less virulent. But one has to think about it analytically.

Finally, and perhaps more loftily, threshold phenomena and coevolutionary phenomena, the population biology and the population genetics of host-virus associations, are typically more complex than has been generally recognized. The associations can, of course, easily maintain polymorphisms, but those polymorphisms can as easily as not be maintained by fluctuating in a cyclic or chaotic way. This conclusion is supported by some recent work on plant populations, and even some work on malaria in New Guinea, with suggestions that we are beginning to observe this type of fluctuation. It is the sort of thing we didn't look for as long as we were still embedded in the Newtonian paradigm that simple deterministic things would be steady. But cyclic or chaotic changes in gene frequency (or other characteristics of the association) are the rule as much as the exception and they form the theater against which this play on thresholds and coevolution is acted out.

ACKNOWLEDGMENTS

This chapter was produced by Stephen Morse from a transcript of my talk at the conference from which this book emerged, and I am grateful to him for his energy and enthusiasm. The work reported here was supported in part by the Royal Society, and by a grant from the National Science Foundation.

REFERENCES

Anderson, R.M., and R.M. May (1979). Population biology of infectious diseases. Nature **280**:361-367 and 455-461.
Anderson, R.M., and R.M. May (1985). Vaccination and herd immunity to infectious diseases. Nature **318**:323-329.
Anderson, R.M., and R.M. May (1988). Epidemiological parameters of HIV transmission. Nature **333**:514-518.
Anderson, R.M., and R.M. May (1991). *Infectious Diseases of Humans: Transmission and Control.* Oxford and New York: Oxford University Press.
Arita, I., J. Wickett, and F. Fenner (1986). Impact of population density on immunization program. J. Hyg. **96**:459-466.
Bartlett, M.S. (1957). Measles periodicity and community size. J. Roy. Stat. Soc. (Ser. A) **120**:48-70.
Levin, S.A., and D. Pimentel (1981). Selection for intermediate rates of increase in parasite-host systems. Am. Natural. **117**:308-315.

May, R.M. (1985). Regulation of populations with non-overlapping generations by microparasites: a purely chaotic system. Am. Natural. **125:**573-584.

May, R.M., and R.M. Anderson (1983). Epidemiology and genetics in the coevolution of parasites and hosts. Proc. Roy. Soc. (Lond.) B **219:**281-313.

May, R.M., and R.M. Anderson (1987). Transmission dynamics of HIV infection. Nature **326:**137-142.

7

Pathogenesis of Viral Infections

BERNARD N. FIELDS

Many virologists, including John Holland, Peter Palese, and Howard Temin among the contributors to this volume, have noted the enormous capacity for viruses to change. If we are faced with the fact that viruses can do virtually anything, why hasn't this enormous diversity wiped out the earth? One of the major issues facing us is why this extreme catastrophe hasn't yet happened.

I think the answer has to lie in the fact that there is an enormous difference in the selective pressures faced by a virus growing in the relatively undemanding environment of cell culture, which illustrates the capacity of a virus to change, and life in the real world, where the virus must survive in a specific environment and as well as within a host, providing the virus with a series of constraints and selective pressures (Tyler and Fields, 1991). When the virus enters a host, there are a series of sequential steps within the host, each of which places further constraints on the virus (Sharpe and Fields, 1985). Because of these constraints, at many points in the life cycle of the virus, much of the potential of the virus to change results in viruses that cannot survive since it will be missing critical properties. We are dealing with a constantly shifting interaction between the virus in the host and its own intrinsic capacity to change.

The viral lifestyle thus places constraints and selective pressures on viral evolution. This lifestyle involves infecting host cells, then using the viral genetic information to direct cellular machinery to make viral products. Unlike other organisms, viruses reproduce themselves or make viral products only when a host cell can do this for them under the genetic control of the virus. Because of this, the host–virus interaction is key to many aspects of viral disease.

Important interactions occur both at the cellular level and at the level of the host organism. The host organism has defense mechanisms including the natural barriers to infection and its immune system. At the cellular level, the capacity of a virus to enter the body by a particular route and to infect a specific cell type will influence the kind of disease caused. Important viral properties include the physical properties of the virus that make it able or unable to infect by a given route, as well as the presence of the appropriate receptors on the cell surface that are needed for the virus to enter the cell (Knipe, 1991). For example, as I will discuss later, a virus must be capable of physically surviving the harsh conditions present in the lumen of the digestive tract and of infecting intestinal epithelial cells in order to infect by the oral route and initiate an infection in the intestine. Factors such as these affect viruses that are extracellular. Other factors, such as those discussed in Chapter 8, can affect expression of a virus inside cells. In addition, host defenses provide major selective pressures on the virus (Murphy and Chanock, 1991). A virus needs to circumvent or subvert host defenses if it is to be a successful pathogen. In some cases, the host immune response can also contribute to disease by causing damage to the host.

Thus when a virus infects a host cell, there are restraints and constraints put on a virus at various levels. At a molecular level, one constraint is whether the proteins that make up the viral structure can assemble, or whether a polymerase needed to copy the viral genetic information can work. At a different level (that of the host), there are constraints such as whether or not the virus is stable enough to pass through the fluids in the stomach or pass through the mucus of the respiratory tract.

Viral virulence—the relative capacity of related viruses to cause disease—therefore involves a few very important features. First, the interplay between a virus, or any microorganism, and a host involves a complicated but relatively ordered series of events. These events are somewhat predictable, depending on the specific environment of the microorganism.

It is somewhat reassuring that although the interplay between virus and host is complicated, it is also ordered. By dividing the series of steps into their components, it is possible to obtain insights into each step and to identify the functions of each component of the virus. Ultimately, when we talk about viral virulence, we need to understand exactly where in their life cycle (i.e., at which step) viruses of different virulence differ among themselves causing them to be more or less virulent.

Because the terms involving viral-host interactions are used in different ways by different people, I would like to define two terms as I (and, I think, most virologists) would use them. These terms are pathogenesis and virulence. Pathogenesis is the interaction of a microbe with a host resulting in an outcome whereby disease occurs. The major point is that it is really the interaction of a microorganism with a host that leads to some kind of tissue injury, in an overt or subtle way leading to disease. Virulence is a more specific term, at least as I think of it. Virulence is relative, and represents the degree of a microbe's capacity to produce disease. Because different viruses can cause different types of disease, I believe that the term virulence should only be used to compare closely related viruses. Giraffes and zebras differ, but it is hard to compare them in a single term. Is HIV more virulent than measles or less virulent than flu?

Why do we rarely talk about *viral virulence factors* as opposed to bacterial virulence factors? With bacteria, we talk about virulence factors, those properties of the microbe that confer ability to cause disease. The reason is that bacterial virulence is a well-established field with many established terms. There are such factors as adhesins or colonizing factors; there are bacterial toxins; there is the ability of bacteria to inhibit phagocytosis by cells involved in host defenses, mediated by specific bacterial products such as surface polysaccharides; there is the ability of bacteria to change and avoid host defenses. These bacterial virulence factors are well defined entities, so why haven't virologists focused more on viral virulence factors?

One major reason is viruses are simpler. Viruses don't make extracellular proteases, or send out extracellular toxins. The virus virulence factors, in essence, are factors that influence parts of the viral life cycle in the host or the host cell. In that sense, viruses are quite different. On the other hand, when a virus infects a cell and the cell sends out a product, whether it be tumor necrosis factor or interferon, maybe we should start thinking of that as the analogy of a bacterial virulence factor, in a sense, if the virus has the capacity to cause a cell to generate a product which itself could cause disease.

Thus when I refer to viral virulence factors, what I mean is factors that influence the relative capacities of virus to produce disease. It is important to note that this capacity is not simply the ability to replicate in a cell, although factors that influence replication may influence virulence. This is worth noting because, classically, viruses often are thought to cause disease by killing cells. While cell killing is an important factor in viral disease, this is not all there is to it. The capacity to cause disease also resides in the capacity of the virus to successfully survive the environment of the portals of entry, to enter cells and undergo primary replication, to spread either to adjacent cells or to distant sites in the host (such as the nervous system), and to enter those distant sites (cell and tissue tropism). Throughout this process, the virus must overcome early host defenses (interferon, macrophages, natural killer cells) to replicate and allow viruses to eventually leave the host to continue its cycle.

Viral infection is complex. Thus, viral virulence is multigenic, which means that the spectrum of changes in a virus influencing differences in viral virulence can't be completely tied to a single gene in the virus. You have to have a "normal" virus in order to undergo all of the various steps involved in the ability to produce disease. However, the inverse, that certain genes do not play specific roles in virulence, is not true. Some genes may play a particular role in virulence, while all the other genes in a particular virus are often important in some other way. Thus by saying certain genes are "virulence determinants" or "virulence genes" does not mean that the others are not important, although sometimes, again, that terminology gets us into trouble.

Defects in virtually any viral gene, under the right circumstances, can weaken, or attenuate, the capacity of the virus to cause disease. There is an enormous literature on attenuation of viruses (Murphy and Chanock, 1991). Strains of viruses used for live virus vaccines are attenuated. Many live virus vaccines are multiple mutants that were generated by continued growth, or passage, in cell culture, and that have genetic lesions of various types. In addition, a variety of viral mutants generated for other purposes are often attenuated in their capacity to produce disease. Examples of two classic vaccines include Sabin polio vaccine, which was generated by passage in cell culture and lost the capacity to spread into the central nervous system and kill neurons, and the Pasteur rabies vaccine, which was passaged in animal brains and can grow in the brain if injected to CNS directly, but cannot spread from the peripheral nerves into the brain to cause disease.

In spite of these examples of the effect of viral mutations causing attenuation, it is worth noting that just because a genetic defect attenuates a virus doesn't necessarily make the affected gene a virulence determinant. We can divide the functions of viral genes into those genes that are specific for replication and transcription, functions that the virus needs to reproduce itself within the restricted intracellular environment ("payload"), versus those genes that are involved in delivering the virus to the host cell ("delivery system"). Certainly, if the virus makes a polymerase that is defective, this will influence virulence. Conversely, something that enhances viral replication, as described by Shenk in Chapter 8, can

Table 7.1. Steps in Virus-Host Interaction

1.	Stability in environment
2.	Entry into host—portal of entry
3.	Localization in cells near portal of entry
4.	Primary replication
5.	Non-specific immune response
6.	Spread from primary site
	Blood
	Nerves
7.	Cell and tissue tropism
8.	Secondary replication
9.	Antibody and cellular immune response
10.	Release from host

make the virus more virulent, but these "payload" properties are very different from these properties involved with the mechanistic ability to deliver a virus ("delivery system") into the nervous system, for a virus where getting into the nervous system may lead to encephalitis. Hence, the delivery system and trafficking is a virulence component.

I would like now to examine specific aspects of how viruses cause disease and how they are controlled. The simplest place to begin is to look at the viral life cycle step by step, at those complex but ordered steps I mentioned earlier (Table 7.1).

A special aspect of viruses is that many viruses persist after entering the host. During persistent infection some of the selective pressures seen in acute infections are not present. But in some of these instances, such as the severe neurological disease SSPE (subacute sclerosing panencephalopathy), caused by a defective variant of measles virus, although the virus is now quite defective and no longer able to initiate an important part of its life cycle, there is certainly a striking impact on the host.

Using the steps outlined in Table 7.1 as a guide, I would like to review briefly the early events of viral entry, into the host and into host cells. What are the selective pressures, based on the few well-studied examples? I will cite a few examples where the causes of virulence, as I have defined the term, have been determined, then briefly mention primary replication, and then briefly consider spread and tropism as other sites in the life cycle that illustrate how viral virulence factors can be expressed.

PORTALS OF ENTRY

Even though there are hundreds or thousands of viruses, there are only a few ways they can enter the host. Therefore, what a new emerging agent would require in order to be able to enter the body through a particular site is almost predictable. The normal portals for viral entry are most commonly the respiratory tract or the gastrointestinal (GI) tract. If a virus is able to bypass these normal sites (for example if it is injected through hypodermic needles), the virus is bypassing what are normal barriers at each portal of entry. For instance, intravenous injection introduces viruses directly into the bloodstream so some of the primary defense mechanisms, the host barriers, are bypassed totally. Similarly, artificially putting viruses into a different portal of entry can bypass a barrier that may normally act as a barrier preventing the virus from entering the host.

The respiratory tract and GI tract have their own microenvironments. And, again, diverse viruses with enormous differences can enter through the same route, but there are some common features.

In infection via the GI tract, a virus must pass through the low pH of the stomach, then encounter the detergent action of bile salts without being dissolved, and then have to infect in tissues where digestion is the rule of the day, where the intestinal contents are designed to break down proteins in order to allow the proteins to enter the circulation.

In general, viruses are not capable of entering the host by the enteric route if they have a lipid envelope, which would be dissolved by the detergent action of bile salts, or if they are sensitive to acid, and would thus not survive the stomach acid.

In the respiratory tract, there is a different microenvironment. There are goblet cells secreting mucus, ciliary motion, and secretory factors present, all creating a very complex mixture that the virus has to adapt to in order to infect respiratory epithelium. In this site, enveloped viruses, such as influenza, fare much better.

What virulence factors affecting sites of entry have been best defined?

Proteases

I have described certain environmental factors that can influence route and type of infection. Other viral factors have been defined. R.G. Webster and colleagues have shown that with a chicken strain of influenza A virus, a single change in the cleavability of the hemagglutinin, one of the viral surface proteins, is associated with an increased capacity for this flu strain to produce pandemics within the avian population (see Chapter 4). The relative susceptibility for specific cleavage in the hemagglutinin protein is necessary for increased virulence. Thus the parent strain is not efficiently cleaved by host proteases and is therefore not very virulent, but a mutation that allows the cleavage to occur results in a highly virulent virus. I consider this one of the best natural examples of how a single amino acid change in a viral protein helps explain differences in virulence between different strains of a virus and why one strain was involved in a pandemic.

There are other instances where viral responses to host proteases act as virulence determinants (Tyler and Fields, 1991). Rotaviruses infect by the GI tract and require cleavage by host proteases in order to activate the rotavirus in the GI tract. The adaptation in response to proteases plays a striking ability in getting rotavirus infection started.

Similarly, proteases have been shown to play a critical role in the activation of reoviruses in the gut, and this property has been genetically mapped to a specific viral determinant (Tyler and Fields, 1991).

In these infections, adding protease inhibitors has an antiviral effect, further providing evidence of how important this response to proteases is in initiating infection. Thus the response of viruses to proteases is one of the most important virulence determinants. It illustrates the close interplay between the microenvironment and ability to initiate infection. It is also true for a number of viruses as a general principle, such as the example I mentioned earlier with influenza.

Spread Beyond the Primary Sites of Replication

Following primary replication, viruses may spread beyond their primary or initial site. The pathways used after entering the host are not well defined for many viruses. Often, viruses enter epithelial cells where they may bind to specific receptors. Epithelial cells line and cover most surfaces of the body, so their proximity and ubiquity to the portal of entry make them a frequent target. Sometimes, a virus may bypass epithelial cells and move in special pathways, such as the intestinal M cell pathway, where some viruses (reovirus, poliovirus) bypass intestinal epithelial cells and move into a type of mononuclear cell in the Peyer's patch of the intestine, where primary replication may take place.

This brings me to the next virulence determinant, interaction with *macrophages* (Mims, 1987). The type of leukocyte known as the macrophage (its precursor in the circulation is called a monocyte) is ubiquitous in many tissues. Many viruses following entry into the host come in contact with macrophages, in the respiratory tract, in the GI tract, or elsewhere. This cell is increasingly recognized as an important early site of growth for systemic viruses, and the capacity of virus to grow in the macrophage, or at least to survive its interaction with the macrophage, may be central in the life cycle of a virus. There are a number of examples, largely descriptive, where the capacity to grow in macrophages in different sites is clearly a viral virulence determinant. For example, with the JHM strain of mouse hepatitis virus, virulent strains are able to grow in macrophages and kill them, but avirulent strains are killed by macrophages. Summarizing a large and sometimes confusing literature, none of which has yet given us a specific mechanism, suffice it to say that macrophages are a key early component in the host defense to many viruses, and the interaction of viruses with macrophages is a critical determinant of the outcome of infection.

Although we do not know what mechanisms determine this outcome, it is likely that, at least in part, the outcome is related to the generation of interferon or other mediators. In addition, macrophages have proteases inside the cell that may inactivate viral particles. This is an important area that needs to be studied at mechanistic levels.

Just as there are a limited number of entry portals, there are also a very restricted number of ways that viruses spread in the host. One way is through the bloodstream, either free in the blood, as in poliovirus, or in association with cells such as mononuclear cells. Hematogenous spread is common for many viruses. The growth in white blood cells may again play a key role, just as it does at primary replication, in regulating spread. We really don't have many insights into genetic determinants of this facet of the life cycle.

The second major pathway of spread for virus is that they can enter nerves, if they have appropriate receptors. Within nerves, viruses enter and move along a physiologic pathway, such as the microtubule based fast axonal transport system used by herpesviruses and reoviruses, or as in the case of rabies, perhaps moving in association with the slow axonal transport pathway (Tyler and Fields, 1991). Such pathways allow neurotropic viruses to enter into the nervous system after infecting a peripheral nerve cell.

The capacity to spread is a critical viral virulence determinant. I have cited the attenuated vaccines against rabies, as one example, and polio as another. These are viruses that can replicate outside the CNS but can't spread very well in the host and have lost the capacity to enter the central nervous system (Murphy and Chanock, 1991). Rabies virus can grow very well in muscle and peripheral tissue, but the rabies vaccine virus has lost the capacity to enter and move through neural pathways, a necessary property to cause the neurologic disease we recognize as rabies. Similarly, we have studied a reovirus mutant that has the same phenotype. It grows peripherally, but it can't penetrate the CNS. This loss of the capacity to move into a target tissue, like the nervous system, or to spread throughout the host, is a very important virulence determinant and is an important property for live attenuated vaccines.

CELL AND TISSUE TROPISM

The next step is a central issue of viral infection, *tropism*, the predilection of virus for specific tissues (see Chapters 8 and 18). There are at least four different types of factors associated with tropism (Tyler and Fields, 1991). The first type is host factors; and clearly age, nutrition, and immunity all play critical roles in the tissue specific injury of viruses.

Second, route of entry is also absolutely critical. If you inject a virus, for example, into the brain it produces lesions in a certain distribution. Put into the mouth, the same neurotropic virus enters different pathways. Put into the lower extremity, it goes up the spinal cord by still different pathways. The importance of route of entry is particularly true for viruses that move through nerves, but also is true for viruses that infect systemically.

The third factor is virus attachment proteins and receptors. A number of virus receptors have recently been identified and this is clearly a field that is just burgeoning. I will address the virus part of it in a moment, but first let me caution you that my saying that receptors and attachment proteins are important does not mean that tissue specific regulatory proteins (discussed in Chapter 8) are not. I cite HIV as one of many examples to point out a virus has to bind to the right receptor, but when it gets into the cell it still has to meet the right environment, and will have to deal with cellular regulatory systems. Both receptors and intracellular environment play critical roles. And again, it points out the problem faced by a hypothetical newly developing agent that may not yet have adapted to meet each of these steps.

Lastly, cellular factors like proteases are important not only at the portals of entry, but also later in the life cycle.

To illustrate these general points, I will discuss a specific example, reovirus, dealing with the issue of tropism (Sharpe and Fields, 1985). There are strains of reovirus that are highly lethal in mice and other strains that are not. A number of years ago we showed that some strains of reovirus, such as Type 1, target to cells in the brain, the ependyma, that are not lethal sites of infection; such strains do not enter or grow efficiently in neurons. The opposite occurs with the much more virulent reovirus Type 3 strains. Reovirus Type 3 is neuronotropic, producing encephalitis. With reovirus Type 3, there is viral antigen in neurons, and there are inflammatory cells, but sparing the ependyma.

This difference of tropism is associated with a striking difference in lethality. With reovirus Type 3, inoculation of one infectious virus particle causes virtually 100 percent mortality in infected mice, while for reovirus type 1, 10^8 infectious particles are not lethal. The reovirus genome is segmented RNA (RNA is separate pieces or segments corresponding roughly to individual genes), and the S1 gene is the determinant responsible for the difference in cell tropism (neurons or ependyma) and hence lethality. The S1 gene codes for the viral hemagglutinin, the viral surface protein responsible for attachment to cells. We know that this is the critical gene because a reassortant virus we made in the laboratory combining nine genes from Type 3 with the S1 gene encoding the hemagglutinin from Type 1 is basically nonlethal, but the reciprocal reassortant that has nine genes from Type 1 with the hemagglutinin gene from Type 3, cases a lethal encephalitis like regular Type 3 virus.

By using resistance to antibody neutralization in cell culture as a selective device, we were able to select mutants that differed from the regular virus by one antigenic site (epitope) in the hemagglutinin. Those mutants grow beautifully in mouse cell line (L cells) in cell culture, so there is nothing wrong with their capacity to enter mouse cells and replicate totally normally. When put into the mouse, in contrast to the wild type which grows to high titer and kills mice, the mutants are strikingly attenuated for lethality, although totally non-defective in cell culture. Thus if certain hemagglutinin functions are mutated, it has no effect on the outcome in cell culture, yet it is strikingly attenuated in the animal. Even more interestingly, a series of mutants of this type showed a fine tuning of tropism; different mutations genetically determine different extent of tissue injury. These mutants differ in single amino acids in certain regions in the attachment region of the hemagglutinin protein (reviewed in Tyler and Fields, 1991).

Let me close by mentioning a few additional factors influencing viral virulence. First of all, interaction with the *immune system* is likely to include very important additional factors of virulence. The viral equivalent of the toxins produced by pathogenic bacteria are the mediators released by infected cells, compounds like tumor necrosis factor, leukotrienes, and interferons. They produce tissue injury and, to me, they are analogous to what the bacteria can do by themselves when they produce toxins.

Second, avoidance of host defense is important for all pathogens. I have mentioned the macrophage, but it is not the only determinant of host defense. One can avoid host defense in a variety of ways. Without reviewing all virus life cycles, I will mention removing or changing T-cell epitopes (antigenic sites recognized by T lymphocytes), which prevents recognition by T cells in the immune system and thus prevents killing of viral infected cells by T cells, and viruses that become latent after getting into cells, thereby not producing viral products that allow the host to recognize the cell as infected.

Finally, aspects of how viruses kill cells are certainly important virulence determinants, but are in general poorly understood at the present. All these areas will offer plentiful research opportunities for the future.

REFERENCES

Knipe, D.M. (1991). Virus-host cell interactions. In *Fundamental Virology* (B.N. Fields and D.M. Knipe, eds.), second ed., Chap. 12 (pp. 267-290). New York: Raven Press.

Mims, C.A. (1987). *The Pathogenesis of Infectious Disease*, third ed., Chap. 4 (pp. 63-91). London and New York: Academic Press.

Murphy, B.R., and R.M. Chanock (1991). Immunization against viruses. In *Fundamental Virology* (B.N. Fields and D.M. Knipe, eds.), second ed., Chap. 15 (pp. 371-404). New York: Raven Press.

Sharpe, A.H., and B.N. Fields (1985). Pathogenesis of viral infections. N. Engl. J. Med. **312**:486-497.

Tyler, K.L., and B.N. Fields (1991). Pathogenesis of viral infections. In *Fundamental Virology* (B.N. Fields and D.M. Knipe, eds.), second ed., Chap. 10 (pp. 191-239). New York: Raven Press.

8

Virus and Cell: Determinants of Tissue Tropism

THOMAS E. SHENK

A number of viruses exhibit a predilection, or tropism, for certain tissues or cell types, sometimes demonstrating considerable selectivity. After infection, the expression of some viruses can also be related to state of the host cell. Anecdotal accounts suggest that some viruses that persist in the body can be influenced by host state, the classic example being cold sores, which are reactivations of latent herpes simplex virus, in synchrony with the menstrual cycle or stress.

While we do not yet have precise answers to the reactivation of herpes, or the events in HIV infection that lead to AIDS, the mechanisms of cellular regulation underlying the tissue tropism and expression of several viruses are beginning to be elucidated. Among the best studied examples to date are several small to medium size DNA viruses, which this chapter will review as a model for understanding the complex interactions between viral regulation and cellular regulation.

TISSUE TROPISM IN SMALL DNA VIRUSES

I will consider primarily two DNA virus families, the papovaviruses and the adenoviruses. The term "papova" refers to the subfamilies of viruses included within the family, namely the papilloma viruses (the "pa" portion of the family name), which cause warts and similar growths and are factors in human cervical carcinoma (zur Hausen, 1989), and the polyoma viruses, named for a virus that causes many different types of tumors in mice. The polyoma subfamily also includes a number of well-studied viruses such as SV40 and several related viruses (JC and BK) that were isolated from humans. (The "va" in the family name is from so-called vacuolating viruses, named for the characteristic effect of SV40 and similar isolates in cell culture; SV40 is now classified in the polyomavirus subfamily.) All papovaviruses are nonenveloped and possess a small DNA genome, which is in a circular form in the virus particle and ranges in size from about 5,000 nucleotides for polyoma to about 8,000-10,000 nucleotides for the papillomaviruses. The adenoviruses, which will be discussed following the papovaviruses, constitute a separate family of DNA viruses. Adenoviruses are considerably larger, possessing a linear DNA genome of about 30,000-40,000 bases, but, like the papovaviruses, the virus particles are also not enveloped. Adenoviruses are very common human pathogens and are frequent causes of conjunctivitis and respiratory infections.

The papillomaviruses exhibit very definite tissue tropisms, being specifically associated with certain types of epithelial cells of the skin and mucous membranes. By contrast, another member of the same family, polyomavirus, gives the appearance of replicating and inducing tumors in virtually every organ of the mouse, and persists in the kidney. A wide variety of tissues of both epithelial and mesenchymal origin is involved, and in fact the name "polyoma" refers to this, poly meaning many and "oma" deriving from the suffix for tumor used in pathology. When further analyzed, part of this diversity is actually due to the fact that various studies have used many different wild type strains of polyomavirus. Individual wild type strains show greater tissue specificity.

SV40 (simian virus 40, originally a monkey virus as the name indicates), is another relative of polyomavirus. While its tissue specificity is unknown, it is known to persist in the kidney in infected monkeys. Because there is extensive information on the molecular biology of SV40, studies on the genetic basis of tissue tropism using SV40 have provided some valuable insights.

All of these viruses possess specialized enhancer-promoter sequences in their DNA. Enhancers are DNA sequences that activate or increase transcription, usually (but not necessarily) at a nearby promoter. A promoter is a sequence in the DNA that is located before the coding information for a gene and functions like a switch. When the gene is activated, the host cell RNA polymerase, which will transcribe the DNA into a messenger RNA (mRNA) copy of the coding information, binds to the promoter to begin transcription. Additional proteins, transcription factors, many of cellular origin, may join in binding at the promoter and help to regulate the process. Activation of a gene is thus often controlled by "turning on" the promoter, which results in transcription from the gene. Regulation of transcription is therefore an important mechanism of gene regulation. A role was demonstrated for the SV40 enhancer-promoter sequences in tissue tropism by testing transgenic (genetically engineered) mice containing the gene for the SV40 tumor (T) antigen, under control of the SV40 enhancer-promoter for that gene. These mice developed tumors in the choroid plexus of the brain, suggesting that this combination of genetic elements conferred a predilection for this cell type (Brinster et al., 1984). This specificity required both of the enhancer-promoter sequences that are located inside the T antigen coding region.

There is clearer evidence for tissue specificity with other papovaviruses. One papovavirus isolated from monkeys, the lymphotropic papovavirus (Brade et al., 1981), was originally isolated from B cells. It has been shown to be able to propagate in both B and T lymphocytes, but in no other cell type. JC virus, a human papovavirus that is the causative agent of PML (progressive multifocal leukoencephalopathy), a rare demyelinating disease of the central nervous system, replicates primarily in oligodendrocytes of the brain.

The adenoviruses replicate in a variety of cells including the epithelium of the respiratory tract, lymphoid cells, conjunctival tissues of the eye, and the gastrointestinal epithelium. Not every adenovirus will replicate in all of these locations. Of the numerous varieties of human adenoviruses, each has its own spectrum of tropisms for some of these locations.

WHAT ARE THE DETERMINANTS OF TROPISM?

The known mechanisms causing viruses to have a predilection for a specific cell or tissue type can be divided into three areas. The first is the site of entry. For a virus to move beyond the site of entry, it will require strategies to evade host defenses and to gain access to channels allowing further dissemination within the body.

A second factor affecting tissue tropism is the role of cellular receptors. In order to infect a cell, a virus needs to be able to get into the interior of that cell. This usually involves a cellular receptor to which the virus can attach to accomplish adsorption. The best known example, of course, is HIV, which attaches to CD4, a surface protein on certain T lymphocytes and other cells. After this step, there are also presumably cellular factors involved in the early intracellular steps, penetration and uncoating of the virus inside the cell.

The third major mechanism encompasses tissue specific cellular factors that are required for transcription (expression of viral genes) and the overall replication of the virus within a cell. The first two mechanisms are discussed in the preceeding chapter, while this third area will be the focus of this chapter. I will concentrate on tissue specific cellular factors required for efficient transcription of these viruses, because this is a promising newly burgeoning area of research.

TRANSCRIPTIONAL REGULATION AS A DETERMINANT

There are numerous examples in the literature demonstrating that tissue tropism, at least for some viruses, is often dependent on transcription factors. It has been known for quite a few years that polyomavirus cannot replicate in undifferentiated teratocarcinoma cells, but can replicate in differentiated cells (Fujimura et al., 1981). Considerable evidence indicates that this is due to enhancer sequences (Katinka et al., 1981; Campbell and Villarreal, 1988). Several mutants of polyomavirus are known that can replicate in the undifferentiated cell (Sekikawa and Levine, 1981; Vasseur et al., 1980). When analyzed, these mutants were found to possess an altered enhancer-promoter region; this region of the viral genome controls expression of the polyomavirus genes. Recent work has provided the key to these observations. Undifferentiated teratocarcinoma cells, in which polyomavirus cannot propagate, have very little of a transcription activity known as AP-1, a host protein that acts in regulating transcription (Kryszke et al., 1987; Wasylyk et al., 1988). In addition to binding to host genes, AP-1 can bind to the polyomavirus enhancer to activate it (Martin et al., 1988; Rochford et al., 1990). The mutant viruses that can replicate in the undifferentiated cell line have in their enhancer regions either additional copies of the binding site for AP-1, enabling the mutant to compete more effectively for the very small amounts of the factor, or multiple copies of other binding sites within the enhancer, presumably so that other transcription factors can be used instead of AP-1 to drive expression of the viral genome. This is a very clear example, identified at the molecular level, of a specific tropism exhibited by polyomavirus.

There has also been some very interesting work on lymphotropism, predilection for lymphocytes, in polyoma and the lymphotropic papovaviruses. Enhancer variants have been shown to determine the ability of polyomavirus to replicate in lymphoid cells. In work by Luis Villarreal and colleagues, the virus acquired lymphotropism when several of the enhancer regions within the polyomavirus genome were amplified and rearranged (Campbell and Villarreal, 1986, 1988). Lymphotropism is not expressed by wild type virus. With the lymphotropic papovaviruses, it has been demonstrated that the enhancer activity of these viruses is restricted to B and T cells. To study a promoter, a reporter gene, such as *cat*, can be appended to a known promoter. The *cat* gene (a bacterial antibiotic resistance gene, but the key point is that its activation can be assessed) causes a detectable product to be made when it is turned on, thereby serving as a "reporter" to indicate when transcription regulated by the promoter it has been attached to has been activated. The monkey lymphotropic papovavirus enhancer-promoter region was appended to the *cat* gene, the construct was introduced into cells, and *cat* activity was tested. Activity was expressed efficiently in B and T cells, but only poorly at best in other cell types (Mosthaf et al., 1985; Erselius et al., 1990). This again leads to the conclusion that this enhancer-promoter combination largely accounts for the infection of B and T cells by the lymphotropic papovavirus.

This line of reasoning is also supported by several experiments inserting recombinant or "foreign" transcriptional regulatory sites into viral genomes. An artificial enhancer, combining components of polyomavirus and Moloney murine leukemia virus, dramatically changed the tissue specificity of polyomavirus (Rochford et al., 1987; Rochford et al., 1991). The recombinant virus replicated specifically in the pancreas, an organ that neither of the parent viruses infected at all. The new enhancer had completely changed the specificity of the polyomavirus.

Similar mechanisms can explain the brain predilection of JC virus. As shown by the late George Khoury and his colleagues at the National Institutes of Health several years ago, activity of the JC virus enhancer is restricted to cells of nerve tissue origin. They were also able to show that a brain cell specific factor, not present in other cultured cells, binds to the enhancer (Feigenbaum et al., 1987). So a number of instances of tissue tropism in DNA viruses can be attributed, at least in part, to the enhancer-promoter region.

It should be noted that this mechanism is not limited to DNA viruses, as there are several examples involving retroviruses. For example, Nancy Hopkins and her colleagues showed that the enhancer domain of a retrovirus can contribute to tropism (Chatis et al., 1983; Speck et al., 1990). Friend murine leukemia virus causes erythroleukemias, affecting the stem cells of both red and white blood cells. Moloney murine leukemia virus, on the other hand, causes T-cell lymphomas. The enhancers of retroviruses are the long terminal repeats (LTR) at the ends of their genomes. A recombinant virus that included elements of the Friend murine leukemia virus but with the LTR sequences of Moloney virus had the tissue tropism of the Moloney virus, causing T-cell lymphomas and not erythroleukemias (Chatis et al., 1983). So retroviruses, as well as DNA viruses, have a component of their tissue tropism determined by their transcriptional signaling apparatus.

ADENOVIRUS TRANSCRIPTION

Some recent work in my own laboratory concerns regulation of transcription in adenoviruses. It illustrates the role of cellular transcription factors in viral transcription and replication, and also shows how factors involved in viral transcription can tie the virus into a key cellular signaling system, specifically the cyclic AMP response system.

Adenoviruses are DNA viruses with genomes considerably larger than those of the papovaviruses. The linear double stranded DNA genome of adenovirus codes for a number of different mRNA transcripts that are made at various times after infection. One key product is the so-called E1A mRNAs that are encoded from a transcription unit at the extreme left end of the viral genome. It has been known for several years that expression of the E1A gene is required to activate transcription from all the other genes. In technical terms, the E1A gene encodes for a transcriptional transactivating polypeptide.

Two principal mRNAs are produced from the E1A gene region (they are actually alternative versions made from a single precursor RNA), encoding proteins of 243 and 289 amino acids each. These two proteins differ in an internal region of 46 amino acids, called conserved region 3, which is absent from the smaller protein. The terminology arose from comparing amino acid sequences of the larger (289 amino acid) E1A protein from a variety of distantly related human adenoviruses. Comparisons revealed that the protein is comprised of portions that differ from virus to virus, and which show only 8 to 10 percent similarity, interspersed with regions that are highly conserved, showing about 50 percent identity between distantly related virus strains. These interspersed regions are designated conserved regions 1, 2, and 3. Each of these conserved regions seems to coincide with a domain on the protein that carries out a specific function, as determined by mutational analysis. Conserved regions 1 and 2 are involved primarily with stimulating DNA replication within the infected cell, causing quiescent cells to be stimulated to undergo cell division. A cell that is actively moving through the cell cycle and is geared up for copying DNA can probably replicate the virus more efficiently; among other things, as will be seen, the virus can utilize the cellular transcription factors.

Conserved region 3 seems to be involved primarily with the activation of transcription of all the other viral genes on the viral DNA. Conserved region 3 has certain interesting features. It contains a single zinc finger, a structural feature of some types of DNA-binding regulatory proteins including several transcription factors. One might speculate that the zinc finger is involved in interaction of the E1A protein with DNA, and, in fact, the protein does seem able to bind to DNA. Also in conserved region 3 is a highly charged portion that has the characteristics of transcriptional activators. These structural features suggest a role for this protein as a transcriptional activator.

As further confirmation, Maurice Green has synthesized the peptide corresponding to conserved region 3. This peptide can transcriptionally activate an E1A responsive gene if gene and protein are microinjected into the same cells (Green et al., 1988). Therefore, conserved region 3 contains all the information necessary for transcriptional activation.

E1A synthesis in the infected cell is carefully controlled, and we therefore thought it would be instructive to examine the E1A control region itself. This region not only has to work inside the cell before E1A protein itself is present, but it is also known that this control region responds to E1A. When the infected cell begins to make E1A protein, this product feeds back on its control region and causes much more of the protein to be made, an apparent transcriptional self-activation. Our strategy for analyzing this process was to look for cellular transcription factors, or other cellular factors, that will bind to the DNA sequences in front of the E1A coding region. We found quite a few; in fact, we stopped when we got to seven.

Focusing on the factor that seemed most abundant, that factor was partially purified and biochemically characterized. Armed with this information, we conducted a computer search for other possible binding sites on the viral DNA. It turned out that there were binding sites for this factor in front of all of the early adenovirus genes with only one exception, the so-called E1B gene (Hardy and Shenk, 1988). The factor itself was identified as a well known cellular factor (Hardy and Shenk, 1988), called the cyclic AMP response element binding protein (CREB). Its binding site on DNA is called a cyclic AMP response element (CRE element). Thus, there are CRE elements in front of E1A and all the adenovirus early genes except E1B. This was exciting because it provided an explanation for how the E1A gene can transcriptionally activate all those other genes, by binding a common factor.

CYCLIC AMP SIGNALING SYSTEMS IN CELLS AND VIRUSES

CREB are considered to be a part of the cellular signaling system involving cyclic adenosine monophosphate (cyclic AMP), which is widely considered one of the central control mechanisms of the cell. Various stimuli, such as the binding of certain hormones to the cell, cause increased intracellular synthesis of cyclic AMP, a famous "second messenger" (the "first messenger" is the original stimulus). Cyclic AMP activates a variety of responses, but the enzymes called protein kinases are thought to be of particular importance. The activities of many key proteins in the cell are regulated, turned on or off, by protein kinases (PK), which regulate them by attaching phosphate groups to certain sites of these proteins. Cyclic AMP activates a specific set of protein kinases, including one known as cyclic AMP-dependent protein kinase (PK A). PK A has been shown to phosphorylate transcription factors, such as CREB, which can then activate genes that contain binding sites for those factors. Intracellular cyclic AMP can be increased artificially by treating cells with dibutyryl cyclic AMP, a derivative that enters the cell and causes the same effects as cyclic AMP, including activating PK A.

Given the finding that the viral DNA has binding sites for proteins related to the cyclic AMP cell signaling system, can these viral genes be activated by dibutyryl cyclic AMP in infected cells? The S49 lymphocyte-like cell line is highly responsive to cyclic AMP. These cells can be infected with an adenovirus, and levels of E4 mRNA (mRNA coding for the E4 protein), an adenovirus product whose gene is activated by E1A, can be assayed 24 hours after infection. When levels of E4 mRNA produced in the absence of added cyclic AMP were compared with E4 levels in cells treated with dibutyryl cyclic AMP for 1 to 5 hours before testing, treated cells showed a considerable increase in the level of E4 mRNA (Engel et al., 1988). Further confirmation was obtained with a mutant line derived from these cells, which does not respond to cyclic AMP because it lacks the PK A activity necessary for many of the actions of cyclic AMP. As expected, adding dibutyryl cyclic AMP to infected cells of this cell line has no effect on the amount of E4 mRNA produced.

What about E1A, which is important in regulation of adenovirus transcription? Is the E1A gene important for this response to cyclic AMP? Treating infected cells with dibutyryl cyclic AMP increased amount of E1A gene transcription. This was confirmed using a virus mutant with the E1A gene deleted. Cyclic AMP treatment of cells infected with this mutant causes an increase, but of considerably less magnitude than if the E1A gene were present. One can calculate relative levels of E4 mRNA, arbitrarily setting the amount produced in the absence of both cyclic AMP and E1A to 1. E1A protein by itself can induce the E4 gene, with a tenfold increase in expression, while cyclic AMP alone causes a fivefold increase. The two together induced a 200-fold increase, an apparent synergy. Unfortunately, unlike what would have been expected, activity of CREB, which should be regulated by the cyclic AMP system, did not change coordinately in treated infected cells. However, another factor, AP-1, was markedly activated (Müller et al., 1989).

The activation of AP-1 is thought to be regulated not by cyclic AMP but by a different protein kinase, protein kinase C (PK C), which normally acts independently of PK A as part of another major cellular regulatory system. The effect of viral E1A with cyclic AMP would appear to be a case of cross talk in which cyclic AMP is causing the activation of AP-1, perhaps indirectly. The data indicate clearly that, whatever the pathway, the end result is activation of AP-1. With S49 cells, we performed an assay to detect the binding of

AP-1 to a small piece of DNA that contains the binding site for the transcription factor. As cells are treated with cyclic AMP, in the absence of E1A, AP-1 binding activity gradually increases to a modest level. Infecting cells with wild type virus, so that E1A is present, greatly enhances the activation of AP-1 binding activity. Several experiments indicate a role for elements of the cyclic AMP response pathway. A compound that inhibits PK A prevented activation of AP-1 in infected S49 cells (Müller et al., 1989). The mutant cell line that lacks PK A gave similar results (Müller et al., 1989).

RELATIONSHIP OF VIRAL ACTIVATION TO HOST CELL STATE

Adenovirus is therefore interacting very closely with the cellular signaling system to regulate activation of all the early viral genes, required for the virus to begin replicating, as well as activating several important cellular genes. Adenovirus tissue tropism is also influenced by the cyclic AMP response system. Cells with high cyclic AMP levels are likely to be more permissive for adenovirus transcription, because they have greater quantities in active form of a key transcription factor that the virus also requires. This increase would presumably lead to enhanced replication of the virus, although I should caution that it is not definitely known in this case that more is better, that more transcription by the virus necessarily translates into enhanced yield. Further study is required on this question.

It is possible to speculate, too, that the relationship of viral expression to the cyclic AMP response system might be especially relevant to adenovirus growth in lymphoid cells, in which the virus has been suggested to establish a persistent infection lasting for months after primary infection. The speculation is based on recent suggestions that lymphocyte activation, for example by interleukin-1, may involve an increase in cyclic AMP. If adenovirus were present in a lymphoid cell undergoing activation, it is conceivable that, as cyclic AMP levels increase, the level of AP-1 would also increase, causing a concomitant enhancement of adenovirus transcription. Speculatively, other stimuli that increase cyclic AMP could have similar effects. In general, since levels of cyclic AMP or of similar mediators can be affected by many different stimuli, such mechanisms could serve to link viral regulation to the state of the host cell.

In conclusion, let us return to the bigger picture. In response to the initial question I posed, "Are interactions with cellular transcription factors an important component of tissue tropism?", the answer is clearly that they are. Evidence includes the inability of polyoma virus to propagate in undifferentiated teratocarcinoma cells that lack the cellular transcription factor AP-1. Further evidence is that one way of overcoming this limitation was by the selection of viral variants that could either compete better for limiting levels of AP-1, or utilize different transcription factors.

These transcription factors are clearly not the only intracellular component to tissue tropism, and the viral enhancer is not the only determinant of tissue specificity, albeit an important component. Thomas Benjamin demonstrated that the variety and locations of polyoma induced tumors in infected mice were determined by two viral factors (Eckhart and Benjamin, 1989). One of these was the enhancer domain, while the other was the coding region for specific polyomavirus gene products. So other viral products are important as well. The various host factors discussed by Fields in Chapter 7, including receptors, proteases, and so on, are clearly operative as well and are important at different levels.

The mechanisms described should give a new appreciation of some of the ways that viruses can link their fate to that of the host cell. It nicely exemplifies Joshua Lederberg's statement, in Chapter 1 of this volume, that the essence of viruses is their entanglement with host cell metabolism. The examples presented here are clear cases of entanglement between the virus and its host cell.

REFERENCES

Brade, L., W. Vogl, L. Gissman, and H. zur Hausen (1981). Propagation of B-lymphotropic papovavirus (LPV) in human B-lymphoma cells and characterization of its DNA. Virology 114:228-235.

Brinster, R., H. Chen, A. Messing, T. van Dyke, A. Levine, and R. Palmiter (1984). Transgenic mice harboring SV40 T-antigen genes develop characteristic brain tumors. Cell 37:367-379.

Campbell, B.A, and L.P. Villarreal (1986). Lymphoid and other tissue-specific phenotypes of polyomavirus enhancer recombinants: Positive and negative combinatorial effects on enhancer specificity and activity. Molec. Cell. Biol. 6:2068-2079.

Campbell, B.A, and L.P. Villarreal (1988). Functional analysis of the individual enhancer core sequences of polyomavirus: Cell-specific uncoupling of DNA replication from transcription. Molec. Cell. Biol. 8:1993-2004.

Chatis, P.A., C.A. Holland, J.W. Hartley, W.P. Rowe, and N. Hopkins (1983). Role for the 3' end of the genome in determining disease specificity of Friend and Moloney murine leukemia viruses. Proc. Natl. Acad. Sci. USA 80:4408-4411.

Eckhart, W., and T.L. Benjamin (1989). Cell transformation and pathogenicity of polyomavirus. In *Common Mechanisms of Transformation by Small DNA Tumor Viruses* (L.P. Villarreal, ed.), pp. 65-73. Washington, D.C.: American Society for Microbiology.

Engel, D.A., S. Hardy, and T. Shenk (1988). cAMP acts in synergy with E1A protein to activate transcription of the adenovirus early genes E4 and E1A. Genes Devel. **2**:1517-1528.

Erselius, J.R., B. Jostes, A.K. Hatzopoulos, L. Mosthaf, and P. Gruss (1990). Cell-type-specific control elements of the lymphotropic papovavirus enhancer. J. Virol. **64**:1657-1666.

Feigenbaum, L., K. Khalili, E. Major, and G. Khoury (1987). Regulation of the host range of human papovavirus JCV. Proc. Natl. Acad. Sci. USA **84**:3695-3698.

Fujimura, F.K., P.E. Silbert, W. Eckhart, and E. Linney (1981). Polyoma virus infection of retinoic acid-induced differentiated teratocarcinoma cells. J. Virol. **39**:306-312.

Green, M., P.M. Lowenstein, R. Pusztar, and J.S. Symington (1988). An adenovirus E1A protein domain activates transcription *in vivo* and *in vitro* in the absence of protein synthesis. Cell **53**:921-926.

Hardy, S., and T. Shenk (1988). Adenoviral control regions activated by E1A and the cAMP response element bind to the same factor. Proc. Natl. Acad. Sci. USA **85**:4171-4175.

Katinka, M., M. Vasseur, N. Montreau, M. Yaniv, and D. Blangy (1981). Polyoma DNA sequences involved in control of viral gene expression in murine embryonal carcinoma cells. Nature **290**:720-722.

Kryszke, M.H., J. Piette, and M. Yaniv (1987). Induction of a factor that binds to the polyoma virus A enhancer on differentiation of embryonal carcinoma cells. Nature **328**:254-256.

Martin, M.E., J. Piette, M. Yaniv, W.J. Tang, and W.R. Folk (1988). Activation of the polyoma virus enhancer by a murine activator protein 1 (AP1) homolog and two contiguous proteins. Proc. Natl. Acad. Sci. USA **85**:5839-5843.

Mosthaf, L., M. Pawlita, and P. Gruss (1985). A viral enhancer element specifically active in human haematopoietic cells. Nature **315**:597-600.

Müller, U., M.P. Roberts, D.A. Engel, W. Doerfler, and T. Shenk (1989). Induction of transcription factor AP-1 by adenovirus E1A protein and cAMP. Genes Devel. **3**:1991-2002.

Rochford, R., B.A. Campbell, and L.P. Villarreal (1987). A pancreas specificity results from the combination of polyomavirus and Moloney murine leukemia virus enhancer. Proc. Natl. Acad. Sci. USA **84**:449-453.

Rochford, R., C.T. Davis, K.K. Yoshimoto, and L.P. Villarreal (1990). Minimal subenhancer requirements for high-level polyomavirus DNA replication: A cell-specific synergy of PEA3 and PEA1 sites. Molec. Cell. Biol. **10**:4996-5001.

Rochford, R., and L.P. Villarreal (1991). Polyomavirus DNA replication in the pancreas and in a transformed pancreas cell line has distinct enhancer requirements. J. Virol. **65**:2108-2112.

Sekikawa, K., and A.J. Levine (1981). Isolation and characterization of polyoma host range mutants that replicate in nullipotential embryonal carcinoma cells. Proc. Natl. Acad. Sci. USA **78**:1100-1104.

Speck, N.A., B. Renjifo, E. Golemis, T.N. Frederickson, J.W. Hartley, and N. Hopkins (1990). Mutation of the core or adjacent LVb elements of the Moloney murine leukemia virus enhancer alters disease specificity. Genes Devel. 4:233-242.

Vasseur, M., C. Kress, N. Montreau, and D. Blangy (1980). Isolation and characterization of polyoma virus mutants able to develop in embryonal carcinoma cells. Proc. Natl. Acad. Sci. USA 77:1068-1072.

Wasylyk, B., J.L. Imler, B. Chatton, C. Schatz, and C. Wasylyk (1988). Negative and positive factors determine the activity of the polyoma virus enhancer α domain in undifferentiated and differentiated cell types. Proc. Natl. Acad. Sci. USA 85:7952-7956.

zur Hausen, H. (1989). Papillomaviruses as carcinomaviruses. In *Advances in Viral Oncology*, vol. 8 (G. Klein, ed.), pp. 1-26. New York: Raven Press.

9

Virus Detection Systems

DOUGLAS D. RICHMAN

The presence of a virus in an infected host can be ascertained either by detecting the virus particle (virion) itself or its components. Detection methods can be classified as open minded (not requiring advance knowledge of the kind of virus sought) or as probe specific (using reagents designed to detect specific viruses) (Richman et al., 1984).

Detection of the virus is open minded when its success is not restricted to any single class or family of virus. Open minded methods include virus isolation and electron microscopy.

Methods to detect viral components or immunity to viral components, in general, are probe specific. There are a few exceptions that I will mention later. To detect antigen or antibody or nucleic acid, one needs to have a specific probe for each, which requires knowledge, specific reagents and methods, before one can detect the desired viral component. For a completely unknown agent this approach obviously has its limitations.

An additional component of viruses that one could look for is virus specific enzyme activity. There are, in fact, some examples of virus specific enzyme activities that can be detected directly in clinical material, the DNA polymerase of hepatitis B, for example. In general, however, detecting activities like reverse transcriptase, viral protease, or neuraminidase has not matched the sensitivity of the other approaches.

An important point to make at the outset is that no positive assay for the presence of the organism proves causality. Disease cannot be attributed to the circumstantial evidence of the organism being present.

Virus isolation became the "gold standard" of virology. It has several limitations. Besides the fact that it is expensive, cumbersome, and requires a certain amount of laboratory expertise, it has the limitation that it will not succeed without a "substrate", namely a permissive host cell. It also requires an effective detection method; one has to be able to know that the virus is in the host cell. One classically looked for cytopathology, virus-induced cell damage, although the detection of HIV was made using the appropriate substrate of peripheral blood mononuclear cells, and a reverse transcriptase assay, with the assumption that a retrovirus was the likely etiologic agent.

Viral isolation in cell culture will not work well if a virus cannot readily be grown in a known or readily available cell type. Examples of this limitation are hepatitis viruses, and most of the gastroenteritis viruses, in which cell culture systems have not been useful in identifying the etiologic agents. Although some agents that fail to grow in cell culture can infect animals, isolation in animals has obvious limitations as well, and even this approach does not work for all human viruses.

When a suitable system is available, virus isolation offers several benefits. First, if it does work, one needs only a single infectious particle, in theory, to be able to detect infection. This amplification of infectivity confers high sensitivity, theoretically surpassing any other method. Isolation also provides specificity; only the virus is amplified. Another benefit is that isolation of the agent permits its characterization and preservation, and it provides reagents for all of the other assays.

Electron microscopy, the other open-minded assay system, is limited by the fact that it is cumbersome, expensive and subject to artifact, but it does have some benefits and it has had utility. It is rapid and it works directly with clinical material if the sample has a relatively high concentration of virions. Examples of new etiologic agents identified this way include many of those agents that could not be identified by cell culture. The gastroenteritis agents, such as Norwalk agent and rotavirus, were first detected by electron microscopy. Hepatitis A was also discovered using immune electron microscopy.

The probe specific methodologies have different limitations and advantages. Antigen or antibody detection methods have been very successful for known agents. However, with the few exceptions that I will mention shortly, the utility of these methods to detect new agents is limited by the fact that success requires either good luck and lots of antigen, examples of this being hepatitis B and the B19 parvovirus, or cross reactivity with a related known agent. Because one has to have a specific probe, either the antigen or the antibody beforehand, antigen or antibody detection is useful only for identifying new agents that are antigenically related to known agents, and one needs either insight or luck to identify what these might be. In the characterization of seal plague virus, Mahy identified the seal virus using antigens for distemper and rinderpest viruses to detect the serologic response in the seals and showed that, in fact, an agent closely related to those viruses was causing the disease in the seals. This success was based on insight into the types of possible agents that could be responsible for the disease.

There are, in fact, some ways in which antigen or antibody detection can be open minded, in which one can look for an antigen or an antibody to an agent without having a specific probe. One useful way is by detecting an unknown antigen in a specimen with convalescent serum. There have been some successful examples of identification of new agents with this approach. The classic one is the Australia antigen in which antigen in the serum of Australian aborigines was discovered by Baruch Blumberg to immunoprecipitate with serum antibodies. It took others to appreciate the fact that this reaction was due to the virus of hepatitis B. Sufficient quantities of antigen were present in the serum for detection without the prior existence of a specific antigen as a probe. A similar phenomenon occurred with the identification of the B19 parvovirus, a very interesting agent which, for very short periods of time, is present in high enough concentrations in serum to be detectable. A third example is rotavirus, which is present in such high concentrations in the stool of children with gastroenteritis, that one can detect the presence of this virus in the stool, by immunoprecipitation or complement fixation using convalescent serum, without having a specific antigen preparation as a probe.

Immunofluorescence or immunohistochemical detection in tissues has been performed in an analogous manner in which acute and convalescent serum are taken, and one looks for antigen detected by the convalescent serum in tissue sections. Notable examples of this are the detection of Hantaan virus, by the Lees and Karl Johnson, using immunofluorescence in the kidneys and other tissues of the infected rodent vectors. Mario Rizzetto in Torino identified the delta antigen, now known to be associated with the delta hepatitis agent (hepatitis D virus), and began to characterize this agent using this technique by examining liver tissue of patients with hepatitis. This approach, of course, is fraught with all of the potential artifactual problems that one can get using uncharacterized reagents, but it has been useful. Immune electron microscopy is an analogous approach in which acute and convalescent sera are used to detect the agglutination of virus in virus-containing samples, usually the stool, by electron microscopy. The identification, in Robert Chanock's laboratory at the National Institutes of Health, of the Norwalk gastroenteritis agents and the hepatitis A virus (by Stephen M. Feinstone) were classic successes with this methodology.

The final example, from Houghton's work with hepatitis C virus, may become one of the more commonly used future approaches to identifying new agents without the prior existence of specific antigen or antibody as a probe. In this method, nucleic acid is isolated from infected patients. DNA clones are prepared from the total nucleic acid extract and introduced into bacteria or cells using a vehicle that allows expression in vitro of any protein products encoded by the DNA. Convalescent serum from the patients is then used to screen for any clones that encode viral antigens (Choo et al., 1989). The DNA clone identified in this manner can now be used to produce both viral antigens for serologic testing (Alter et al., 1990; Kuo et al., 1989), and probes for nucleic acid analysis of the virus (Choo et al., 1989).

The detection of virus specific nucleic acid has been used extensively only in the last decade or so (Richman and Wahl, 1986). It has several potential benefits. For many known viruses and virus families, there is considerable information regarding their nucleic acid sequences. These sequence data permit the design of probes with any desired specificity, ranging from strain to species to genus to family, depending upon the sequence that one selects. Secondly, technologies for molecular cloning and oligonucleotide synthesis permit preparation of unlimited amounts of standardized reagents.

The limitation of this approach, at least at present, is an appropriate assay format. Standardization is still difficult. Slight modification of the conditions can yield great increases in signal for which proper quantitative controls may be difficult to establish. This is probably true with almost any assay, but despite these limitations, with nucleic acid detection techniques a lot of people have been able to design experiments to detect almost anything they wanted to for any disease.

Using HIV as the example, I will now discuss approaches to detection of nucleic acid. In general, at least three approaches have been used for detection. The first is in situ hybridization. This has not been very useful, to date, for primary detection and diagnosis of new agents, but it is useful for studies of pathogenesis. The second method is the detection of nucleic acid extracted directly from clinical specimens. As described elsewhere in this volume, Mahy used this technique with seal plague virus. The third approach is detection of nucleic acid extracted from clinical specimens following genome amplification. This has been the subject of considerable recent interest, especially methods involving amplification of the nucleic acid by the polymerase chain reaction (PCR). I will now describe some examples of each.

Several examples with HIV demonstrate the utility of immunohistochemical staining for viral antigen and in situ hybridization to detect viral nucleic acid. The pathogenesis of the dementia in HIV infection has been of great interest. By histopathology, all that was originally seen were vague inflammatory cells or occasional multinucleated giant cells, without any clear mechanisms of disease. Several groups, beginning about 5 years ago, have demonstrated that the only cells consistently infected in the central nervous system are macrophages. These cells comprised the multinucleated giant cells; by various immunohistochemical staining or in situ hybridization techniques, the cells in the brain that were infected with HIV were shown to be almost exclusively macrophages. I should mention that Ashley Haase, using the related animal lentivirus visna as an example for HIV, established a lot of the standards for this art form. I am afraid that in many ways it is still more a form of art than science.

The detection of nucleic acid by extraction and detection of nucleic acid in nitrocellulose or in other solid phase assays, reacting with a known nucleic acid probe, is one approach people have found more useful for diagnosis. If one extracts nucleic acid from peripheral blood mononuclear cells, or if one examines HIV infected cultured cells, there are over a thousandfold more copies of viral RNA than DNA; this result implies that for HIV, detection of RNA is going to prove more sensitive than detecting DNA (Richman et al., 1987). In fact, the direct detection of DNA in tissues is very difficult with HIV, requiring the extraction of extremely large quantities of tissue. But in about 70 percent of seropositive patients it is possible to directly detect viral RNA extracted from a sample of peripheral blood mononuclear cells containing about a million cells, while controls remain negative (Richman et al., 1987). With infected cell lines one can detect between 10 and 100 infected cultured cells.

This is not particularly useful since the serologic test detects 100 percent of these same patients, and so people have gone on to consider amplification by polymerase chain reaction (PCR) for greater sensitivity (Guatelli et al., 1989). Using these enzymatic DNA amplification techniques, one can almost double the quantity of target sequences with each round of amplification, this successive doubling leading to tremendous increases, typically a millionfold to a billionfold over the course of the 30 to 35 rounds of amplification usually used. There are number of variants of this approach with different formats, but all employ the same principle, using a bacterial DNA polymerase to enzymatically amplify target DNA sequences, such as a viral DNA, in a clinical sample. For viruses whose genomes are DNA, such as parvoviruses or herpesviruses, PCR would therefore work with the viral genome directly. For most RNA viruses, one first has to convert the viral RNA genome to a DNA copy, termed complementary DNA (cDNA), before amplification. This conversion is carried out in vitro using the enzyme reverse transcriptase, which is purified from a retrovirus. Retroviruses, like HIV, are RNA viruses that have their own reverse transcriptase and use it during their life cycle in the cell. For PCR detection of these viruses, there is a choice: you can use as the target for PCR the viral DNA forms found in infected cells, or can perform the cDNA in vitro before beginning the amplification.

With HIV, if one uses a reverse transcriptase step before the amplification, one gets significantly more signal than if one just amplifies the DNA directly. So the reverse transcriptase step is useful in detecting HIV nucleic acid in cells. This is a corollary of something I mentioned earlier, that there are a lot more copies of RNA sequences of the retroviruses present than there are copies of their DNA sequences. One has a prior amplification, if you will, of RNA in infected cells. This is true in both culture and in patients.

This is useful for retroviruses, but for most other viruses discussed in this book, an initial reverse transcription step is going to be essential because most of the viruses we are interested in have only RNA copies represented in infected cells.

A second point is that one can take either a host cell DNA that exists in a single copy in the cell, such as the gene for β-globin, or an RNA, such as the messenger RNA from β-actin or HLA genes, and use these as a standard by co-amplifying. This has two purposes. First, it serves as a control to show that, in fact, the extraction and amplification are working. Second, it can potentially be used as a denominator to quantitate nucleic acid by determining ratios. This may have some utility in the future, since one limitation of PCR right now is that it isn't quantitative. However, for both RNA and DNA, it has recently been possible to get almost straight line standard curves with cell culture material, quantitating the number of copies, or the number of infected cells, using a ratio of HIV to globin copy number (Guatelli et al., 1989).

This quantitative approach works consistently with cell culture material. As soon as one examines clinical material with similar methods, the relative efficiencies of coamplifications become so variable that the reliability of this methodology has not yet been proved.

In addition to quantitative PCR using coamplification of β-globin or other genes, quantitative methods have been developed in which radiolabeled PCR primers are used; incorporated radioactivity is then counted to provide a measure of product produced (Daar et al., 1991; Pang et al., 1990; Zack et al., 1990). Another method, limiting dilution, has also been used to quantify PCR, for example to determine copy number of HIV provirus in infected cells (Psallidopoulos et al., 1989; Schnittman et al., 1989). Quantitation is performed by making serial dilutions of the DNA sample, performing the PCR on all of these samples, and determining the greatest dilution that will still give a PCR product. Quantitative endpoint is determined by comparing results with dilutions of standards containing known copy numbers of HIV DNA.

Many modifications have been developed to enhance the capabilities of PCR for various applications (Erlich et al., 1991). Additionally, methods have recently been published for PCR in situ, potentially combining the sensitivity of PCR with the ability of in situ hybridization to allow visualization of the cells harboring the target nucleic acid sequence (Haase et al., 1990; Nuovo et al., 1991a; Staskus et al., 1991). PCR is performed on the intact tissue or cell sample, followed by in situ hybridization to detect the desired nucleic acid sequence. The PCR amplification prior to in situ detection could greatly increase the sensitivity of the latter (Haase et al., 1990; Nuovo et al., 1991a; Staskus et al., 1991). The method could be combined with cytochemical techniques for further identification of the positive cells by additional markers.

I will conclude by summarizing the potential applications of PCR to human retroviruses and, by extrapolation, to other new and emerging viruses. The potential uses of PCR are many. With regard to HIV, using the methodologies of today, virtually 100 percent of individuals who are infected can be detected with antibody assay, with culture of peripheral blood, or with PCR. However, the use of PCR to detect infected people is limited, since it is very much more difficult to perform than ELISA, the standard test for antibody.

With the current methodology, the use of PCR is restricted to a small subset of people, antibody negative subjects. Who are these people? Clearly, the most important subgroup is perinatally infected children because many of them may be seropositive on the basis of passive maternally acquired antibody, and to discriminate which infants are truly infected among offspring of seropositive mothers has some real utility. In that case, for identifying either antibody positive subjects who may not be infected, or to identify those belonging to a subset of perinatally infected children who never develop an antibody response, PCR may be very useful.

Are there adults who are antibody negative? There are two possible situations where this may be of practical use. One is for people in that short window between infection and antibody response. The second is that very small subset of people who, for other reasons, have not developed an antibody response. Although the publicity about it far exceeds its practical importance, it is nevertheless of some potential interest.

I think PCR will find more general use as more convenient quantitative PCR assays are developed. Then it will be extremely useful in measuring nucleic acid load or quantity in clinical material, to help to characterize changes during therapy or change of disease status, and to assess amounts of virus in different cells and tissues to help explain pathogenesis and transmission.

PCR would probably be more useful in other retrovirus infections, such as HTLV. One purpose for which PCR has already proved useful is to demonstrate the presence of virus, especially in certain diseases in which detecting the antibody response, or isolating the virus, is much more difficult to document than it is with HIV. For example, in HTLV-associated myelopathy, or tropical spastic paraparesis, PCR has been useful in characterizing people with this sort of disease who are HTLV infected and discriminating these conditions from other diseases.

Another example with HTLV comes from work by at least two groups, Beatrice Hahn and George Shaw at the University of Alabama and Irvin S.Y. Chen and his group at the University of California, Los Angeles. These groups have shown that of the fairly large numbers of HTLV-I seropositive people in the United States, there are some populations that have relatively high seroprevalence rates when tested by ELISA tests containing HTLV-I antigen. These assays were thought to identify fairly large pockets of HTLV-I infection in certain subsets in this country, most of whom are primarily injectable drug users, but including people identified through wider serosurveys in the southeastern United States. However, these researchers have shown, by using PCR, that at least 90 percent of the drug users who are positive by those serologic assays are, in fact, infected with HTLV-II and not HTLV-I. This was documented by using PCR with probes that could distinguish these two agents.

A final example shows the potential of PCR for identifying unknown viruses, and also illustrates the need for caution in interpreting results. Multiple sclerosis has been a candidate viral disease virus for over a generation. Various investigators have identified several viruses for this, none of which has conclusively proven to be the etiologic agent. A recent candidate has been HTLV-I or an HTLV-I related agent. Several groups have used PCR to try to identify HTLV-I sequences in the brain tissue of people with multiple sclerosis. One group published a positive result using PCR. A second group has asserted that the same primer pair used by the other group to identify HTLV-I in the brain specimens from patients with multiple sclerosis, in their hands gives consistently positive results with all specimens. They believe that endogenous sequences are probably present and cross react with the primer pairs that were identified.

This case exemplifies both the benefits and the limitations of new approaches for new agents. The potential application of PCR for the identification of new agents is just beginning. But this case also demonstrates the potential for pitfalls and problems. I think that rigorous scientific method, requiring independent confirmation of results and multiple analytic approaches, is the only way it will be possible to get true answers, to separate fact from artifact.

REFERENCES

Alter, H.J., R.H. Purcell, J.W. Shih, J.C. Melpolder, M. Houghton, Q.-L. Choo, and G. Kuo (1990). Detection of antibody to hepatitis C virus in prospectively followed transfusion recipients with acute and chronic non-A, non-B hepatitis. N. Engl. J. Med. 321:1494-1501.

Choo, Q.-L., G. Kuo, A.J. Weiner, L.R. Overby, D.W. Bradley, and M. Houghton (1989). Isolation of a cDNA clone derived from a blood-borne non-A, non-B viral hepatitis genome. Science 244:359-362.

Daar, E.S., T. Moudgil, R.D. Meyer, and D.D. Ho (1991). Transient high levels of viremia in patients with primary human immunodeficiency virus type 1 infection. N. Engl. J. Med. 324:961-964.

Erlich, H.A., D. Gelfand, and J.J. Sninsky (1991). Recent advances in the polymerase chain reaction. Science 252:1643-1651.

Guatelli, J.C., T.R. Gingeras, and D.D. Richman (1989). Nucleic acid amplification *in vitro*: The detection of sequences with low copy numbers and application to the diagnosis of HIV-1 infection. Clin. Microbiol. Rev. 2:217-226.

Haase, A.T., E.F. Retzel, and K.A. Staskus (1990). Amplification and detection of lentiviral DNA inside cells. Proc. Natl. Acad. Sci. USA 87:4971-4975.

Kuo, G., Q.-L. Choo, H.J. Alter, G.L. Gitnick, A.G. Redeker, R.H. Purcell, T. Miyamura, J.L. Dienstag, M.J. Alter, C.E. Stevens, G.E. Tegtmeier, F. Bonino, M. Colombo, W.-S. Lee, C. Kuo, K. Berger, J.R. Shuster, L.R. Overby, D.W. Bradley, and M. Houghton (1989). An assay for circulating antibodies to a major etiologic virus of human non-A, non-B hepatitis. Science 244:362-364.

Nuovo, G.J., F. Gallery, P. MacConnell, J. Becker, and W. Bloch (1991a). An improved technique for the *in situ* detection of DNA after polymerase chain reaction amplification. Am. J. Pathol. 139:1239-1244.

Nuovo, G.J., P. MacConnell, A. Forde, and P. Delvenne (1991b). Detection of human papillomavirus DNA in formalin-fixed tissues by *in situ* hybridization after amplification by polymerase chain reaction. Am. J. Pathol. 139:847-854.

Pang, S., Y. Koyanagi, S. Miles, C. Wiley, H. Vinters, and I.S.Y. Chen (1990). High levels of unintegrated HIV-1 DNA in brain tissue of AIDS dementia patients. Nature 343:85-89.

Psallidopoulos, M.C., S.M. Schnittman, L. M. Thompson III, M. Baseler, A.S. Fauci, H.C. Lane, and N.P. Salzman (1989). Integrated proviral human immunodeficiency virus type 1 is present in CD4+ peripheral blood lymphocytes in healthy seropositive individuals. J. Virol. 63:4626-4631.

Richman, D.D., D.C. Redfield, P.H. Cleveland, M.N. Oxman, and G.M. Wahl (1984). Rapid viral diagnosis. J. Infect. Dis. 149:298-310.

Richman, D.D., and G.M. Wahl (1986). Nucleic acid probes to detect viral diseases. In *Concepts in Viral Pathogenesis*, II (A.L. Notkins and M.B.A. Oldstone, eds.), pp. 301-309. New York: Springer Verlag.

Richman, D.D., J.A.McCutchan, and S.A. Spector (1987). Detecting human immunodeficiency virus RNA in peripheral blood mononuclear cells by nucleic acid hybridization. J. Infect. Dis. 156:823-827.

Schnittman, S.M., M.C. Psallidopoulos, H.C. Lane, L. Thompson, M. Baseler, F. Massari, C.H. Fox, N.P. Salzman, and A.S. Fauci (1989). The reservoir for HIV-1 in human peripheral blood is a T cell that maintains expression of CD4. Science 245:305-308.

Staskus, K.A., L. Couch, P. Bitterman, E.F. Retzel, M. Zupancic, J. List, and A.T. Haase (1991). *In situ* amplification of visna virus DNA in tissue sections reveals a reservoir of latently infected cells. Microb. Pathog. 11:67-76.

10

New Technologies for Virus Detection

DAVID C. WARD

In the previous chapter, Richman has given an overview of the various methods for viral detection that are available, ranging from the immunological to nucleic acid hybridization. Apart from the "gold standard" culture methods, it appears at the moment that the most sensitive methods are based on nucleic acid hybridization for detecting viral genetic sequences, particularly with the application of polymerase chain reaction (PCR) to amplify target sequences.

I will discuss here three other emerging techniques that could be applied to the analysis of viral infection. One of these methodologies involves fluorescent optical imaging, particularly using confocal microscopy, with the idea of obtaining information on virus integration, viral latency, and, in general, for detecting within intact cells a single copy of a viral genome. One often desires quantitative data (a plaque assay, for example, is quantitative and not merely qualitative), and fluorescent optical imaging techniques have this advantage.

The second methodology is chemiluminescent enzymology, the development of substrates for enzymes that can be detected by the emission of light and are linear over a 10 millionfold range. Such methodology can be used to amplify the detection signal in enzyme immunoassays.

Third, I will then describe briefly another method for increasing the sensitivity of detection, based on amplification of specific sequences by the RNA replicase (RNA copying enzyme) from the bacteriophage Qβ. In distinction to PCR, which is a target amplification system, the Qβ system is a signal amplification system with the potential to amplify the detection signal attached to a particular target sequence about a billionfold in 30 minutes or less. This methodology was originally developed by Fred Russell Kramer at the New York Public Health Research Institute and Leslie Orgel at the Salk Institute (Kramer and Lizardi, 1989; Lizardi et al., 1988; Lomeli et al., 1989). We have been experimenting with some of these methodologies in our laboratory, and I will briefly summarize some of our experience and point out some of the relative advantages and disadvantages of these methods.

Other than viral isolation in culture, and because of the polymerase chain reaction, one of the most sensitive methods for detecting a viral entity is by hybridization based assays. All these hybridization assays are based on the "double helix", the strong and specific attraction between a given nucleic acid sequence and another piece of nucleic acid containing a sequence of bases complementary to the first sequence. Forming the double helix in this way is called hybridization. The nucleic acid sequence we want to detect is usually called the "target" sequence; the piece of nucleic acid, usually DNA but sometimes RNA, that we use to detect the target is called the "probe". A viral probe can be made from a known viral nucleic acid extracted from infected cells, or it can be a viral DNA cloned in bacteria or yeast cells, or, once the nucleotide sequence is known, may be made synthetically. As Richman mentioned in his chapter, by varying the conditions of hybridization, what we call the stringency of the reaction, one can detect either highly specific individual viral entities or whole families or genera of viruses.

In theory, the sensitivity of a technique like in situ hybridization, in which individual cells are examined microscopically for the presence of the target nucleic acid as detected by hybridization with probe, is to the level of a single infected cell. Ashley Haase and others have in fact managed to use hybridization methods for detecting single infected cells in tissues.

Another type of nucleic acid hybridization technique is the filter based assay, in which nucleic acids are extracted from the potentially infected cells, immobilized on a solid support such as nitrocellulose filter paper, and reacted with the probe on this solid support. Common formats include the Southern blot and hybridization dot blot; the level of sensitivity with existing methodologies is between 100,000 and 500,000 target molecules. Solution hybridization methods, carrying out the reactions in liquid medium instead of on filter paper, have similar sensitivity in the absence of an amplification step (in the range of 100,000 or more target molecules). With an amplification reaction, such as PCR, to increase the number of target molecules before detection, sensitivity is 10 to 100 target molecules or an equivalent number of bacterial or viral genomes. The ability to amplify specific genes from a single sperm cell has been reported, for example. So this methodology has the potential to detect single viral genomes.

Partly because of the Human Genome initiative and partly because of our longstanding interest in nuclear topography and structure, my own laboratory has been interested recently in developing methods for the detection of single copy genes, genes present in one set per cell. Our major approach, confocal microscopy, is the high tech approach; I will discuss it first. The two others will be lower tech, more easily applied in the field.

The high tech approach uses a laser scanning confocal microscope to detect fluorescent labeled hybridization probes. The instrument is a highly modified version of a regular epifluorescence microscope, which is standard equipment in most diagnostic laboratories for techniques like immunofluorescence. The microscope is equipped with a suitable laser (in our instrument, an argon ion laser). The laser will fire a beam into a black box, a piece of equipment known as a wobbler laser scanning head, which takes the laser beam and scans it across the specimen on the microscope stage. Scanning times are typically fractions of milliseconds for most specimens. One is looking for a fluorescent signal in the specimen; typically this would be a probe with a fluorescent dye attached to visualize the probe. One can scan a sample very rapidly to detect a fluorescent signal; filtered photomultiplier tubes are used to detect the emitted light. The signal from the detector goes through a computer, which digitizes the signal and visually displays the fluorescence on a video screen.

Aside from the speed of scanning a sample—it can scan a sample for the fluorescent probe much faster than is possible by eye—the advantage of this type of instrumentation is that it can perform direct photon counting, counting individual photonic events of light emitted from the fluorescent probe. This provides quantitative data on the hybridization. The word confocal in the description of this system means that the emitting light and the detector system are at the same focal plane, which provides a method of optically sectioning cells or tissues without having to physically slice them for examination. The equipment allows the operator to optically cut a cell into 100 pieces, look at the fluorescence in each of the 100 pieces, and then reconstruct the whole cell in three dimensional space by computer.

Its initial use, in our own laboratory, has been to map genes. It has been a powerful technique for gene mapping, and has potential application for defining virus integration sites in various latently infected cells. By hybridizing probes with any suitable label, to metaphase chromosome preparations, for example, from human or mouse cells, almost any desired gene can be identified. Biotin is a very useful label. The protein avidin binds tightly to biotin. Thus, probes labeled with biotin can be detected directly by adding avidin that has been tagged with a fluorescent dye and looking for the fluorescence of the bound avidin. The chromosomes are counterstained by the DNA binding dye propidium iodide, which makes the rest of the DNA appear red, in contrast to the yellow or green of the specific fluorescent signal.

One can use this method for any genetic sequence that has been cloned. One does not have to worry about repetitive sequences, which are generally present in probes, or, if one is using viral sequences, about a viral sequence that may cross hybridize to human DNA, because these signals can readily be suppressed by the addition of normal human DNA as a competitor for nonspecific binding. We have used this method to detect several genes, including single copy genes on human chromosomes 11 and 21, and the gene for the mouse T cell marker Thy-1. In each case, not only can you see this particular clone on the chromosome, but you can see the two fluorescent dots on the interphase nuclei indicating the two single copies of these genes, one on each chromosome. They look like worms with glowing eyes.

A major advantage of confocal microscopy is that all of the information is digitized and can be displayed on the video screen. In addition, calculations are possible. With a computer mouse cursor, touching the ends of the chromosomes or the sides of the chromosome on the screen will immediately cause the computer to display numbers for the length and width of the chromosome in micrometers. You can draw a line through a chromosome, passing the cursor through a signal, and the computer will instantly plot on an insert the number of photons at each pixel, or position, along this line. One can directly quantitate the number of photons in each pixel. The computer calculates intensities and gives the map coordinates on the chromosome.

We have been using this to make physical linkage maps of the human genome, using cloned genes obtained from various collaborators. Testing different clones, randomly hybridized, but localized to known chromosomes, we can very easily walk our way down and look at genes that span the entire chromosome. This is good for high resolution mapping. Some of the genes we have mapped this way on chromosome 11 include various oncogenes such as H-*ras* and the *ets*-1 oncogene, and a variety of other specifically known genes, as well as random cloned genes (Lichter et al., 1990).

Although all we have here are banded chromosomes, one could easily identify chromosomes by coupling fluorescent hybridization with various fluorescent banding techniques used in classical cytogenetics, such as chloroquine banding or DAPI banding. One can also do banding by hybridization.

One can score, literally, hundreds of chromosome spreads. The overall hybridization time is 3 to 5 hours, or overnight if one feels lazy. So as many as 20 or 25 samples can be processed overnight, making it possible to screen fairly large populations of cells. We can do about 50 of these a week. In a matter of about 2 months, Peter Lichter, working in my laboratory, has mapped about 250 gene sequences on various human and mouse chromosomes using this optical method.

More recently we have begun to look at some virus integration sites. Marcello Siniscalo, at the Sloan-Kettering Institute, provided us with a variety of human cell lines that have been transformed by adenovirus. Probing with adenovirus 5 (Ad 5) DNA and looking at hybridization of the Ad 5 DNA to chromosomes, we find a signal at the telomeric region of the short (p) arm of chromosome 1, at region 1p3,5. A second preferential site for adenovirus integration into human DNA is at 1p1,3 region.

Classically, chromosome spreads are done on cells in the metaphase stage of the cell cycle. Similarly, we can quantitate viral integration directly in cells during interphase. For example, in an interphase cell that contains adenovirus integrated into the cellular DNA, one can often see two copies (one per chromosome) of the adenovirus integrated into the cell nucleus. Using a different labeling strategy, one can also see some cells that have four copies of adenovirus integrated into the nuclei, showing very early events in viral infection. In similar studies with C127 mouse cells that were transfected with bovine papilloma virus and have become transformed as a result, we can see individual viral genomes in the nucleus of each cell and can quantify as well as analyze the distribution of individual viral genomes.

We have also examined various human cell lines that have been transformed by adeno-associated virus (AAV), a parvovirus. Kenneth Berns' group at Cornell University Medical College had examined integration of AAV into chromosomal DNA by cloning junction regions around the integration site, and found that the flanking sequences were different in each of the half a dozen or more clones that they obtained. That is, the human DNA flanking the AAV integration site had different sequences in each of the transformed human lines. However, taking a larger piece of flanking DNA, in this case about 5 to 8 kilobases, and mapping those larger pieces on human chromosomes by this method, we find that in each case all of the AAV is integrated at a unique site on chromosome 19 (Kotin et al., 1991). So the virus, although it does not have a unique sequence adjacent to its integration site, uniquely integrates in a small region covering a few kilobases on a specific region of chromosome 19. We can see this also by probing with the flanking sequence.

Now this technique is not yet a standard or routine laboratory test. But the idea is to develop a technology that can be used to study, for example, retroviral integration sites. We are in the process of building piezoelectric optical scanners, which are very fast, and which could optically section a cell in a tenth of a second, and with x-y coordinate movers be able to detect a single cell infected with an integrated HIV provirus by scanning 10^5 or 10^6 cells in real time analysis. Although this is too specialized and expensive to be a run of the mill laboratory technique, this technology could be applied to the analysis of very rare events, particularly as more sophisticated computer and optical analysis systems are developed. We would hope eventually to be able to analyze viral genomes in cells in the same way that a laboratory currently uses rapid blood screens for determining white blood cell or platelet counts.

Since this is a fluorescent detection method, one can go trough multiple fluorochromes with different colors to analyze several different things simultaneously in the same sample. We are in the process of scaling up to distinguish eight different fluorescent dyes simultaneously. We have already managed to differentiate four such probes to physically order various genes on human chromosome 11, distinguishing the β-globin gene, which is near the telomere, at the end of the p arm of chromosome 11, and three other randomly selected genes for which we have cloned DNA probes and which we can physically link by these measurement methods (Lichter et al., 1990). By going to multiple fluorochromes, it potentially becomes possible to look at the relationships between viral genes, or expression of viral gene transcripts, or interrelationships between helper viruses and dependent viruses, as with adenovirus and AAV, or many other parameters that govern gene structure and expression.

So much for high tech. However, there are other types of new methodologies for amplifying the signal in a detection assay, and some are more accessible. As one example, I would like to mention another quantitatable methodology based on chemiluminescence, which was published several years ago (Coyle et al., 1986; Matthews et al., 1985). This luminescent method uses Luminol and rate enhancers such as p-phenylphenol to amplify the standard ELISA detection system, which often uses the enzyme horseradish peroxidase, by turning it into a photon emitter. Usually, such enzymes are detected by a color reaction, but, in the presence of these compounds, the horseradish peroxidase reaction causes light to be emitted. The detection sensitivity, at least by luminometry, which counts photons, was a reasonably good comparison with the standard colorimetric or radioactivity measurements of approximately 10^5 or 10^6 molecules. Detection times were also relatively short. Besides ELISA detection, applications for this technology include detection systems for the sorts of studies done by in situ, dot blot, or filter hybridization methods.

For this type of application, one often uses film to detect the signal. We found that the method as published by Matthews was not readily adapted to detection using conventional films in place of a luminometer. While we could get very rapid detection to an acceptable level, about one picogram of target, representing approximately 200,000 molecules, increasing exposure time, even by twentyfold, did not give a signal for a sample that was just half as concentrated. This is due to a film phenomenon called low light intensity reciprocity failure, which prevents any image from forming if photon flux is too low. More recently, commercial suppliers such as DuPont-New England Nuclear have developed other enhancers and films that do not suffer the same degree of reciprocity failure. Without advocating any particular product, the point is that such methods can lower the minimal detectable signal in a hybridization assay to below 0.1 picogram, approximately 10,000 target molecules or less, increasing detection sensitivity between fifty- and one hundredfold. This opens up new applications for sequencing and other molecular biological tools.

A second and more recent approach is a different kind of chemiluminescent emitter, based on dioxetane chemistry, which was originally developed by investigators at Wayne State University (Pollard-Knight et al., 1990), and is now under commercial development by companies called Lumigen and Tropix. Chemically, these emitters are very restricted dioxetane rings, using an adamantyl group to stabilize this four-membered ring. These compounds can be modified to detect directly specific enzymes used in ELISA systems. For detecting alkaline phosphatase, a derivative of adamantyl dioxetane has been synthesized that contains a benzoid ring with a phosphate; the phosphate is removed by the alkaline phosphatase, yielding an unstable hydrolysis product that gives off light in the 480 to 500 nanometer range as it decomposes.

This methodology, like the peroxidase detection system mentioned previously, can give approximately a one hundredfold increase in sensitivity of detection compared with presently used enzyme substrates. Other enzyme substrates based on dioxetane derivatives are being developed. All of these should provide linear detection over six to seven orders of magnitude, and with sensitivity, in standard research assay formats, down to approximately 10,000 molecules.

Another, entirely different kind of signal amplification system is based on Qβ replicase. We have been working with this system for bacterial detection, but it is equally applicable to viral detection and, indeed, viral applications are being developed commercially. Fred Russell Kramer had worked on the RNA replicase enzyme of the bacteriophage Qβ (Kramer and Lizardi, 1989). This remarkable viral RNA polymerase rapidly and faithfully copies the Qβ genomic RNA. However, there are various smaller RNA molecules that are also replicated by the enzyme. One such RNA, 220 nucleotides in length, is called the midi-variant (MDV) Qβ molecule. It has a high degree of secondary structure because portions of the 3' and 5' ends of the molecule are base paired to each other. More important for us, it contains two sequences, which are the only two signals that are required for recognition of an RNA by Qβ replicase. Qβ replicase will replicate this molecule or Qβ RNA, but no RNA molecule lacking these recognition sequences. The doubling time of this RNA by Qβ replicase is 13 seconds. So one can exponentially amplify this molecule very quickly by incubation with Qβ replicase. In work by Leslie Orgel, seeding a reaction with 1,000 molecules (10^{-20} moles) of RNA recognized by the replicase, the enzyme can build up to 200 nanograms within 30 minutes, an astounding amplification of well over a billionfold.

The original Qβ enzymes that were used in Orgel's and Kramer's studies were contaminated with a trace amount of midi-variant RNA. This trace contamination caused background that limited the detectability because, over time, the trace RNA was amplified so much it began to show. This endogenous background has now been eliminated by using a pure cloned Qβ replicase. The corresponding DNA sequence for the Qβ MDV RNA has been cloned, again in Kramer's laboratory, in appropriate vectors, and with various linkers to allow attaching specific DNA probe sequences to this clone of the midi-variant RNA (Kramer and Lizardi, 1989; Lizardi et al., 1988). Qβ replicase will recognize these chimeric molecules and make copies of them. Different probes that have been inserted include one for *Plasmodium falciparum*, the cause of falciparum malaria, and viral probes for HIV and cytomegalovirus. We have also used probes for the bacteria *Hemophilus influenzae* and *Neisseria meningitidis*.

A company called Gene-Trak Systems is developing this technology commercially, with probes for HIV and cytomegalovirus. To take advantage of this particular amplification system, we have combined different approaches. Basically, after hybridizing the target DNA or RNA and the probe, there are various hybridization and washing steps to cleanly separate the input DNA or RNA from the probe; after this, the remaining probe, with the Qβ signal attached, is then amplified by the enzyme. The amplified RNA can readily be detected colorimetrically or fluorometrically, quantitatively if desired. Using this approach, we have been able to detect between 50 and 100 *Hemophilus influenzae* per ml of cerebrospinal fluid in real life experiments.

This is a signal amplification method, rather than a target amplification (PCR is an example of a target amplification system). Because it is a signal amplification method, it is subject to background, and various background reduction methods, involving cycles of hybridization, washing, and separation steps, are necessary to keep background low. However, this method also is applicable to standard immunoassays, such as an indirect immunoassay using a biotinylated second antibody. One can then incubate with avidin-Qβ RNA to bind the biotinylated antibody, add the replicase nucleotides, and achieve amplification that reflects the binding of the secondary antibody.

There are therefore a variety of ways, of which these are a

sample, whereby one can use light emission or amplifiable molecules to increase the detectability of viral or bacterial pathogens in diagnostic applications. With further refinements such methods are useful to many broader applications, including the sensitive and rapid detection of new and emerging viruses.

REFERENCES

Coyle, P.M., G.H.G. Thorpe, L.J. Kricka, and T.P. Whitehead (1986). Enhanced luminescent quantitation of horseradish-peroxidase conjugates. Application in an enzyme-immunoassay for digoxin. Ann. Clin. Biochem. **23**:42-46.

Kotin, R.M., J.C. Menninger, D.C. Ward, and K.I. Berns (1991). Mapping and direct visualization of a region-specific viral DNA integration site on chromosome 19q13-qter. Genomics **10**:831-834.

Kramer, F.R., and P.M. Lizardi (1989). Replicatable RNA reporters. Nature **339**:401-402.

Lichter, P., C.-j. Chang Tang, K. Call, G. Hermanson, G.A. Evans, D. Housman, and D.C. Ward (1990). High-resolution mapping of human chromosome 11 by in situ hybridization with cosmid clones. Science **214**:64-69.

Lizardi, P.M., C.E. Guerra, H. Lomeli, I. Tussie-Luna, and F.R. Kramer (1988). Exponential amplification of recombinant-RNA hybridization probes. Bio/Technology **6**:1197-1202.

Lomeli, H., S. Tyagi, C.G. Pritchard, P.M. Lizardi, and F.R. Kramer (1989). Quantitative assays based on the use of replicatable hybridization probes. Clin. Chem. **35**:1826-1831.

Matthews, J.A., A. Batki, C. Hynds, and L.J. Kricka (1985). Enhanced chemiluminescent method for the detection of DNA dot-hybridization assays. Anal. Biochem. **151**:205-209.

Pollard-Knight, D., A.C. Simmonds, A.P. Schaap, H. Akhavan, and M.A.W. Brady (1990). Nonradioactive DNA detection on Southern blots by enzymatically triggered chemiluminescence. Anal. Biochem. **185**:353-358.

11

Assessing Geographic and Transport Factors, and Recognition of New Viruses

ROBERT E. SHOPE AND ALFRED S. EVANS

Twenty-three years ago one of us wrote a paper called "The instant-distant infections" (Evans, 1966). It was concerned with many of the same issues we are considering here—namely the geographic emergence of new or unusual organisms, usually in some distant area, and new instant transport, often via modern jets, to susceptible persons in our country.

We shall discuss the assessment of geographic and transport factors at five levels involved in the emergence of viruses and subsequent host-virus interactions. These are shown in Table 11.1. The first level is the evolution of the virus in nature. In the second level, the agent has evolved, but effective human contact has not yet occurred. Usually we do not know about the agent at this point, with some exceptions. The third level is the effective exposure, leading to human infection and resulting in a new disease. This is termed "new disease; new agent." A fourth level, which we are not sure exactly fits in this sequence, involves viruses that are previously latent, or nonpathogenic agents that produce disease in compromised hosts. This has been termed "old agent" disease. Finally, we shall discuss more extensively the known viruses in search of diseases or known diseases in search of viruses, or the "accidental tourist," that is, unknown viruses in search of unknown diseases.

Agents evolve in geographic and ecologic isolation and then they are transported to human communities when humans enter the habitat of the virus, or by vertebrate or arthropod vectors that move into the human community. One of the concepts we need to keep in mind is that viruses evolving in indigenous hosts often cause an inapparent infection. There are some exceptions to this, but it is a good general rule. When the viruses are transported to the new ecosystem, or to the new geographic area, or to the new host, they often then appear as new diseases. The corollary is obvious, that in order for these diseases to appear, we need receptive soil; we need to have the appropriate transport mechanism and an appropriate portal of entry into susceptible hosts, to receive the virus.

In 1969 we were stimulated by some electron micrographs of F.A. Murphy to recognition of a set of viruses that caused severe encephalitic disease in Africa. One of the set was Mokola virus (Shope et al., 1970) associated with fatal human encephalitis in Ibadan, Nigeria (Familusi et al., 1972) and first isolated in a virus search program of the Rockefeller Foundation and the Nigerian Government. Later, Mokola virus was again associated with encephalitis in cats and a dog in Zimbabwe (Foggin, 1982). Another of the set was Duvenhage virus from the brain of a farmer in South Africa bitten on the lip by a bat (Meredith et al., 1971). Murphy's pictures said these were rabies virus, but our serologic evidence told us otherwise. These were viruses that had evolved with rabies virus in Africa in shrews and bats respectively; they were related to rabies, but different enough to emerge as new agents.

We were concerned that these agents might appear as pathogens outside of Africa. Our concern was reinforced in 1981 with the report of a Duvenhage-like virus in bats in Europe (Schneider and Meyer, 1981), and the death in 1985 of a Finnish bat researcher after being bitten by a bat. The Duvenhage-like virus was isolated postmortem. This may be an example of a virus that evolved in Africa and was transported to Europe, perhaps by bats on boats from Africa. The transportation may have been recent or in the more distant past.

We want to emphasize that the recognition of the cause of death in the Finnish bat researcher depended on prior studies in Africa. The ability to make rapid identification was a direct result of the foresight of programs such as those of the Rockefeller Foundation in collaboration with foreign governments in establishing virus search projects in tropical Africa, and an indirect result of the reference

Table 11.1
Levels of Virus Emergence and Interaction Between Host and Virus*

Level 1:	The virus evolves in a natural ecosystem
Level 2:	The virus has evolved; contact between virus and human has not effectively been accomplished
Level 3:	The virus contacts the host, causes infection resulting in disease (new virus, new disease)
Level 4:	A virus that was previously latent or nonpathogenic causes disease in compromised host (old virus, new disease)
Level 5:	The known virus is in search of disease; or the known disease is in search of a virus; or the unknown virus is in search of the unknown disease (accidental tourist)

*Modified from Evans, 1990.

Table 11.2   Concepts of Virus Geographic and Transport Factors*

1. Viruses evolve in isolated ecosystems and focal geographic areas, and are transported by arthropods, and wild and domestic animals to human communities, or humans travel to the isolated ecosystems

2. Viruses evolving in indigenous hosts usually cause inapparent infection

3. When viruses enter new ecosystems, new geographic areas, or new hosts, they often cause newly recognized diseases

4. Receptive soil (nonimmune host) and appropriate transport are needed for viruses to emerge

5. Virus diseases are often missed because of the umbrella of malaria

6. New viruses should be sought in old diseases

*Modified from Evans, 1990.

functions at the Centers for Disease Control and universities supported by the National Institutes of Allergy and Infectious Diseases, the Department of Defense, and the World Health Organization.

Once a new virus has emerged, a number of factors are involved in its transport and subsequent host interactions. Some of these principles are shown in Table 11.2. Their transport to local susceptibles in urban areas can be by several routes to which we shall return later.

Viruses that cause only inapparent infection in their indigenous host may result in new diseases in a new host from which epidemics can start. There are three ingredients needed: a new agent, a group of susceptibles, and effective transport. As W.G. Downs has so well emphasized (Downs, 1975) in his paper "Malaria: the great umbrella", the presence of the malaria parasite in a febrile patient does not always indicate a causal relationship. Some other virus or microbe may be the true cause of the fever. "Challenge the diagnosis," he says, and in his days in Trinidad this philosophy and vigorous laboratory studies led to the identification of several agents new to that area such as Oropouche virus, dengue and yellow fever. Similarly in Africa, French workers at the Institut Pasteur and others have recognized Tataguine, Ilesha, Zika, and even Lassa fever viruses from febrile patients, the viruses often hiding under the umbrella of malaria, since all patients also had malarial parasitemia.

Table 11.3 summarizes factors involved in the transport of emerging or new viruses to susceptible hosts. Tourist travel, and exploration into the air, soil, and ocean involve possible exposure to new infectious agents. Secondly, the great human migration from rural and remote areas into larger communities and urban settings brings with it new infectious agents that can then spread into susceptible human populations. Similarly, wild mammal, bird, or insect spread to more crowded areas results in the introduction of new agents.

Some human change in a local setting such as a new dam, water storage containers, or the collections of old tires can provide the means of amplifying the growth of an arthropod vector. The increasing use of animals or animal organs in the laboratory can introduce a new agent into susceptible laboratory personnel as occurred with Marburg virus infection (Martini and Siegert, 1971); the use of donor organs such as dura mater or corneas can lead to Creutzfeldt-Jakob disease or rabies in recipients of these donor tissues. As the demand for such donor organs increases, the "organ hunter" may venture into remote sources where nondetectable agents, such as non-A-non-B hepatitis, slow viruses, and new retroviruses may lurk. Finally, new routes or portals of entry of infection, either by invasive procedures or by behavioral changes may lead to new clinical syndromes.

Some recent examples of new or recrudescent viral diseases and possible reasons for their emergence are listed in Table 11.4. The human immunodeficiency virus and its devastating clinical result, AIDS, is the most striking example and probably a major motivation for this conference. While the origin of HIV is not clear, a zoonotic origin, migration from rural to urban areas, prostitution, and return of infected travelers to more developed areas such as the United States is a possible scenario. Here, from its presumed beginning in Africa, the spread of the virus was enormously enhanced by homosexual and intravenous drug activities in settings that involved multiple partners. Spread by venereal means and by dirty needles created rapid vectoring of the virus through new portals of entry. These factors, plus an incubation period of some 11 years to clinical disease resulted in wide seeding of the infection before it, and its methods of transmission were recognized. The behavioral patterns of its unfortunate victims and a political environment in which

Table 11.3   Some Contact Factors Favoring Emergence of Viruses*

Factor	Examples
1. Exploration	Tropics, ocean depths, space, archeological diggings
2. Human travel	Migration from rural settings to cities
3. Animal movements	Transport to new ecological situations; contact with new susceptibles
4. Transport of arthropods	Flight, by wind, by birds or airplanes, on people or domestic animals, in food, as eggs in tires
5. Organ movement	Organs for human transplant or for tissue culture
6. New entry portals	New or old viruses enter by new route of inoculation because of alterations in human behavior or invasive medical procedures

*Modified from Evans, 1990.

Table 11.4

Examples of New, Transported, or Recrudescent Virus Diseases*

Disease	Area (Year)	Risk Factors
AIDS	USA (1981 on)	Introduction of HIV-1; homosexual and IV spread
Argentine hemorrhagic fever	Argentina (1958)	Rodent exposure, corn harvest
Bolivian hemorrhagic fever	Bolivia (1959)	Rodent exposure in houses
Ebola hemorrhagic fever	Zaire and Sudan (1976)	Patient contact; needle spread
Epidemic polyarthritis and rash (Ross River disease)	Pacific Islands (1979)	Introduction of viremic human; exposure to mosquitoes
Lassa fever	Nigeria (1969)	Hospital exposure
	Liberia, Sierra Leone (1970 on)	Rodent exposure
Marburg disease	Germany, Yugoslavia (1967)	Monkeys imported from Africa; exposure to monkey organs
	South Africa (1975)	Exposure to index case
Rift Valley fever	Egypt (1977)	Unexplained spread from Sudan (wind, imported camels, sheep?); exposure to mosquitoes, contact with sheep and cattle blood
	Mauritania (1987)	Opening of dam; mosquito exposure
Yellow fever	Nigeria (1986 on)	Introduced from sylvan source; spread by viremic travelers; mosquito exposure

*Modified from Evans, 1990.

prompter action for its recognition and control were not taken were certainly factors enhancing the spread of the epidemic.

The other examples shown in Table 11.4 represent much more local outbreaks such as Argentine and Bolivian hemorrhagic fevers, in which exposure to infected rodents in the fields or the homes was a critical factor in their emergence. Ebola fever spread via contact with infected patients and use of unsterilized needles.

Epidemic polyarthritis and rash, a mosquito-borne illness more recently called Ross River disease, was known in Australia for decades; in 1979 it spread like wildfire through the Pacific Islands

Both exposure to hospital patients and to rodents were involved in Lassa fever outbreaks. Marburg disease has already been mentioned and emphasizes the cautions that must be observed in a vaccine production facility and in the laboratory. The appearance of Rift Valley fever in Egypt in 1977, presumably transported from the Sudan, seems due to a number of possible factors originating in a local Sudanese outbreak, and carried either by wind (Sellers et al., 1982), mosquitoes, or infected sheep or camels to the north. Ten years later, another epidemic of Rift Valley fever presented in Mauritania. This time, the Diama Dam was opened at the mouth of the Senegal River in an area where the virus was present, but the disease was not encountered often enough to be recognized. The completion of the dam created conditions for mosquito propagation that probably accounted for the epidemic.

Yellow fever during the past several years has occurred in Nigeria and probably represents the biggest epidemic in recent history, with case fatality rates over 50%. The population at risk is over 20 million in the epidemic area. About two million of these have been vaccinated, but presumably either not enough vaccine was available, there was a break in the cold chain, or the logistics did not permit reaching a larger population.

Sometimes we are fooled into thinking a virus has been introduced into a new area, only to find an indigenous virus is causing a newly recognized disease. This happened recently when we were called upon by the Animal and Plant Health Inspection Service (APHIS) of the U.S. Department of Agriculture to help investigate outbreaks suspected of being foreign animal diseases. In January 1987, we were notified (G. Combs and W. Garnett, personal communication) that there was a massive epizootic in sheep in Texas and Nebraska. The disease was arthrogryposis and hydranencephaly (AGH) in which the lambs are born dead and/or malformed.

In other parts of the world this condition is known to be caused by Akabane virus, a virus originally isolated from mosquitoes by A. Oya in Japan 30 years ago (Oya et al., 1961), and identified in our laboratory as a Simbu group virus in the family Bunyaviridae. It was a virus in search of a disease for a decade until it was shown to cause AGH in Japan, Australia and Israel. The virus infects the ewe during the fifth week of gestation, passes the placenta and damages the embryonic tissue. Infection at any other period of gestation does not cause disease.

The APHIS scientists suspected that Akabane had been introduced to Texas by sheep imported from Australia or New Zealand, and that it had then spread to Nebraska. The USDA had placed the affected areas in quarantine.

We received sheep sera from Texas and Nebraska and, with R. Yedloutschnig of APHIS at Plum Island, tested for Akabane and the other Simbu group viruses in the United States, Buttonwillow and Mermet. These tests were negative, but we also tested for Cache Valley virus, a virus in the same family as Akabane, and which was known to cause fever (but not known to cause AGH) in sheep and cattle in Texas.

By now you have guessed the result. The ewes giving birth to AGH lambs were positive to the Cache Valley antigen. This finding led to an extensive investigation of the relationship of Cache Valley virus to the outbreak (Chung et al., 1990). We now know that the entire outbreak in both Texas and Nebraska was associated with Cache Valley infection, not the exotic pathogen, Akabane. The USDA was able to lift the quarantine because Cache Valley virus is an indigenous agent distributed from Canada to Mexico.

This was the first recorded widespread AGH epizootic in the United States as far as we know, although sporadic AGH attributed to toxic plants or to bluetongue virus infection has been recorded frequently. The Cache Valley virus is neither new, nor transported.

What happened in 1987 to cause the outbreak? The virus is present every year in mosquitoes. The rains were heavy in 1986 and the mosquito population was abundant. The sheep were probably mostly nonimmune. The high prevalence of mosquitoes coincided with the fifth week of gestation (August or September 1986) and Cache Valley virus infection of large numbers of ewes at just the right time led to disease the following January.

Not only are new viruses or new diseases emerging, but also the tools are emerging to recognize them. Candidate diseases are shown in Table 11.5. Of the acute diseases, we think that Kawasaki disease presents the most interesting challenge (Kawasaki et al., 1974). Some aspects of this syndrome, such as the immune response, suggest a retroviral etiology; others such as the leukocytosis and peeling rash suggest a bacterium or toxin; while the coronary artery aneu-

Table 11.5   Diseases and Syndromes Seeking a Virus Etiology

Disease	Possible Candidate Virus
Alzheimer's disease	? Slow virus
Insulin dependent diabetes	? Coxsackie B7
Kawasaki disease	? New retrovirus
Multiple sclerosis	?? HTLV-I
Rheumatoid arthritis	? EBV
Sarcoidosis	?
Systemic lupus erythematosus	?

Table 11.6   Early Detection of New Viruses and New Diseases*

- Establish sentinel surveillance and serological units in high risk areas for emerging viruses (these units should be supported, if possible, by a high level laboratory, or at least a rapid transport system to one); monitor and collect blood samples and secretions from febrile illnesses

- Prepare a mobile team and laboratory under the Centers for Disease Control or the World Health Organization, staffed by highly trained microbiologists, epidemiologists, entomologists, and other scientists, prepared to leave on a moment's notice to investigate an outbreak of disease anywhere in the world

- Set up a "red alert"reporting system for hospitals, especially in high risk areas, to report unusual cases or epidemics

---

*Modified from Evans, 1990.

rysms found in some 15-20% of the cases resemble an autoimmune phenomenon. Among central nervous syndromes, multiple sclerosis and Alzheimer's disease remain major etiological challenges. But virologists in search of the agents, beware! The pathway in the past has been strewn with false leads and disappointed hopes.

Let us give two examples from the research of one of us (ASE) of how seroepidemiological studies led to new observations. In the first, a health survey of 1,000 persons in Bridgetown, Barbados was carried out in 1972. The sera were stored until 1986, when HTLV-I tests became available. Testing in conjunction with the National Cancer Institute revealed that 4.2% of the population had already been infected with HTLV-I (Reidel et al., 1989), 8 years prior to the discovery of the virus. VDRL reactions had been determined in 1972; comparison of HTLV-I reactivity with the previously done VDRL showed an association, and suggested sexual transmission of HTLV-I virus.

In the second example, a serological survey had been done on 637 persons with varying degrees of exposure to zoonotic agents (Thompson and Evans, 1965). One of the antigens that was included in the Wisconsin survey was California encephalitis virus. In 1943, W.McD. Hammon and W.C. Reeves had discovered the virus in mosquitoes of California and associated it with three cases of encephalitis in children (Hammon and Reeves, 1952). Since then, no further human cases had been found in California or elsewhere.

Antibody to California encephalitis virus was found in 26% of the Wisconsin sera. There was an unusually high prevalence in sera of young men working in forestry camps, and in persons who recovered from CNS infections.

A 4-year-old girl had died of encephalitis in a LaCrosse hospital. An initial attempt to isolate a virus from her brain failed. The following year, now with the knowledge of the association of California encephalitis antibody with CNS disease, Thompson and his colleagues tried again to isolate the virus. This time they succeeded. Isolation of the LaCrosse virus led to development of a diagnostic test, and subsequently to recognition of the importance of LaCrosse encephalitis as perhaps the most common endemic arboviral CNS disease in the United States. This example shows how results of a serological survey can lead to the discovery of a "new" disease (although the disease is not really new, only newly recognized).

Finally, some of the approaches to the surveillance of new viruses and virus/host interactions are shown in Table 11.6. The recognition and reporting of unique febrile diseases and of disease outbreaks is a crucial first step. From a laboratory standpoint the continual investigations of disease in sentinel individuals and in high risk populations in sentinel geographic areas is important. The establishment of an ongoing virological investigation of all febrile disease in a few selected areas of Africa, Latin America, and Asia, preferably through a sophisticated on-site laboratory, is highly desirable. This might be a study of febrile disease in a well-equipped, mobile laboratory. The resources of such a laboratory should be available at all times for the Centers for Disease Control and/or the World Health Organization and laboratories of other nations to investigate outbreaks of infectious disease wherever they occur. The field sites should be staffed with virologists, bacteriologists, parasitologists, epidemiologists, entomologists, and a veterinarian who is a specialist in infectious disease. A red alert reporting system should be established for health centers in high risk areas, where unusual epidemics or individual cases would be reported.

In the United States a cadre of well-trained infectious and tropical disease physicians is needed to recognize and study severe febrile diseases occurring in travelers returning from high risk areas. This need has been documented by a recent study (Institute of Medicine, 1987). The recent death from Lassa fever in a U.S. citizen returning from Nigeria highlights this need (Holmes et al., 1990). The routine serologic monitoring of groups such as missionaries, the Peace Corps, and the military prior to and after assignment to remote areas may reveal emerging new viruses and diseases.

In overseas settings the United States already has the tools available for the surveillance and identification of new viruses and new diseases, but we have lost some of our valuable overseas laboratories. The U.S. Public Health Service closed the NIH Middle America Research Unit in Panama followed by closing the NIH Pacific Research Unit in Hawaii. The U.S. Army has closed its field facility in Malaysia. After debate, Congress failed to include funds for the Gorgas Memorial Laboratory in Panama in its 1992 budget. This historic listening post for virus diseases now appears doomed. What is required are continuing virus studies in tropical and subtropical areas. These in the past have usually been justified on the basis that they were contributing knowledge on known problem diseases, but future investigators should be indulged, and better yet, encouraged to survey for baseline virus spectra and investigate new syndromes that might be viral. We must know what diseases and pathogens are there. Our national policy for two decades for at least one disease, yellow fever, has been surveillance in the United States to recognize the first imported case (Sencer, 1969). We need to rethink our policy. If we wait for the diseases to come to our own shores, that will be too little and too late.

REFERENCES

Chung, S.I., C.W. Livingston Jr., J.F. Edwards, R.W. Crandell, R.E. Shope, S.A. Shelton, and E.W. Colisson (1990). Evidence that Cache Valley virus induces congenital malformations in sheep. Vet. Microbiol. **21**:297-307.

Downs, W.G. (1975). Malaria: the great umbrella. Bull. N.Y. Acad. Med. **51**:984-990.

Evans, A.S. (1966). The instant-distant infections. J. Am. Med. Womans Assoc. **21**:210-216.

Evans, A.S. (1990). Challenges to the epidemiology of infectious diseases in the next decade. In *Advances in Brucellosis Research* (L.J. Adams, ed.), Chap. 21 (pp. 321-337). College Station, Tex.: Texas A & M University Press.

Familusi, J.B., B.O. Osunkoya, D.L. Moore, G.E. Kemp, and A. Fabiyi (1972). A fatal human infection with Mokola virus. Am. J. Trop. Med. Hyg. **21**:959-963.

Foggin, C.M. (1982). Atypical rabies virus in cats and a dog in Zimbabwe. Vet. Rec. **110**:338.

Hammon, W.McD., and W.C. Reeves (1952). California encephalitis virus, a newly described agent. I. Evidence of natural infection in man and other animals. Calif. Med. **77**:303-309.

Holmes, G.P., J.B. McCormick, S.C. Trock, R.A. Chase, S.M. Lewis, C.A. Mason, P.A. Hall, P.A., L.S. Brammer, G.I. Perez-Ordonoz, M.K. McDonnell, J.P. Paulissen, L.B. Schonberger, and S.P. Fisher-Hoch (1990). Lassa fever in the United States. N. Engl. J. Med. **323**:1120-1123.

Institute of Medicine (1987). *The U.S. Capacity to Address Tropical Infectious Disease Problems*. Washington, D.C.: National Academy Press.

Kawasaki, T., F. Kosaki, S. Okawa, I. Shigematsu, and H. Yanagawa (1974). A new infantile acute febrile mucocutaneous lymph node syndrome (MLNS) prevailing in Japan. Pediatrics **54**:271-276.

Martini, G.A., and R. Siegert (eds.) (1971). *Marburg Virus Disease*. New York and Berlin: Springer-Verlag.

Meredith, C.D., A.P. Rossouw, and H. Van P. Fraag Koch (1971). An unusual case of human rabies thought to be of chiropteran origin. S. Afr. Med. J. **45**:767-769.

Oya, A., T. Okumo, T. Ogata, I. Kobayashi, and T. Matsuyama (1961). Akabane, a new arbovirus isolated in Japan. Jpn. J. Med. Sci. Biol. **14**:101-108.

Reidel, D.A., A.S. Evans, C. Saxinger, and W.A. Blattner (1989). A historical study of human T lymphotropic virus type 1 transmission in Barbados. J. Infect. Dis. **159**:603-609.

Schneider, L.G., and S. Meyer (1981). Antigenic determinants of rabies virus as demonstrated by monoclonal antibody. In *The Replication of Negative Strand Viruses* (D.H.L. Bishop and R.W. Compans, eds.), pp. 947-953. New York: Elsevier/North Holland.

Sellers, R.F., D.E. Pedgley, and M.R. Tucker (1982). Rift Valley fever, Egypt 1977: Disease spread by windborne insect vectors? Vet. Rec. **110**:73-77.

Sencer, D.J. (1969). Health protection in a shrinking world. Am. J. Trop. Med. Hyg. **18**:341-343.

Shope, R.E., F.A. Murphy, A.K. Harrison, O.R. Causey, G.E. Kemp, D.I.H. Simpson, and D.L. Moore (1970). Two African viruses serologically and morphologically related to rabies virus. J. Virol. **6**:690-692.

Thompson, W.H., and A.S. Evans (1965). California encephalitis virus studies in Wisconsin. Am. J. Epidemiol. **81**:230-244.

12

Phylogenetic Moments in the AIDS Epidemic

GERALD MYERS, KERSTI MacINNES, AND LYNDA MYERS

INTRODUCTION

By 1983, several laboratories had identified and isolated the etiologic agent of AIDS, the retrovirus now denoted HIV, and by 1985
nucleotide sequences derived from those early isolates were reported. This molecular information was available in time to address
a flurry of speculations and allegations concerning the sudden emergence of the AIDS virus. In 1986, two avirulent strains of herpes
simplex virus were discovered to have generated a lethal recombinant in vitro (Javier et al., 1986), and this quickly touched off
speculation that the AIDS virus may have been similarly generated
in nature or in a testtube. Such speculations contributed to a worldwide climate of anxiety and created a potential for dissemination of
false and misleading information. In light of this, we at the HIV
Sequence Database and Analysis Project (an NIH-funded project at
the Los Alamos National Laboratory), recognized the immediate need for
an investigation of the molecular facts pertinent to the origin of AIDS.

Of the many ways to inquire into the evolutionary origins of an
organism or pathogen, a comparative study of genetic sequences is
the most incisive, since the sequences constituting the genome are
unique for each species and, in some cases, for each individual in a
species. The HIV genome, which consists of a single molecule, is
approximately 9,700 nucleotides in length, a length more than adequate for precise identification of the virus. Thus in 1985, we set out
to classify the newly determined nucleotide sequences of HIV by
performing a computer search of all known genetic sequences that
were stored in international databases. The sequences of HTLV-III
and LAV, as they were called then, were compared to approximately
six million bases of mammalian, plant, and viral sequences with the
result that no similarity could be found. The search for close relatives
was repeated again in 1986 when there were nine million bases in

120

libraries and again in 1988 when there were over fifteen million bases. This inquiry has shown that if HIV arose in recent time as a recombinant of two or more viruses, naturally or through human agency, it came from viruses that have not been characterized, that is from genetic sequences that are not in the international databases. A growing body of circumstantial evidence—outlined below—argues that HIV has not arisen in recent decades as a recombinant of any viruses, known or unknown.

An equally provocative early speculation about the origin of AIDS was that it arose from a monkey virus that had recently crossed species lines. Unfortunately, this possibility was brought forward more than once in terms that were unnecessarily offensive to Africans, on the one hand, and not helpful to AIDS researchers on the other hand. In what follows we will present what we believe to be a more informed hypothesis positing a simian origin of AIDS. Arguments for this hypothesis will entail tracking HIV and SIV (simian immunodeficiency viruses) nucleotide sequences into the past, but before we turn to that project, we will mention some features of the onset of the AIDS pandemic which are of central importance for any discussion of the origin of AIDS.

EPIDEMIOLOGICAL SNAPSHOTS

Early seroepidemiological and clinical data reveal two especially perplexing features of the onset of the AIDS pandemic:

First, all available evidence suggests that AIDS appeared suddenly and concurrently in the United States and Africa, the two major centers of the pandemic. AIDS was first recognized in the United States in the spring of 1981. The retrospective examination of sera collected in the late 1970s in association with hepatitis B studies in San Francisco, Los Angeles, and New York City, suggests that for the most part HIV-1 entered the U.S. population sometime in the mid-1970s (Jaffe et al., 1985; Stephens et al., 1986). Thus, for example, stored sera of nearly one thousand Los Angeles patients having either acute or chronic hepatitis were examined for HIV antibodies and the earliest sample in which antibodies were detected was from 1979 (DeCock et al., 1987). Although there is the intriguing report of a young man from St. Louis who presented AIDS-like symptoms in 1968, and whose tissues, stored upon death in 1969, have tested positive for antibodies, confirmation of HIV infection by PCR analysis and sequencing has not been possible up to now. A review of serosurveys associated with dengue fever in the Caribbean likewise found that the earliest evidence of HIV in Haiti comes from 1979 samples (Pape et al., 1987).

A similar and virtually concurrent epidemiological record is found in the other large center of the pandemic, Africa. While the seroepidemidemiologic and clinical data are limited, the available facts, summarized in Figure 12.1, also point to a relatively recent eruption of AIDS there (Piot et al., 1988).

In Africa, just as in St. Louis, there is evidence of an exceptionally early case of AIDS: a 1959 seropositive sample from Kinshasa that was, unfortunately, never tested for virus (Nahmias et al., 1986). However, sera sampled in 1970 that were taken from 805 healthy women in the same city revealed only two positives, while the 1980 sampling of a smaller group revealed fifteen (Desmyter et al., 1986). Sera from 659 persons examined in connection with a 1976 outbreak of Ebola fever in rural Zaire produced five HIV positives. Of these, the one confirmed positive (it is well known that false positives increase with time of storage of serum samples) was known to have recently lived in Kinshasa where she may have worked as a prostitute (Getchell et al., 1987). The HIV-1 virus isolated from that stored 1976 sample is the oldest molecular specimen that we have (Srinivasan et al., 1989).

From nearby Congo, sera of 340 pygmies were collected between 1975 and 1978. These people are in direct contact with monkeys, which they hunt and eat. None of the sera from these pygmies has been confirmed HIV positive (Rouzioux et al., 1986). And in South Africa, 3,500 samples were taken from the black miner population between 1970 and 1974 as part of a pneumococcal vaccine study. At most, two of these (both unconfirmed) were HIV positive. Yet by 1986, nearly four percent of the subpopulation of miners from Malawi were found to be positive (Sher et al., 1987). In urban Somalia to the north, there is no evidence of HIV prior to 1983 (Titti et al., 1986). And an extensive study of prostitutes and patients at STD clinics in Nairobi revealed low prevalence of HIV positives in 1980 that rose to 60% in some groups by 1985 (Piot et al., 1986). By 1991, the World Health Organization estimated that six million adults were HIV infected in Africa, with some countries showing seroprevalence rates of greater than 10% (Palca, 1991).

These serological studies all point to a sudden recent spread of HIV by travelers and prostitutes in central Africa that was undoubtedly facilitated by the road running from outside Kinshasa, Zaire to Mombasa, Kenya (Fig. 12.1; Conner and Kingman, 1988). Thus, AIDS appeared suddenly and concurrently in the United States and Africa, the two major centers of the pandemic.

The second feature of the AIDS epidemic that is especially intriguing is the fact that two major foci of AIDS are manifest in Africa: HIV-1 disease in central and southern Africa and HIV-2 disease in West Africa. Although there is a paucity of retrospective data pertaining to HIV-2 that would show how closely the onset of the HIV-2 epidemic coincided in time with that of HIV-1, available evidence suggests that the temporal onset of the two epidemics may

AFRICA

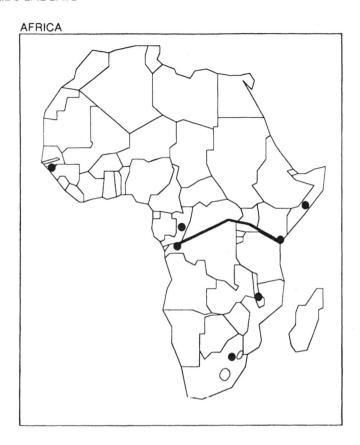

Figure 12.1 A computer-generated map of Africa showing sites for which retrospective serosurvey data, discussed in the text, are available. The main highway connecting Kinshasa, Zaire (in the west) to Mombasa, Kenya (in the east) is shown as pointed out by Conner and Kingman (1988).

have been separated by years but hardly by several decades. Through review of serological samples from an investigation of Lassa fever in Guinea Bissau, Fultz and coworkers concluded that the seroprevalence of HIV-2 in West Africa, which was 6% in 1986, could have been no higher than 1% in 1980 (Fultz et al., 1987). There was no evidence of HIV-1 in West Africa until recently when a case of dual HIV-1/HIV-2 infection was reported from Ivory Coast (Rayfield et al., 1988). Without evidence to the contrary, we may assume for the sake of inquiry that AIDS has been a "twofold epidemic," that HIV-1 disease and HIV-2 disease came forward at about the same time.

This brief epidemiological snapshot of the early years of the AIDS pandemic leaves us with two major questions: (1) What is implied by the suddenness and virtual simultaneity of onset of the epidemics in the United States and in Africa? (2) Under what presumption can the twofold (HIV-1 and HIV-2) epidemic in Africa be understood? We will turn to these questions now.

EVIDENCE FOR THE SIMIAN ORIGIN OF AIDS

In a succinct review entitled "The simian-human connection",
Doolittle (1989) has summarized two recently popular hypotheses
concerning the origin of HIV. The first is that HIV-2 (the second type
of human AIDS-causing virus discussed above) derives from the
mangabey virus. In support of this hypothesis is the fact that the
nucleotide sequence of the mangabey virus proves to be closely
homologous with HIV-2 sequences (Hirsch et al., 1989; Marx et al.,
1991), and the fact that the natural habitat of the mangabey overlaps
West Africa, the region of the HIV-2 epidemic (Hirsch et al., 1989;
Marx et al., 1991; Johnson et al., 1991). The second currently popular
hypothesis presented by Doolittle, which we shall see is less likely,
is that the other type of human AIDS-causing virus, HIV-1, recently
arose from viruses expected to be found in an extensive population
of SIV-positive green monkeys inhabiting sub-Saharan Africa
(Hendry et al., 1986; Kanki et al., 1985; Johnson et al., 1991). How
plausible are these hypotheses taken together? They require at least
two distinct accidents of cross-species transmission over apparently
the same time period.

Duesberg's challenge to the conclusion that HIV is the cause of
AIDS raises precisely this problem: "It is highly improbable that
within the last few years two viruses that are only 40% sequence-
related would have arisen that could both cause the newly defined
syndrome AIDS. ... [S]ince viruses, like cells, are the products of
gradual evolution, the proposition that within a very short evolutionary time, two different viruses capable of causing AIDS would
have evolved or crossed over from another species is highly improbable" (Duesberg, 1989).

While Duesberg's conclusion that HIV is not the cause of AIDS
seems unwarranted for many reasons that we will not explore here,
the logical improbability that he mentions must be faced. In order to
do this, we shall make use of phylogenetic trees constructed from
homologous gene sequences with the help of a computer. Figure
12.2 presents an example of a phylogenetic tree that has been built
from representative *gag* gene sequences of the now known five types
of primate immunodeficiency viruses, namely HIV-1 and the related
SIV from a chimpanzee (IV); HIV-2 and its close relatives SIV-
macaque and SIV-mangabey (I); SIV_{AGM} (African green monkey)
(III); SIV_{mnd} (mandrill) (V); and SIV-Sykes (II). Only a few representatives of the first three types are shown for sake of simplicity. Some
very interesting SIV_{AGM} sequences from West African green monkeys, as well as some HIV-2 sequences from rural Liberia, cannot be
included because they have been sequenced over only a small portion of the *pol* gene (Allan et al., 1991; Hahn, 1990). Their relevance
to this inquiry will be discussed below.

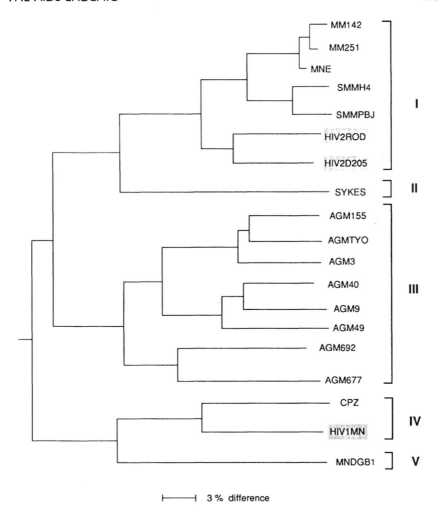

Figure 12.2 Molecular phylogenetic analysis of representative primate immu-nodeficiency viral *gag* p24 gene sequences: I, HIV-2 and related SIV's, in particular SIV-smm from the sooty mangabey; II, SIV-Sykes; III, SIV-AGM's (grivet, vervet, and tantalus species); IV, HIV-1 and the closely related SIV-cpz from a Gabonese chimpanzee; V, SIV-mnd (mandrill isolate). For the sake of clarity, only a small number of the known HIV-1 and HIV-2 sequences are shown; these are high-lighted. The phylogenetic tree was generated from 648 homologous nucleotide sites (of which 416 were variable), as described in Hirsch et al. (1989) and Myers et al. (1991). Only the horizontal branch lengths should be used with the bar scale to estimate percent differences. The tree was rooted at the midpoint of the greatest patristic distance (PAUP, version 2.4.2).

The tree analysis begins with alignment of homologous nucle-otide sequences. By restricting attention to just single-base changes in a relatively conserved coding sequence such as the retroviral *gag* gene, we can be reasonably confident about an unambiguous alignment. The cluster analysis program takes as input the alignment and infers the minimal evolutionary path for the set of sequences. The "parsimony" assumption (that the minimal evolutionary path has been followed) is appropriate for conditions of rapid mutation and recent divergence from some common ancestry. By conducting similar analyses for the several major genes of these primate immunodeficiency viruses, we can corroborate the results. That is to say, in absence of genetic recombination, a phylogenetic tree for the *pol* gene sequences will be congruent with a tree for *gag* gene sequences. Branch lengths will vary, of course, because differing selective forces are at play, but the overall topology of the trees should be invariant (excepting recombination). The branching order can be further evaluated by a statistical procedure known as "bootstrap" analysis (Felsenstein, 1988).

As is apparent from Figure 12.2, phylogenetic tree analysis of the five known types of viruses causing human and simian AIDS implies a common ancestor for these viruses and strongly supports the hypothesis of the simian origin of AIDS. Particular attention is called to the HIV-2 and related SIV sequence group, or clade. Recently, a viral sample taken from an asymptomatic person living in rural Liberia has been found to map with the *pol* gene sequences of the mangabey (not shown in Fig. 12.2; Hahn, 1990), providing strong evidence that immunodeficiency viruses can be transmitted to humans from nonhuman primates. In light of this molecular evidence, the theory of a simian origin of AIDS has been gaining widespread acceptance (Daniel et al., 1988; Hirsch et al., 1989; Doolittle, 1989; Doolittle et al., 1990; Huet et al., 1990; Desrosiers, 1990; Gilks, 1991; Karpas, 1990; Johnson et al., 1991; Myers et al., 1992).

Although the overall picture presented in Figure 12.2 agrees in general with the cluster analyses of other investigators, some of which have been based upon a different algorithm, or even upon amino acid rather than nucleotide sequences (Smith et al., 1988; Yokoyama et al., 1988; Sharp and Li, 1988; Tsujimoto et al., 1989; Doolittle et al., 1990; Gojobori et al., 1990; Miura et al., 1990; Johnson et al., 1991), the exact branching order of the various types of primate immunodeficiency viruses whose sequences have been analyzed through cladistic analysis has encountered some ambiguities, depending upon the mode of analysis and the coding sequence under investigation. For example, the tree presented in Figure 12.2 links the SIV_{AGM} sequences more closely with the HIV-2's than with the HIV-1's, while only the chimpanzee viral sequence is closely linked to the type 1 HIV sequences. Furthermore, the chimpanzee viral sequence is not so closely related to the type 1 human virus as the mangabey virus is to the type 2 human viruses. Interestingly, one human viral isolate, an HIV-1 from Cameroon, is known to be more divergent from all other HIV-1's than is the SIV_{cpz} in Figure 12.2

(DeLeys et al., 1990; Vanden Haesevelde et al., 1991).

Doolittle's results (Doolittle, 1989; Doolittle et al., 1990), on the other hand, suggest a closer relationship between SIV_{AGM} sequences and HIV-1, and he has taken this result (as noted above) to support the hypothesis of an origin of HIV-1's from the green monkey reservoir. Tree analyses are typically performed on *gag* and *pol* coding sequences or amino acid sequences. Other modes of cluster analysis based upon envelope and regulatory protein sequences argue for a closer relationship between the AGM's and the HIV-2/ SIV's (Gojobori et al., 1990; Myers et al., 1992). With the recently discovered SIV-Sykes and SIV-AGM *tantalus* and *sabaeus* variants available for reevaluation of this question, not to mention the baboon and chimpanzee viral isolates now being sequenced, it should soon be possible to resolve much of this ambiguity.

A "BIG BANG" OF AIDS?

Attention should be drawn to the fact that phylogenetic tree analysis seems to suggest that there was a single point of radiation for the SIVs and thus ultimately for the HIVs that emerged from them. This may imply a special and decisive phylogenetic moment in the history of AIDS, what might be called a "big bang": it is as if several major types of the primate immunodeficiency viruses represented in Figure 12.2 emerged simultaneously and perhaps recently from a common ancestor. Most analyses to date, irrespective of the exact branching order of the primate immunodeficiency viruses, have implied this single point of radiation. This has been schematized in Figure 12.3 (Sharp and Li, 1988; Tsujimoto et al., 1989; Doolittle et al., 1990; Johnson et al., 1991).

Is the "big bang of AIDS" real or merely an artifact of the sequence analysis? Is the single point of radiation shown in Figure 12.3 actual or virtual? There is some reason to believe that the convergence of the evolutionary lines on a single point could be merely a consequence of "mutational saturation," or "noise accumulation" (Kirchhoff et al., 1990). The high rate of nucleotide substitution documented in Table 12.1 (below) implies that multiple events, creating so-called "character-conflict", and back-mutation are likely to be complicating the computer analysis, thereby casting a shadow over the distal evolutionary record of the primate lentiviruses. The unusual base composition—high adenine, low cytosine content—of HIV's and SIV's further complicates phylogenetic analyses of the "deep branches" (Sidow and Wilson, 1990). The situation has some formal parallel with the current uncertainty surrounding the theory of a cosmological big bang: radical homogeneity (mutation rates and

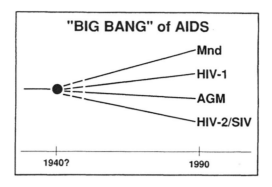

Figure 12.3 Hypothesis of a single nonhuman primate ancestral virus for four of the currently recognized five types of immunodeficiency viruses. The results shown in Figure 12.2, as well as results based upon several different analyses (see text), are suggestive of a common point of evolutionary radiation, that cannot be more recent than 50 years ago, the minimum lookback time for HIV-1 divergence from HIV-2. Alternatively, this point of radiation may be merely virtual, the consequence of mutational saturation and/or nonhomogeneous rates of nucleotide substitution (as discussed in the text).

energy radiation) and radical heterogeneity (different genomic features and galactic distributions) are both observed, and the final interpretation of the respective first moments awaits some definitive insight or discovery. Fortunately, viral relics are easier to come by than cosmic relics, and for this reason a reasonably complete understanding of the evolution of AIDS viruses may be imminent.

While it cannot be said yet whether or not all AIDS-related viruses have a single common ancestor, there is evidence that their emergence was, on an evolutionary timescale, sudden and dramatic, a first decisive moment in the emergence of AIDS. For instance, descendants of African green monkeys brought to the Caribbean as early as the sixteenth century are not seropositive (Hendry et al., 1986). To our knowledge, no feral hosts for the simian immunodeficiency viruses have been found in South America or Asia. Only captive macaques, for example, have been found to be infected, and these undoubtedly contracted the virus from captive mangabeys. At least eight infected African nonhuman primate species are known to exist for which sequence data is still to be obtained and analyzed, among which are the baboons, colobus monkeys, guenons, and talapoins (Johnson et al., 1991).

In the third section of this paper we concluded with some certainty that the human AIDS-causing viruses have a simian origin, and in this section suggested with less certainty but significant probability that the first simian AIDS-causing viruses emerged sometime within the last few hundred years, that is quite suddenly on the scale of evolutionary time. If this is the case, what light does it shed upon the two questions that we posed at the end of the second section, namely the suddenness and virtual simultaneity of the onset of the AIDS epidemic in its major centers less than 2 decades ago, and the apparent simultaneity of the emergence of HIV-1 disease and HIV-2 disease? In order to address these questions more precisely, we will turn our attention in the next section to the time frame for the recent evolutionary development of the human AIDS-causing viruses.

DATING THE PHYLOGENETIC TREE

Tree analyses, such as Figure 12.2, do not provide explicit information about the time required for the evolutionary process being mapped by the molecular sequences. Additional hypotheses are needed. One way to estimate the time implicit in a tree is to assume a representative mutation rate, for example, a typical retroviral rate (known to be at least a millionfold higher than the rate for mammalian nuclear genes). Alternatively, the tree can be calibrated or "resolved" through the inclusion of samples acquired at different times. Both strategies have been adopted by various investigators, and a brief summary of the findings as they pertain to the divergence of HIV-1 from HIV-2 are given in Table 12.1.

The analytical results of sequence analysis performed by several groups using different strategies and different viral sequences have been in remarkable agreement. All of the estimates in Table 12.1,

Table 12.1   HIV-1/HIV-2 Divergence Time Estimates

Base Substitution Rates (per site per year)	Basis	HIV Divergence Time (minimum years)	Reference
0.0005	Murine retroviral *gag* genes	280	Yokoyama et al., 1988
0.0116	HIV-1/2 *env* genes	40	Smith et al., 1988
0.001	HIV *pol* genes	150	Sharp and Li, 1988
0.0008	Ovine lentiviral *pol* genes	203	Querat et al., 1990

however, presuppose a molecular clock: reasonably uniform rates of nucleotide substitution observed over a relatively short time period—5 to 40 years, approximately—are assumed to apply in the more distant past. There is some reason to think that this assumption may not be valid in relation to some of the feral SIV's (Allan et al., 1991; Myers et al., 1992). Moreover, if the phenomenological rate constant is a function of the number of infected individuals—"epidemic-driven variation"—then the actual divergence time could be much further back in time. In fact, by almost every other assumption, the divergence time will be greater than the estimates summarized in Table 12.1. On the other hand, even the radically lower estimate for the minimal divergence time—40 years (Fig. 12.3)—for the simian ancestors of HIV-1 and HIV-2 does not help us understand why these viruses first appeared in humans only within the last 2 decades (as discussed in the section Epidemiological Snapshots, above). Furthermore, the phylogenetic record does not provide a satisfactory explanation for the enigma of two virtually simultaneous cross-species transmissions.

DUAL CROSS-SPECIES TRANSMISSION

Can any more be said at this time about the second decisive moment in the AIDS pandemic, the twofold introduction of virus into human hosts? Assuming (with greater confidence now) a simian origin for the AIDS viruses, and acknowledging the improbability that the two independent and virtually simultaneous cross-species transmissions took place naturally (i.e., without human intervention), we will consider several contexts in which human accients might have occurred and that could explain the coincidence that we have been calling, for lack of better description, the twofold epidemic. First, there was a sharp increase in the exportation of monkeys from Africa in the 1960s, largely for purposes of medical research. This entailed extensive handling of captured animals (Conner and Kingman, 1988). Second, there was also in the 1960s a valiant push to vaccinate Third World populations. In particular, many countries began using live polio vaccines in the spring of 1960, creating some small but finite opportunity for introduction of passenger viruses through contaminated vaccine lots, as in fact happened with SV-40. A great potential for amplification of infections, natural or accidental, exists in the use of contaminated needles.

Short of discovering SIV-infected lots of vaccines prepared in the 1960s, it seems unlikely that a clear verdict regarding these possible modes of transmission will ever come forward. Blomberg and coworkers (1990) have recently documented cross-reactivities of normal human sera with capsid proteins of diverse simian retroviruses, suggesting a way to evaluate some of these potential modes of transmission. Such antibodies probably have arisen as a result of accidental exposure to simian retroviral antigens, although molecular mimicry cannot be ruled out. To the extent that the putative twofold cross-species transmission resulted from increased handling of animals and use of unsterile needles, there exists the disturbing prospect of future transmissions out of the large, qualitatively diverse pools of simian immunodeficiency viruses that are now being discovered.

There is, to keep the record straight, no evidence supporting any of the human accident hypotheses beyond the circumstantial evidence outlined above. And the possibility of uncovering long-established but highly isolated endemic sources in humans—the so-called "lost tribe" hypothesis—for which Hahn (1990) has provided a bit of evidence in relation to the HIV-2 epidemic in West Africa, cannot be dismissed at this time.

MOLECULAR EPIDEMIOLOGY

Sampling and sequencing of HIV-1 up to the present has provided a surprisingly coherent geographical picture of the viruses responsible for the major part of the pandemic: envelope gene sequences from Zairean samples have been clustering together and sequences from U.S. isolates have been clustering together. This neat segregation of viral forms, which is testimony to the "newness" of AIDS, is doomed to be transitory. By 1992, at least 5 distinct subtypes of HIV-1 could be identified, based upon *gag* and *env* coding sequences, in major centers of the pandemic. At least 2 of these 5 forms of HIV-1 are now known to be cocirculating in Thailand, and another two forms in Brazil; thus, it is only a matter of years, at most a decade, before a redistribution of HIV-1 variants is achieved. In the face of the extreme diversity of HIV-1 and HIV-2, and because of the limited sampling thus far (until recently all African HIV-1 samples had been taken from Kinshasa), several international programs of molecular epidemiology have been mounted; now we have sequenced samples from Gabon, Cameroon, Uganda, Kenya, and South Africa, to name some of the sites under study. The results of these programs will be especially important for the vaccine trials that are anticipated.

The random sampling and sequencing to date—molecular snapshots so to speak from HIV-1 samples representing some of the earliest infections—presents a sobering picture of what has to be expected in the future from these emerging viruses. These sequence studies have revealed that viruses with envelope gene sequences differing by 0% to 6% are typical of clones from a single patient (intrapatient variation), while viruses with sequences differing by 6% to 12% have been characteristic of samples from different patients (interpatient variation) in the United States up to 1985. In the 1990-1991 investigation of a Florida dentist and the patients to whom he apparently transmitted virus in the course of invasive oral procedures (Morbidity and Mortality Weekly Report of 18 January, 1991, published by the U.S. Centers for Disease Control), viral samples at large in the Florida population were found to differ by up to 19%(Ou et al., 1992).

This more recent sampling of descendants of the earlier forms in the United States (there is little evidence of significant migration of new forms into the United States between 1985 and 1990) implies that the average interpatient distance appears to be increasing at approximately 1% per year. This rough calculation is in fairly good agreement with the envelope nucleotide substitution rates reported in several recent studies involving other cohorts as well as single individuals (reviewed in Myers and Pavlakis, 1992). Since it is inevitable that both viral migration and recombination will be making significant contributions to the total diversity over a longer period of the pandemic, the value of 1% per year for single base changes should be regarded as a minimum rate.

There is no clear evidence to date that individuals can be dually or multiply infected with the same type of immunodeficiency virus; if superinfection can naturally occur, it should soon become apparent with the Thai and Brazilian samples that are now under investigation. HIV-1 envelope gene sequences that differ by 40% are known to exist for highly divergent viruses found in the United States and Africa. The extraordinary variation of AIDS viruses, observed especially in human and captive animal populations, may be a paradigmatic example of non-steady state evolution, or "bottom-heavy cladism" resulting from a recent ecological breakthrough (as stated by Gould et al., 1987, "Clades diversify rapidly in ephemeral times of unusual opportunity").

Tracking human immunodeficiency viruses is not a futile task. Precisely because these retroviruses vary so rapidly, we discover all the more quickly the conserved and invariant properties of their genes and proteins (Myers et al., 1991). The design of antiviral agents will be enormously facilitated by the fact that these viruses, unlike more conservative microbes, are unable to keep the essential elements of their genomes a secret.

SUMMARY AND CONCLUSION

The preceding discussion has suggested the following results:

1. Phylogenetic tree analysis points strongly to a simian origin of the human immunodeficiency viruses. This conclusion is cor-

roborated by cluster analyses done by many other investigators.

2. The five (or more) major types of viruses that infect simians and cause AIDS in humans may have emerged from a common ancestor at about the same time. This arguably first phylogenetic moment of the AIDS epidemic, which may be likened to the "big bang", cannot explain the sudden and concurrent appearance of human AIDS in the known centers of the epidemic, beyond accounting for a very large and diverse reservoir of nonhuman primate immunodeficiency viruses present in Africa at the onset of the pandemic.

3. The divergence of the type 1 and type 2 human AIDS viruses may have taken place as recently as 40 years ago, though most estimates would place it at 150 to 250 years ago. While this is a relatively short time on an evolutionary scale, even the minimum 40-year figure is too long to explain the sudden and concurrent emergence of the epidemic in its major centers only as recently as the late 1970s.

4. In brief, neither the hypothetical "big bang" nor the range of possible dates for divergence of HIV-1 from HIV-2 accounts for the "improbable" simultaneous cross-species transmission of both HIV-1 and HIV-2 that apparently occurred.

5. These perplexing facts might be explained by two possible avenues of cross-species transmission that occurred in the 1960s: the widespread use in Africa of needles in association with vaccination programs (and possibly of live virus vaccines cultured on monkey tissue), and the sharp increase in exportation of monkeys from Africa, largely for medical research, which entailed extensive handling of captured monkeys. There is no direct evidence for either of these possibilities, however the transmission of virus in 1988 from an infected dentist to five of his patients painfully reminds us that human accidents can be primary avenues for viral emergence.

6. Sampling and sequencing projects now underway will provide additional information about variations in the nucleotide and protein sequences of the AIDS-causing viruses and their rate of change. This will throw light not only on the evolutionary history of these viruses, but on their likely future.

ACKNOWLEDGMENTS

Vanessa Hirsch and Phillip Johnson, of Georgetown University and the National Institute of Allergy and Infectious Diseases of the National Institutes of Health in the United States, kindly provided prior to publication the sequences for the Sykes

and *tantalus* viral isolates analyzed in Figure 12.2. The HIV Sequence Database and
Analysis Project is funded by the AIDS Division of the National Institute of Allergy
and Infectious Diseases through an interagency agreement with the U.S. Department of Energy (LAUR 89-3408).

REFERENCES

Allan, J. S., M. Short, M.E. Taylor, S. Su, V.M. Hirsch, P.R. Johnson, G.M.
    Shaw, and B.H. Hahn (1991). Species-specific diversity among simian
    immunodeficiency viruses from African green monkeys. J. Virol.
    65:2816-2828.
Blomberg, J., E. Vincic, C. Jönsson, P. Medstrand, and R. Pipkorn (1990). Identification of regions of HIV-1 p24 reactive with sera which give "indeterminate"
    results in electrophoretic immunoblots with the help of long synthetic peptides. AIDS Res. Hum. Retroviruses **6**:1363-1372.
Conner, S., and S. Kingman (1988). *The Search for the Virus.* London:
    Penguin.
Daniel, M. D., Y. Li, Y.M. Naidu, P.J. Durda, D. K. Schmidt, C.D. Troup, D.P.
    Silva, J.J. MacKey, H.W. Kestler III, P.K. Sehgal, N.W. King, Y. Ohta, M.
    Hayami, and D.C. Desrosiers (1988). Simian immunodeficiency virus
    from African green monkeys. J. Virol. **62**:4123-4128.
DeCock, K. M., J.C. Niland, H.P. Lu, V. Edwards, C. Shriver, J.W. Mosley,
    et al. (1987). Human immunodeficiency virus infection in patients with
    hepatitis B virus and hepatitis delta virus infections in Los Angeles,
    1977-1985. Abstract MP.84, Third International Conference on AIDS,
    Washington, D.C., 1-5 June 1987.
De Leys, R., B. Vanderborght, M. Vanden Haesevelde, L. Heyndrickx, A.
    van Geel, C. Wauters, R. Bernaerts, E. Saman, P. Nijs, B. Willems, H.
    Taelman, G. van der Groen, P. Piot, T. Tersmette, J.G. Huisman, and H.
    Van Heuverswyn (1990). Isolation and partial characterization of an
    unusual human immunodeficiency retrovirus from two persons of
    west-central African origin. J. Virol. **64**:1207-1216.
Desmyter, J., P. Goubau, S. Chamaret, and L. Montagnier (1986). Anti-
    LAV/HTLV-III in Kinshasa mothers in 1970 and 1980. Abstract S17g,
    Second International Conference on AIDS, Paris, 23-25 June 1986.
Desrosiers, R. C. (1990). A finger on the missing link. Nature **345**:288-289.
Doolittle, R. F. (1989). Immunodeficiency viruses: The simian-human connection. Nature **339**:338-339.
Doolittle, R. F., D.-F. Feng, M.A. McClure, and M.S. Johnson (1990).
    Retrovirus phylogeny and evolution. In *Retroviruses. Strategies of Replication* (R. Swanstrom and P.K. Vogt, eds.), pp. 1-18 [Current Topics in
    Microbiology and Immunology, 157]. Berlin and New York: Springer-
    Verlag.
Duesberg, P. H. (1989). Human immunodeficiency virus and acquired
    immunodeficiency syndrome: Correlation but not causation. Proc. Nat.
    Acad. Sci. U.S.A. **86**:755-764.
Felsenstein, J. (1988). Phylogenies from molecular sequences: Inference and
    reliability. Ann. Rev. Genet. **22**:521-565.
Fultz, P. N., W.M. Switzer, C.A. Schable, R.C. Desrosiers, D. Silva, and J.B.

McCormick (1987). Serologic evidence for infection by HIV-2 in Guinea Bissau in 1980. Abstract MP.72, Third International Conference on AIDS, Washington, D.C., 1-5 June 1987.

Getchell, J.P., D.R. Hicks, A. Srinivasan, J.L. Heath, D. A. York, M. Malonga, D.N. Forthal, J.M. Mann, and J.B. McCormick (1987). Human immunodeficiency virus isolated from a serum sample collected in 1976 in central Africa. J. Infect. Dis. **156**:833-837.

Gilks, C. (1991). AIDS, monkeys and malaria. Nature **354**:262.

Gojobori, T., E.N. Moriyama, Y. Ina, K. Ikeo, T. Miura, H. Tsujimoto, M. Hayami, and S. Yokoyama (1990). Evolutionary origin of human and simian immunodeficiency viruses. Proc. Natl. Acad. Sci. USA **87**:4108-4111.

Gould, S. J., N.L. Gilinsky, and R.Z. German (1987). Asymmetry of lineages and the direction of evolutionary time. Science **236**:1437-1441.

Hahn, B. H. (1990). Biologically unique SIV-like HIV-2 variants in healthy west African individuals. In *Retroviruses of Human A.I.D.S. and Related Animal Diseases* [Proceedings of the Fifth Cent Gardes Colloquium, Paris, Oct. 29-31, 1990] (M. Girard and L. Valette, eds.), pp. 31-38. Lyon: Fondation Marcel Mérieux.

Hendry, R.M., M.A. Wells, M.A. Phelan, A.L. Schneider, J.S. Epstein, and G.V. Quinnan (1986). Antibodies to simian immunodeficiency virus in African green monkeys in Africa in 1957-62. Lancet ii:455.

Hirsch, V. M., R.A. Olmsted, M. Murphey-Corb, R.H. Purcell, and P.R. Johnson (1989). An African primate lentivirus (SIV$_{sm}$) closely related to HIV-2. Nature **339**:389-392.

Huet, T., R. Cheynier, A. Meyerhans, G. Roelants, and S. Wain-Hobson (1990). Genetic organization of a chimpanzee lentivirus related to HIV-1. Nature **345**:356-359.

Jaffe, H.W., W.W. Darrow, D.F. Echenberg, P.M. O'Malley, J.P. Getchell, V.S. Kalyanaraman, R.H. Byers, D.P. Drennan, E.H. Braff, J.W. Curran, and D.P. Francis (1985). The acquired immunodeficiency syndrome in a cohort of homosexual men. Ann. Int. Med. **103**:210-214.

Javier, R.T., F. Sedarati, and J.G. Stevens (1986). Two avirulent herpes simplex viruses generate lethal recombinants in vivo. Science **234**:746-748.

Johnson, P., G. Myers, and V.M. Hirsch (1991). Genetic diversity and phylogeny of nonhuman primate lentiviruses. In *AIDS Research Reviews*, vol. 1 (W.C. Koff, F. Wong-Staal and R.C. Kennedy, eds.), pp. 47-62. New York: Marcel Dekker.

Kanki, P.J., J. Alroy, and M. Essex (1985). Isolation of T-lymphotropic retrovirus related to HTLV-III/LAV from wild-caught African green monkeys. Science **230**:951-954.

Karpas, A. (1990). Origin and spread of AIDS. Nature **348**:578.

Kirchhoff, F., K. Dieter Jentsch, B. Bachmann, A. Stuke, C. Laloux, W. Lüke, C. Stahl-Hennig, J. Schneider, K. Nieselt, M. Eigen, and G. Hunsmann (1990). A novel proviral clone of HIV-2: biological and phylogenetic relationship to other primate immunodeficiency viruses. Virology **177**:305-311.

Marx, P.A., Y. Li, N.W. Lerche, S. Sutjipto, A. Gettie, J.A. Yee, B.H. Brotman, A.M. Prince, A. Hanson, R.G. Webster, and R.C. Desrosiers (1991). Isolation of a simian immunodeficiency virus related to human immunodeficiency virus type 2 from a west African pet sooty mangabey. J. Virol. **65**:4480-4485.

Miura, T., J.-i. Sakuragi, M. Kawamura, M. Fukasawa, E.N. Moriyama, T. Gojobori, K.-i. Ishikawa, J.A.A. Mingle, V.B.A. Nettey,   H. Akari, M. Enami, H. Tsujimoto, and M. Hayami (1990). Establishment of a phylogenetic survey system for AIDS-related lentiviruses and demonstration of a new HIV-2 subgroup. AIDS 4:1257-1261.

Myers, G., and G.N. Pavlakis (1992). Evolutionary potential of complex retroviruses. In *The Retroviridae* (J.A. Levy, ed.), vol. 1, pp. 51-104. New York: Plenum.

Myers, G., B. Korber, J.A. Berzofsky, R.F. Smith, and G.N. Pavlakis (1991). *Human Retroviruses and AIDS 1991.* Theoretical Biology and Biophysics, Los Alamos National Laboratory, Los Alamos, N.M. 87545.

Myers, G., K. MacInnes, and B. Korber (1992). The emergence of simian/human immunodeficiency viruses. AIDS Res. Hum. Retroviruses 8:373-386.

Nahmias, A.J., J. Weiss, X. Yao, F. Lee, R. Kodsi, M. Schanfield, T. Matthews, D. Bolognesi, D. Durack, A. Motulsky, P. Kanki, and M. Essex (1986). Evidence for human infection with an HTLV-III/LAV-like virus in central Africa. Lancet i:1279-1280.

Ou, C.-Y., C. A. Ciesielski, G. Myers, C.I. Bandea, C.-C. Luo, B.T.M. Korber, J.I. Mullins, G. Schochetman, R.L. Berkelman, A.N. Economou, J.J. Witte, L.J. Furman, G.A. Satten, K.A. MacInnes, J.W. Curran, H.W. Jaffe, Laboratory Investigation Group, and Epidemiologic Investigation Group (1992). Molecular epidemiology of HIV transmission in a dental practice. Science 256:1165-1171.

Palca, J. (1991) The sobering geography of AIDS [News Article]. Science 252:372.

Pape, J.W., M.E. Stanback, M. Pamphile, R. Verdier, M.-M. Deschamps, W.D. Johnson Jr., et al. (1987). Pattern of HIV infection in Haiti: 1977-1986. Abstract M.8.6, Third International Conference on AIDS, Washington, D.C., 1-5 June 1987.

Piot, P., F.A. Plummer, M. Rey, E.N. Ngugi, C. Rouzioux, J.O. Ndinya-Achola, L.J. D'Costa, G. Vercauteren, et al. (1986). Retrospective seroepidemiology of AIDS virus infection in Nairobi populations. Abstract S10a, Second International Conference on AIDS, Paris, 23-25 June 1986.

Piot, P., F.A. Plummer, F.S. Mhalu, J.-L. Lamboray, J. Chin, and J.M. Mann (1988). AIDS: an international perspective. Science 239:573-579.

Querat, G., G. Audoly, P. Sonigo, and R. Vigne (1990). Nucleotide sequence analysis of SA-OMVV, a visna-related ovine lentivirus: phylogenetic history of lentiviruses. Virology 175:434-447.

Rayfield, M., K. DeCock, W. Heyward, L. Goldstein, J. Krebs, S. Kwok, S. Lee, J. McCormick, J.M. Moreau, K. Odehouri, G. Schochetman, J. Sninsky, and C.-Y. Ou (1988). Mixed human immunodefiency virus (HIV) infection in an individual: demonstration of both HIV type 1 and type 2 proviral sequences by using polymerase chain reaction. J. Infect. Dis. 158:1170-1176.

Rouzioux, Ch., G. Jaeger, F. Brun-Vezinet, M.C. Dazza, M.A. Rey, L. Montagnier, G. Charmot, et al. (1986). Absence of antibody to LAV/HTLV-III and STLV-III (mac) in pygmies. Abstract 378, Second International Conference on AIDS, Paris, 23-25 June 1986.

Sharp, P. M., and W.-H. Li (1988). Understanding the origins of AIDS viruses. Nature 336:315.

Sher, R., E. Antunes, B. Reid, and H. Falcke (1987). HIV antibody prevalence in black miners between 1970-1974. Abstract MP.42, Third International Conference on AIDS, Washington, D.C., 1-5 June 1987.

Sidow, A., and A.C. Wilson (1990). Compositional statistics: an improvement of evolutionary parsimony and its application to deep branches in the tree of life. J. Mol. Evol. 31:51-68.

Smith, T. F., A. Srinivasan, G. Schochetman, M. Marcus, and G. Myers (1988). The phylogenetic history of immunodeficiency viruses. Nature 333:573-575.

Srinivasan, A., D. York, D. Butler Jr., R. Jannoun-Nasr, J. Getchell, J. McCormick, C.-Y. Ou, G. Myers, T. Smith, E. Chen, G. Flaggs, P. Berman, G. Schochetman, and S. Kalyanaraman (1989). Molecular characterization of HIV-1 isolated from a serum collected in 1976: nucleotide sequence comparison to recent isolates and generation of hybrid HIV. AIDS Res. Hum. Retroviruses 5:121-129.

Stevens, C.E., P.E. Taylor, E.A. Zang, J.M. Morrison, E.J. Harley, S.R. de Cordoba, C. Bacino, R.C.Y. Ting, A.J. Bodner, M.G. Sarngadharan, R.C. Gallo, and P. Rubinstein (1986). Human T-cell lymphotropic virus type III infection in a cohort of homosexual men in New York City. JAMA 255:2167-2172.

Titti, F., A. Aceti, P. Verani, G.B. Rossi, K. Bile, and A. Sebastiani (1986). Seroepidemiologic screening for antibodies to HTLV-III/LAV in Somalia. Abstract 380, Second International Conference on AIDS, Paris, 23-25 June 1986.

Tsujimoto, H., A. Hasegawa, N. Maki, M. Fukasawa, T. Miura, S. Speidel, R.W. Cooper, E.N. Moriyama, T. Gojobori, and M. Hayami (1989). Sequence of a novel simian immunodeficiency virus from a wild-caught African mandrill. Nature 341:539-541.

Vanden Haesevelde, M., J.L. Decourt, L. Heyndricks, B. Vanderborght, E. Saman, R. DeLeys, G. van der Groen, and H. Van Heuverswyn (1991). Molecular cloning and complete sequence analysis of a highly divergent African HIV isolate. Abstract M.A.1157, Seventh International Conference on AIDS, Florence, 16-21 June 1991.

Yokoyama, S., L. Chung, and T. Gojobori (1988). Molecular evolution of the human immunodeficiency and related viruses. Mol. Biol. Evol. 5:237-251.

13

Arthropod-Borne Viruses

THOMAS P. MONATH

There are now over 520 registered arthropod-borne viruses ("arbo-viruses") (Karabatsos, 1985). Of these, approximately 100 cause disease in humans and another 25 are pathogenic for domesticated animals. At least 20 of these viruses fulfill the criteria for "emerging viruses", in the sense that they appear in epidemic form at unexpected times or at periodic and generally unpredictable intervals. Each of these diseases, of which I will discuss only a few examples, presents very interesting epidemiological and ecological features.

Two patterns of emerging arboviral diseases may be defined. One pattern has been the appearance of a hitherto undescribed virus, a novel agent, which first appears in epidemic form. In this case we may presume that an evolutionary change was responsible for this emergence. Kyasanur forest disease, Rocio encephalitis, and o'nyong-nyong represent possible examples. In another section of this book, James Strauss discusses the example of Western equine encephalitis, a virus that also appears to have arisen this way. However, most examples of emergence really are explained by increased geographic distribution, frequency, size, or severity of epidemics of viral diseases that have been around for a long time, rather than by newly evolved viruses. In order to understand why these diseases emerge we need first to consider their ecology and epidemiology.

FACTORS INFLUENCING ARBOVIRUS TRANSMISSION

A unique feature of arbovirus infections is their multifactorial epidemiology (Monath, 1988/1989). At least five variables directly or indirectly influence the rate at which arboviruses are transmitted in nature and thus underlie the emergence of epidemic spread. These are virus, vector, wild vertebrate hosts, humans, and environmental factors. The interactions between these elements of arbovirus transmission cycles are complex. Environmental factors profoundly influence cycles of transmission, mostly by effects on the vectors themselves, as will become apparent later.

138

Arboviruses have natural enzootic maintenance cycles involving one or more species of blood-feeding arthropod vector and vertebrate host that develop viremic infections and serve to amplify transmission. Depending on the virus, the vector may be either a mosquito, other biting flies, or ticks, and vertebrate hosts wild mammals, birds, or even reptiles. Maintenance cycles are generally silent in the sense that the hosts themselves rarely demonstrate any signs of illness. This fact makes surveillance of these infections and prediction of epidemics a very difficult challenge.

The maintenance cycle is usually fairly stable and involves horizontal spread of virus between vector and host in the maintenance cycle. However, in addition to this cycle, many viruses are also adapted for survival over periods that are adverse to activity of the arthropod vector itself, such as tropical dry seasons or temperate zone winters (Reeves, 1979). Vertical transmission, in which the virus is carried transovarially, through the eggs or larvae of infected vectors, is the most notable of these mechanisms. If the rate of transovarial transmission is high, or if a large population of female mosquitoes contribute infected ova at the end of a transmission season, emergence of epidemic transmission may be favored in the succeeding year.

Under circumstances of amplified transmission in the primary enzootic cycle, viruses may spill over to humans or domesticated animals, the clinical hosts for these agents, with an ensuing epidemic or epizootic (an epizootic is the same as an epidemic, but among animals rather than people). The vectors responsible for spread to humans or domesticated animals are often different from those involved in the primary enzootic maintenance cycle. In certain circumstances infected humans themselves, or domesticated animals, may have enough virus in their blood to infect mosquitoes or ticks or other arthropods with the result that there is interhuman spread by the agency of still other vector species. The term "viremic host" refers to any host species that maintains sufficient virus in the blood to infect a blood-feeding arthropod belonging to a competent vector species.

I mentioned the five principal elements involved in arbovirus transmission. Alterations in one or more of these principal elements of the arbovirus transmission cycle can have dramatic effects. Changes in the viral genome induced by intramolecular events, or gene reassortment, can result in virus strains capable of producing increased virus levels in the blood, or increased disease expression in the host, or antigenic variants that escape herd immunity, or even increased infectibility for arthropod vectors. Although there are many examples of genetic variation among the arboviruses, the epidemiological significance of these changes remains largely obscure. To my knowledge there is no clear, documented example of the emergence of an arbovirus epidemic that has been the result of a mutational or recombinational event. However, we are only now beginning to use tools of molecular biology to address these important questions.

In the case of the arthropod, alterations in a variety of biological attributes of the vector may be responsible for the emergence of epidemic disease. They include increases in the vector population density or the proclivity of a vector to bite hosts; increased movement or dispersal such that a virus is spread over long distances; or an increase in the genetically determined competence of the vector for transmitting the agent. Rapid fluctuations in vertebrate host populations (seen in some rodents and other species with high population turnovers), long-range dispersal (typical of migrating birds), and changing levels of population immunity may profoundly affect arbovirus transmission and favor virus amplification and emergence of epidemics.

Environmental changes influence arbovirus transmission by their effects on vectors and hosts. Those that increase the opportunity for breeding of insects with aquatic larval stages, such as increased rainfall, flooding, snow melt, irrigation practices, and so on, are obvious factors in the occurrence of arbovirus outbreaks. But other environmental and climatic changes are less readily understood. In the case of St. Louis encephalitis at northern latitudes in the United States, epidemic years are characterized by low temperatures during the spring, and by high persistently elevated temperatures during the summer months when the epidemics occur (Monath, 1975). The elevated temperatures may shorten the reproductive cycle of mosquitoes, as well as decrease the extrinsic incubation period. But it is not at all clear how low temperatures during the spring contribute to transmission of this agent. In another example, dengue fever, elevated temperature greatly shortens the extrinsic incubation period of dengue virus in the mosquito, increasing the rate of arbovirus transmission. In fact, high temperatures seem to be the predominant factor for the emergence of dengue epidemics in Southeast Asia (Watts et al., 1987).

Some environmental factors are even more obscure. The appearance of St. Louis encephalitis epidemics in the United States follows approximately a 10- or 11-year cycle, which seems to correspond with the nadir of sunspot activity and very little else that can be definitely identified. There underlying factors responsible have not been identified.

APPEARANCE OF NOVEL VIRUSES

There are three principal examples of arboviruses that first appeared in the setting of an epidemic disease: Kyasanur Forest disease, o'nyong-nyong, and Rocio encephalitis.

Kyasanur Forest disease (KFD) is a severe hemorrhagic disease that first appeared in 1956-1957 in southern India in the form of an epizootic affecting monkeys, followed by human cases. At first it was feared that yellow fever had invaded Asia, but a series of classical investigations revealed that a new flavivirus transmitted by ticks was responsible (Work, 1958). Did KFD emerge as a mutant or recombinant virus? If so, were potential precursor viruses, related agents, present in the same geographic area where this disease first occurred? The answer to that is no, although there are some antigenically related agents some hundreds of miles away, but not in the same area. Ecological factors, including deforestation, cattle grazing, and an increased opportunity for tick density were probably responsible for the appearance of this disease, which has persisted as an endemic infection since that time. The virus was probably circulating silently in ticks and rodent hosts; ecological changes provided an opportunity for amplified transmission, and human encroachment in this altered environment led to the emergence of epidemic disease.

O'nyong-nyong, an alphavirus, appeared in epidemic form in Uganda in 1959, and rapidly affected millions of people over a wide area extending south to Malawi (Haddow et al., 1960). The disease is characterized by fever, lymph node swelling, and severe joint pains, hence the name, which means "swelling". There was a potential precursor virus, an antigenically closely related alphavirus called chikungunya, which was endemic (and occasionally epidemic) in East Africa. Unlike KFD, there did not appear to be major ecological or demographic changes that could explain the emergence of o'nyong-nyong, and the virus persisted for a relatively brief period of time. If o'nyong-nyong arose from chikungunya, the genetic change may have altered the vector specificity, favoring transmission by the ubiquitous malaria vector, *Anopheles* (chikungunya is transmitted by *Aedes* mosquitoes), while retaining the ability to produce high viremias in humans, the host for both viruses. The origin of this outbreak is a question that could now be addressed by molecular biology.

The third example, a flavivirus named Rocio, seems even more plausible as a newly evolved virus. Rocio emerged in 1975 in an epidemic of encephalitis in Brazil (Iversson, 1989). There were suitable precursor viruses in the same area in which Rocio arose. The virus has not persisted, which lends further support to the hypothesis that Rocio represented the evolution of a novel agent.

Rocio virus appeared in the Santista lowlands just south of São Paulo in the Ribeira Valley, and caused an epidemic that persisted over a 2-year period, 1975-1976. There were no precedents and the disease has not appeared since. The presumed transmission cycle involves wild and possibly domestic birds as the viremic vertebrate host, and mosquitoes, principally *Aedes scapularis* and possibly *Psorophora ferox*. Humans were infected and became ill with encephalitis. There were about 1,000 cases, of which approximately 10% were fatal, but humans did not take part in perpetuating the transmission cycle.

What about precursor viruses in this environment? The flaviviruses are grouped on the basis of reactions in classical serologic tests, which involve antibody reactions. The most closely related viruses are cross-reactive in neutralization tests, so that antibodies to one virus will also inactivate a closely related virus. There is a complex of flaviviruses that includes many important human pathogens, such as St. Louis encephalitis, a virus that occurs in this area of Brazil. Rocio virus itself is related by other tests to St. Louis encephalitis, but antibodies do not cross-neutralize. Rocio is also related to Ilheus virus, another virus that has long cocirculated in the same region, which is a rare cause of human disease. Both St. Louis encephalitis and Ilheus viruses were known to be associated with the same species of mosquitoes and vertebrate hosts (birds) that were responsible for the spread of Rocio virus during the outbreak in 1975-1976, so that there may have been opportunities for genetic interchange. In addition, there did not appear to be any clear environmental change, and no human-, vector-related or wild vertebrate-related factors that could have explained the emergence of this epidemic. We may hypothesize that this virus arose, possibly from one or both of these precursor agents, but this question, too, needs to be addressed by molecular biology.

EMERGENCE OF VIRUSES DUE TO EPIDEMIOLOGIC AND ECOLOGIC CHANGES

Other examples illustrate a far more frequent situation: emergence of diseases that have been around for some time, but are increasing in distribution, frequency, or severity. A number of possibilities may explain such events, including introduction of the virus from a distant focus; the introduction of an exotic, more efficient vector species; the introduction of immunologically susceptible animal or human hosts into an endemic area; altered environmental conditions in the endemic area that favor an increased rate of virus transmission; and, finally, the emergence of altered virus strains.

Consider a disease called Oropouche fever, which produces a nonfatal but incapacitating illness with fever, headache, muscle pains, and occasionally meningitis. The virus is a member of the genus *Bunyavirus* of the family Bunyaviridae. The virus was first isolated in Trinidad in about 1957, but since the early 1960s has been the cause of intense outbreaks involving tens of thousands to hundreds of thousands of cases in the Amazon region of Brazil, including some rather remote areas (LeDuc and Pinheiro, 1989). A 1980 outbreak, with over 200,000 cases, was typical. Incidentally, the virus has recently surfaced elsewhere, with the first epidemic of Oropouche outside Brazil identified in Panama in late 1989.

What are some of the factors responsible for these outbreaks? An important element in Brazil is the opening of the Amazon region to colonization. Human populations have increased dramatically and with human populations comes both subsistence and cash crop agriculture. A prominent cash crop is cacao, the hulls of which are deposited in piles outside buildings. These piles and other vegetational detritus associated with human habitation provides breeding sites for the vector, a biting midge called *Culicoides paraensis*. In the epidemic transmission cycle of this virus, humans are effective viremic hosts and *Culicoides* gnats are the principal vectors. This vector and human hosts have been recently superimposed on the primordial and as yet undefined forest cycle of the virus involving possibly mosquitoes as vectors and monkeys and sloths as vertebrate hosts. The appearance of epidemics is thus related to colonization of the Amazon region, the cultivation of cacao, and environmental changes that increase the density of the *Culicoides* and their interaction with humans. Increased communication and movement of viremic humans may also play a role in spread of the virus and emergence of epidemics.

In Chapter 5, Karl Johnson mentioned Rift Valley fever. This virus is a member of the *Phlebovirus* genus of the family Bunyaviridae. It produces a lethal infection of cattle and sheep, high rates of abortion, 90% lethality in newborn lambs, and also a severe illness of humans, in many cases characterized by hemorrhagic fever, hepatitis, encephalitis, and retinitis. The distribution of Rift Valley fever is confined to sub-Saharan Africa, epizootics occurring in association with periods of high rainfall having been described throughout much of this region. There have been two human epidemics, one in 1977-1978 in Egypt, which is outside of the endemic region, and the other more recently in Mauritania. Work by Davies, Linthicum and their colleagues has shown a clear association between periods of elevated rainfall, and the appearance of Rift Valley fever epizootics in East Africa (Davies et al., 1985). They showed that the ecological basis for these outbreaks was related to a curious geological formation, shallow depressions in the ground called *dambos*, which are dry throughout much of the year, but fill with water during periods of extended rainfall and produce large numbers of flood water *Aedes* mosquitoes. Linthicum artificially flooded a dambo of about 1,800 square meters and out of this little patch of land was able to find over two million pupae and nearly a million adult mosquitoes belonging to the principal vector species of Rift Valley fever. Moreover, Rift Valley fever virus was isolated from both male and female mosquitoes reared from larvae from both naturally flooded and artificially flooded dambos. After many years of speculation and unrewarding study, the maintenance mechanism of this virus was elucidated: The virus was shown to persist by vertical transmission of the agent in flood water *Aedes* mosquitoes. During periods of extended rainfall, *Aedes* vectors reached sufficient population density to infect viremic hosts, cattle and sheep. Under appropriate circumstances this could lead to a vector-borne epidemic with ancillary spread of the virus by many other mosquito species, as well as by contact and aerosol between animals and humans. Linthicum is now using remote sensing by satellite photography and radar as a surveillance tool to define the distribution of dambo breeding sites and to predict Rift Valley fever epidemics. Indeed, the most recent episode of Rift Valley fever, in Mauritania in 1987, was predicted by remote sensing. Construction of a dam there resulted in the emergence of floodwater and irrigated rice fields producing high densities of vectors.

Could a new property of the virus itself have been responsible for epidemic Rift Valley fever? There has been considerable research on the antigenic and biological properties of a large number of Rift Valley fever virus strains isolated in Africa. Rift Valley fever virus, like other Bunyaviridae, has a genome in three segments that can reassort genetically. The strain of Rift Valley fever virus isolated from the 1978 epidemic in Egypt (responsible for several hundred thousand human cases and much serious disease) did appear to have unique biological properties. For example, unlike other strains of the virus isolated elsewhere and usually associated with less severe disease, the Egyptian strain appeared more virulent; it could infect and kill rat liver cells (hepatocytes), was lethal for laboratory rats and, most remarkably, was resistant to the actions of interferon, a natural antiviral agent produced by the infected host (Anderson and Peters, 1988; Peters and Anderson, 1981). This suggests the possibility that the virus itself may have been an important additional factor in the emergence of this epidemic disease in Egypt.

My final example is dengue virus. It has already been mentioned as an important disease. Dengue, which is caused by one of four viruses or serotypes, designated dengue 1, 2, 3, and 4, belonging to the family Flaviviridae, occurs in two clinical forms: classical dengue fever, a self-limited febrile disease with joint pains, rash and fever, and dengue hemorrhagic fever, a more severe and potentially lethal form.

The transmission cycle of dengue includes principally interhuman spread by the agency of several *Aedes* vectors, but most importantly *Aedes aegypti*, which breeds in water containers in close association with humans. There is also a natural forest cycle, the epidemiological importance of which is presently unknown, involving monkeys and treehole-breeding mosquitoes.

Dengue fever is an expanding or emerging disease. If one charts the distribution of epidemic dengue fever in 1979 and in 1989, one readily appreciates its expansion throughout much of Central and South America, Australia, southern China, and East Africa during that decade.

In the Americas, the interval between dengue epidemics has gradually shortened to the point where, since the late 1970s, there are major epidemics every year. Moreover, a cocirculation of multiple serotypes of the virus has appeared for the first time in this hemisphere. This pattern is reminiscent of the situation that preceded the appearance of dengue hemorrhagic fever in Southeast Asia.

Dengue hemorrhagic fever in Asia, an emerging disease, occurred for the first time in the late 1950s, and now epidemics of large size are an annual event. Thousands of cases are officially reported annually in Thailand, Vietnam, Burma, and elsewhere in Southeast Asia (Gubler, 1991).

What are the factors responsible for this emergence? Has the virus changed? Is there any evidence to support the notion that virulent strains of dengue virus are emerging and could explain these events?

There has been considerable effort in recent years to examine a large library of dengue viruses by oligonucleotide fingerprinting and now some limited gene sequencing is being done. Indeed, there is great genetic variation in dengue virus, and evidence for genetic drift in individual countries over time. In some cases, identical genetic variants have appeared in different widely dispersed locations, suggesting an original source of introduction. Unfortunately, because of the absence of an animal model to study virulence, genetic variation cannot, at present, be associated with the emergence of epidemic disease or severe (hemorrhagic) forms of dengue.

Human (host) factors are more apparent determinants of the emergence of dengue and dengue hemorrhagic fever. Acquired immunity seems to be an important element because it has been repeatedly demonstrated that individuals who have sustained one dengue virus infection, and who were later superinfected with a heterologous serotype, are at higher risk of developing dengue hemorrhagic fever and dengue shock syndrome. The present cocirculation of multiple serotypes in the Caribbean, which results in immunological sensitization and increases the risk of severe disease, mimics events in the 1950s when hemorrhagic dengue emerged in Southeast Asia. Indeed, major outbreaks of dengue hemorrhagic fever have recently emerged in the Americas (in Cuba in 1981, in Venezuela in 1990, and in Brazil in 1991).

Urbanization, with great concentration of people in close association with the *Aedes aegypti* vector, is a very important factor in the emergence of this disease. Water storage practices are largely responsible for dense populations of the mosquito. Throughout the developing world, where dengue is a major problem, water is stored in open vessels, where *Aedes aegypti* lays its eggs and undergoes larval development. The superimposition of disposable containers (bottles, tires, and other receptacles that hold rainwater) in expanding urban environments greatly increases the opportunity for vector breeding.

Dengue virus is spread by viremic humans. The dramatic increase in air travel since the 1960s, counted in billions of passenger miles, is a factor in the emergence of outbreaks and in the spread of this virus around the world.

Another very important factor in the emergence of dengue epidemics has been the reinvasion of tropical America by *Aedes aegypti*, which had been eradicated from much of South America due to intensive vector control efforts earlier in this century. Efforts up until the early 1970s by the Pan American Health Organization and member countries maintained that *Aedes aegypti*-free status, which has been dramatically reversed in the 1980s, with recolonization of coastal Brazil, Paraguay, central Bolivia, Peru and Ecuador, and parts of Colombia. This has been followed by large dengue epidemics in these same locations, with several million cases occurring during the 1980s. An important point, that has also been noted by Shope, is the potentially increased hazard due to urbanization of yellow fever in these areas (Monath, 1991).

Another factor that has not yet been responsible for the emergence of dengue, but may well be important in the future, has been the invasion of an exotic vector *Aedes albopictus*, the so-called Asian tiger mosquito, into the Americas (Craven et al., 1988; Gubler, 1991). This species is involved in the spread of dengue epidemics in parts of Southeast Asia, China, and the Seychelle Islands. Since 1985, it has mounted separate invasions and colonizations of the United States and Brazil. From an original entry point near Houston, Texas, *Aedes albopictus* has now spread throughout 18 states in the United States. In many parts of the United States this mosquito is now displacing *Aedes aegypti* in our cities.

Aedes albopictus invaded the United States by means of containerized cargo ships, which were used to import used automobile and truck tires from Asia, many of which contained rainwater prior to loading. Millions of used tires are imported into the United States each year, but there was a rather dramatic increase in this trade about the time of the invasion. *Aedes albopictus* larvae were discovered in tires coming into the United States, with about 20 tires infested per 10,000. These tires are transported around the United States where they are recapped, but about 20 percent are not recappable and wind up in enormous storage piles, mostly outdoors.

The *Aedes albopictus* strains in the United States and Brazil have been tested for their vector competence. Experiments were conducted at the Centers for Disease Control (CDC) laboratory in Fort Collins, Colorado, at Notre Dame University, and at the U.S. Army Medical Research Institute of Infectious Diseases. Although differences were observed between mosquito strain and virus pairs, *Aedes albopictus* proved capable of transmitting dengue, yellow fever, Mayaro, Venezuelan equine encephalitis, and other pathogenic viruses.

Recently, several viruses have been recovered from wild-caught *Aedes albopictus* in the United States. The most important of these from the standpoint of human and veterinary health is Eastern equine encephalomyelitis (EEE), a severe disease of low incidence in the United States. Human infections with EEE virus are relatively rare, in part because the enzootic vector (*Culiseta melanura*), responsible for transmitting the virus between wild birds, is not attracted to humans as a source of blood. Multiple strains of EEE virus were recovered from *Aedes albopictus* in central Florida in 1991 (Niebylski et al., 1992), raising the fear that involvement of an avid human-biting mosquito in virus transmission could increase the risk of human (and equine) infection.

PREVENTION AND CONTROL OF ARBOVIRUS EPIDEMICS

What are the prospects for prevention of these emergent epidemics? The risk of introduction of certain viruses from distant foci has dramatically increased with the expansion of air travel. Those viruses that cause viremias in human beings at levels high enough to infect mosquito species of worldwide distribution (e.g., *Aedes aegypti, Culex pipiens*) are the agents likely to be spread by this means. These include dengue, yellow fever, chikungunya, Mayaro, and possibly Rift Valley fever and Oropouche. Even the most optimistic of us who think about the public health implications realize that interceding in the movement of viruses by limiting movement of people is an unrealistic possibility.

I have not really discussed transport of infected vectors, but there are examples in which this may occur by natural means that would be very difficult to interdict. The movement of African horse sickness and Western equine encephalitis viruses by long-distance transport of vectors caught in high-altitude wind currents has been postulated to explain outbreaks of these diseases (Craven et al., 1988; Gubler, 1991).

Introduction of exotic vector species, especially those whose breeding sites are artifacts moved around by humans, such as automobile tires and plants, is theoretically preventable by public health measures, but once introduced such exotic species may be very difficult to control.

Altering the immune status of the human population or domestic animals seems to be a realistic goal, and considerable effort is being expended on the development of appropriate vaccines. It should be mentioned, however, that yellow fever is still an important epidemic disease with hundreds of thousands of cases occurring in Africa in intermittent outbreaks, despite the availability of a very effective, safe vaccine. The public health commitment to preventive immunization has often lagged far behind technical successes in vaccine development.

Altered environmental conditions in the endemic area, which favor increased rates of virus transmission and emergence of epidemics, may be under human control, such as the construction of water resource projects and irrigation schemes. More attention is required in the assessment of environmental impacts of such projects on the potential for vector-borne diseases.

Finally, we clearly need to understand much more about the role of molecular variation in viruses and to build surveillance systems that examine and understand the possible significance of changes in viral genomes.

REFERENCES

Anderson, G.W. Jr., and C.J. Peters (1988). Viral determinants of virulence for Rift Valley fever (RVF) in rats. Microb. Pathog. 5:241-250.

Craven, R.B., D.B. Francy, D.A. Eliason, et al. (1988). Importation of *Aedes albopictus* (Skuse) and other exotic mosquito species into the United States in used tires from Asia. J. Am. Mosq. Contr. Assoc. 4:138-142.

Davies, F.G., K.J. Linthicum, and A.D. James (1981). Rainfall and epizootic Rift Valley fever. Bull. WHO 63:941-943.

Gubler, D.J. (1991). Dengue hemorrhagic fever: a global update. Virus Info. Exch. Newslett. 8:2-3

Haddow, A.J., C.W. Davies, and A.J. Walker (1960). O'nyong nyong fever: an epidemic virus disease in East Africa: Introduction. Trans. R. Soc. Trop. Med. Hyg. 54:517-521.

Iversson, L.B. (1989). Rocio encephalitis. In *The Arboviruses: Epidemiology and Ecology* (T.P. Monath, ed.), Chap. 40 (vol. 4, pp. 77-92). Boca Raton, Fla.: CRC Press, Inc.

Karabatsos, N. (ed.) (1985). *International Catalogue of Arboviruses Including Certain Other Viruses of Vertebrates*, third ed. San Antonio, Tex.: American Society of Tropical Medicine and Hygiene.

LeDuc, J.W., and F.P. Pinheiro (1989). Oropouche fever. In *The Arboviruses: Epidemiology and Ecology* (T.P. Monath, ed.), Chap. 36 (vol. 4, pp. 1-14). Boca Raton: CRC Press, Inc.

Monath, T.P. (1975). Epidemiology. In *St. Louis Encephalitis* (T.P. Monath, ed.), Chap. 6 (pp. 239-312). Washington, D.C.: American Public Health Association.

Monath, T.P. (ed.) (1988/1989). *The Arboviruses: Epidemiology and Ecology* (4 vols.). Boca Raton: CRC Press, Inc.

Monath, T.P. (1991). Yellow fever - Victor, Victoria? - Conqueror, Conquest - Epidemics and research in the last 40 years and prospects for the future. Am. J. Trop. Med. Hyg. 45:1-43.

Niebylski, M.L., J.P. Mutebi, G.B. Craig, et al. (1992). Eastern equine encephalitis virus associated with *Aedes albopictus* — Florida, 1991. Morbidity and Mortality Weekly Reports 41:115,121.

Peters, C.J., and G.W. Anderson Jr. (1981). Pathogenesis of Rift Valley fever. In *Rift Valley Fever* [Contrib. Epidemiol. Biostat., 3] (T.A. Swartz, M.A. Klingberg, and N. Goldblum, eds.), pp. 21-41. Basel: S. Karger.

Reeves, W.C. (1979). Overwintering of arboviruses. Progr. Med. Virol. 17:193-220.

Watts, D.M., D.S. Burke, B.A. Harrison, R.E. Whitmire, and A. Nisalak (1987). Effect of temperature on the vector efficiency of *Aedes aegypti* for dengue 2 virus. Am. J. Trop. Med. Hyg. 36:143-152.

Work, T.H. (1958). Russian spring-summer virus in India—Kyasanur forest disease. Progr. Med. Virol. 1:248-277.

14

Hantaan (Korean Hemorrhagic Fever) and Related Rodent Zoonoses

JAMES W. LeDUC, J.E. CHILDS, G.E. GLASS, AND A.J. WATSON

Human disease due to hantaviral infections first came to the attention of western medicine during the Korean Conflict, when a mysterious "new" disease, Korean hemorrhagic fever, was seen among the United Nations forces. Over 2,000 U.S. troops were infected, and many deaths occurred (Earle, 1954). In spite of intense investigations by some of the most prominent medical scientists of the era, the causative agent could not be identified, and it wasn't until 1976, just over a decade ago, that the etiologic agent was finally discovered.

Dr. Ho Wang Lee and his colleagues, working in Seoul, Korea, was the first group to isolate the virus that causes Korean hemorrhagic fever (Lee et al., 1978). They named it Hantaan virus in recognition of the Hantaan River, which transects the endemic region of Korea near the demilitarized zone. The virus was isolated from lung tissues of the striped field mouse, *Apodemus agrarius*. This very common animal is now recognized as the major rodent host of that virus.

Within a year or two of its initial isolation, Hantaan virus was adapted to growth in cell culture, allowing development of an indirect immunofluorescence (IFA) test for serologic testing and laboratory investigations (French et al., 1981). Infected cells, stained with fluorescent-labeled antibodies and examined microscopically, show a characteristic cytoplasmic stippling, common to all Hantaan viruses.

This IFA test is part of the real history of the virus because there is a significant cross-reactivity using that test between all of the recognized Hantaan-related viruses, which we now know are distinct viruses in themselves. These viruses collectively form the genus *Hantavirus* of the family Bunyaviridae. During the past decade we have witnessed a dramatic increase in our understanding of this group of viruses, leading to recognition that they are very widely distributed and likely to be responsible for human disease in many parts of the world where they are not now recognized.

The availability of both the virus and the serologic test allowed experimental infection of natural rodent hosts to be undertaken. And through these studies, one of the key characteristics of the Hantaan viruses was discovered. When Hantaan virus is experimentally inoculated into seronegative (uninfected) *Apodemus agrarius*, a brief viremia ensues. Subsequently, however, Hantaan viral antigen is detected for weeks to months in many major organs, but most importantly, infectious virus is shed in saliva and feces, and especially urine, perhaps for the duration of the rodent's life (Lee et al., 1981). This virus shedding occurs in spite of the presence of antibody in the serum, which can be detected by both IFA and virus neutralization tests. Thus, the infected rodent becomes a persistent source of infectious virus and we suspect that most human infections occur through aerosolized virus excreted in infected rodent urine and feces.

Human disease in Asia is closely associated with the basic biology of the rodent host *Apodemus agrarius*. Because of this, there is a marked seasonal distribution of cases. Most cases occur during the late fall and early winter and this temporal pattern is seen throughout Korea, China, and into the eastern portions of the former Soviet Union.

Hantaan virus accounts for over 100,000 cases of disease in China alone, and its incidence is probably underreported. Several regional names have been proposed for human disease due to hantaviral infections. In the case of Asian forms, Korean hemorrhagic fever and epidemic hemorrhagic fever have been used most often. Recently, however, the World Health Organization has endorsed a single name, hemorrhagic fever with renal syndrome (HFRS), to be used as a generic term to cover all forms of hantaviral disease.

The typical clinical HFRS in Asia generally progresses through either a moderate or severe picture, with relatively well defined successive stages. These are, in order, the febrile, hypotensive, oliguric, diuretic, and convalescent stages (Earle, 1954). The major signs and symptoms typically seen in each stage are, respectively, fever, shock, renal impairment, relative hypervolemia, and fluid and electrolyte imbalance. Most patients also have a characteristic facial flushing, especially visible along the neck. A petechial rash is usually seen, but it is often limited to the axilla. As an additional hemorrhagic sign, ecchymosis is frequently seen among the severely ill patients. Scleral injection, bloodshot eyes, is also not uncommon.

Most of the clinical characteristics of the disease, however, are due to the marked kidney damage, which may progress to complete renal failure and death. This includes unique and characteristic damage to the renal medulla.

We have recently completed a two-year double-blind, placebo-controlled efficacy trial of the antiviral drug Ribavirin for the treatment of epidemic hemorrhagic fever in China. This study offered us the opportunity to examine nearly 300 acutely ill patients, and to optimize our diagnostic techniques as well as to evaluate the drug (Xiang et al., 1988). For this study we selected enzyme immunoassay (ELISA) as the most appropriate technique to yield a rapid diagnosis, and we tried to measure specific hantaviral antigen as well as IgM and IgG antibody to Hantaan. We were uniformly unsuccessful in our attempts to detect Hantaan viral antigen in serum from acutely ill patients. But we did find that virtually all patients had high titers of IgM antibody on admission. Since IgM is the first class of antibody made during an infection, followed later by an IgG antibody response, these findings indicate that infection was recent. Consequently, we have targeted our diagnostic test development on efforts to measure Hantaan viral specific IgM antibodies. This has proved successful, not only with the disease due to prototype Hantaan virus, but also to the other forms of HFRS.

Without going into a great deal of detail about the drug trial itself, let me just say that Ribavirin appears to be efficacious in preventing death due to Hantaan viral infection if it is administered early in the course of disease, with best results obtained among those whose treatment is started on or before day four. Fifty-seven patients were enrolled in the first year of the study, and 187 in the second year. Pooling the results from the 2 years, 10 deaths occurred among the 108 patients receiving placebo, while only 3 died among 123 patients treated with the drug. This difference is statistically significant ($P<0.04$).

The drug also appeared to markedly reduce morbidity and frequently decreased the time patients spent at each stage of illness. As one example, treatment substantially reduced levels of serum creatinine (an indication of kidney damage) among treated patients, as compared to those receiving placebo. Ribavirin clearly has a place in the treatment of HFRS, especially if patients can be diagnosed and treatment initiated early in the course of their illness (Xiang et al., 1988).

Nephropathia epidemica is a less severe form of HFRS that is found in Scandinavia, the western part of the former Soviet Union, and Europe. This disease was first described in the medical literature during the 1930s, at least in the Scandinavian medical literature, and the similarities between it and the Asian forms of HFRS have also been known for some time (Gajdusek, 1962).

Consequently, in the context of our theme on emerging viruses, this is not a new disease. It was, however, a direct result of the successful isolation of Hantaan virus that the causative agent of nephropathia epidemica, Puumala virus, was identified. Clinically, without going into detail, nephropathia epidemica is very similar to the Asian forms, with renal dysfunction a prominent characteristic, but without the serious hemorrhagic manifestations and marked mortality characteristic of Hantaan viral infections in Asia.

Some hantaviruses do, indeed, represent emerging virus diseases. An apparently new virus, at least new in terms of our recognition, was recently discovered in the Balkans. For the past several years we have been collaborating with Dr. Tony Antoniadis in Thessaloniki, Greece, to investigate HFRS. Although the disease was not recognized in Greece prior to our studies, we now know that there is a very severe form of the disease in the northwestern provinces. This form has a significant renal involvement which often leads to death (LeDuc et al., 1986a).

For the 27 Greek patients studied in detail, the disease was very severe and more closely resembles the disease due to Hantaan virus seen in Asia, rather than the milder nephropathia epidemica found in Scandinavia and other parts of Europe. The bottom line is that the mortality rate here is about 15 percent versus 1 percent for nephropathia epidemica in Scandinavia and around 5 to 10 percent for Hantaan induced infections in Asia.

We have succeeded in isolating a hantavirus from a sick Greek patient and have shown it to be antigenically similar to prototype Hantaan virus, although sufficiently distinct to allow specific recognition (LeDuc et al., 1986a; Antoniadis et al., 1987). We proposed the name Porogia virus for this particular agent. Recent studies in Yugoslavia, Bulgaria and Albania suggest that this virus, or closely related viruses, occur in these countries as well and are probably responsible for major outbreaks of HFRS that were recorded over the past several decades.

Unlike the late fall-early winter seasonality typical of both Hantaan and Puumala viruses, most cases seen in Greece occur during the warmer months of the year; cases peak around August. Investigations of the natural host of this virus indicate that the rodent *Apodemus flavicollis* (the common yellow-necked field mouse) is the most likely reservoir for Porogia virus.

To summarize briefly, then, with regard to the hantaviruses discussed so far, three distinct hantaviruses are recognized, which are regionally associated with HFRS. Hantaan virus is found in Asia and is responsible for a moderate to severe form of HFRS locally named Korean hemorrhagic fever or epidemic hemorrhagic fever. Puumala virus, found in Scandinavia, the western Soviet Union, and much of Europe, causes a less severe form of HFRS called nephropathia epidemica. Porogia virus, and perhaps some other closely related viruses, are found in the Balkan Region and these cause a very severe form of HFRS.

Seoul virus, another distinct hantavirus that is associated with domestic rats, adds another dimension to the picture. The story of Seoul virus begins in the early 1980s and, again, Ho Wang Lee and his colleagues in Korea played a prominent role in its discovery. With the aid of the IFA test developed for Hantaan virus, they diagnosed HFRS among patients who resided in the urban centers of Korea, far from the recognized endemic region of Korean hemorrhagic fever (Lee et al., 1982). The patients were city dwellers, people with no history of travel outside the city. When attempts were made to collect small rodents around patients' houses, no *Apodemus* could be found. However, domestic rats were present. Captured rats were examined and both viral antigen and antibody to what appeared to be Hantaan virus were detected using IFA techniques. Both *Rattus norvegicus* and *R. rattus*, captured in a variety of different neighborhoods in Seoul and other Korean cities, were positive. For example, of 477 captured *R. norvegicus* tested, 63 were antibody positive and 37, or about half of these, were also antigen positive.

Subsequent study with more specific techniques, namely neutralization tests, however, showed that the virus in domestic rats was, in fact, an agent closely related to prototype Hantaan virus, but distinct. This virus was named Seoul virus after the Korean city where it was first isolated.

Soon thereafter my own group, in collaboration with several others, began a global serosurvey of domestic rats to determine the distribution of this newly recognized virus. Antibody positive rats were found in many parts of the world, suggesting that the virus itself was not new, but rather our ability to detect it had changed (LeDuc et al., 1986b). Many antibody positives were found in North America and South America, as well as in Africa, Australia, Asia, and Europe.

We then focused our efforts locally to investigate the maintenance of this virus among domestic rats in the United States. Many of our studies were conducted in inner city neighborhoods in Baltimore, although similar conditions exist in any number of cities in the United States. In the alleyways of the inner cities, litter and trash abound; rat burrows are associated with these piles of litter. We have studied hantaviruses in the rat populations in these neighborhoods of Baltimore for several years now, and we have found Seoullike viruses especially common among rats in this environment (Childs et al., 1987). We have used the name Baltimore rat virus (BRV) for the local Seoul-like hantavirus.

We have isolated strains of Seoul-like virus from rats captured there, and we have monitored the hantaviral antibody prevalence rates in these populations. Tabulating percent seropositive by body mass groupings, which is a good estimator of rat age, about a third of the animals in the lowest mass group, that is, the youngest age group, have antibody to hantaviruses (Childs et al., 1985; Childs et al., 1987). We suspect that this is maternal antibody, which is lost over the next several weeks. There is a dip in prevalence rates, to about 10% in rats weighing about 200 grams, which are slightly older. As the rats age, the prevalence rates increase until virtually all (>80%) are seropositive in the largest rats, which represent the oldest age group. Male and female rats follow virtually the same track.

With such an abundance of infected rats coexisting with the resident human population, and recognition in Asia that Seoul virus is capable of causing overt human disease, 2 years ago we began a study to attempt to document acute hemorrhagic fever with renal syndrome in Baltimore residents.   In a prospective study from January 1986 to October 1988 with inpatients and outpatients at the Johns Hopkins Hospital, patients were tested for quantitative 24-hour urine protein, as an indicator of kidney damage, and had a blood sample drawn, to test for prior infection. All patients with proteinuria greater than 250 milligrams per 24 hours were selected for further study. As a control, we also included two patients per week who had proteinuria of less than 150 milligrams per 24 hours and had blood work done on these patients. Patients were excluded if they were actively undergoing chemotherapy for cancer or treatment of HIV, although a history of either of these alone was not a basis for exclusion. Sera were screened by ELISA for both IgM and IgG antibodies to hantaviruses. Suspect positives were confirmed by Western blot and the identity of the infecting virus was determined by virus-specific plaque reduction neutralization tests in tissue culture. Although we examined a total of 1,669 sera from 1,148 individuals, we failed to identify any with evidence of acute hantaviral infection. We did, however, find 15 patients with antibody to the local strain of hantavirus, the Seoul-like virus, that we had isolated from captured rats in Baltimore. Let me emphasize that these people had antibody to the same virus that we have isolated from the domestic rats captured in the same neighborhoods in Baltimore (Childs et al., 1988; Glass et al., 1990).

While we were disappointed in not being able to document acute disease in that study, we were struck by the fact that many of the seropositive persons suffered from chronic renal disease or hypertension, or both. Consequently, we went back to this same study population and conducted a type of case-control study (Glass et al., 1990). For purposes of this study we called all of those serologically positive for virus as cases. We then randomly selected 5 seronegative patients from the same patient population, to serve as controls for each case. Controls were matched for age to within 3 years, and also for sex. The medical records were then reviewed by a nephrologist without prior knowledge of the patients' serologic status. Based on clinical records, the nephrologist made a clinical diagnosis. Again, there were 15 seropositives, all of whom were infected with the local strain of rat associated hantavirus, and none of whom had a history of foreign travel. The seropositives represented 10 women and 5 men; 13 were black and 2 were white. We found no significant differences between the seropositive cases and the matched seronegative controls with regard to race, age, occupation, location of residence, or clinical measurement such as blood pressure, serum creatinine, or proteinuria. We did, however, find significant differences in the prevalence of chronic renal disease, including hypertension and a history of cerebral vascular accident. These conditions were significantly more prevalent among those seropositive to hantaviruses as compared to their matched seronegative controls. This was not due just to differences in health. Rates of diabetes, for example, were not significantly different. When we looked closely at the specific causes of chronic renal disease, we found that the association was specific for hypertensive renal disease, but not for the other common causes of chronic renal disorder.

When we originally set up this study, we did not specifically control for race. And even though the final matching did not differ significantly between the seropositives and the seronegatives with regard to race, there was a larger percentage of blacks among the seropositives than among the seronegatives. Realizing the known increased frequency of hypertension and cerebral vascular accidents among blacks, we conducted a substudy in which only black seropositives and seronegatives were considered. The study was exactly as outlined initially, but only 3 seronegative controls were used for each seropositive case.

The association originally detected in the initial study was still evident when only blacks were considered. As mentioned earlier, these results are very preliminary and still under analysis. However, the results, if confirmed, have some startling implications, since they could well represent the first recognition of what might appear, to the general public, to be a new emerging virus disease.

Some obvious questions immediately come to mind. Could hantaviral infections account for a portion of the chronic renal disease and hypertension so well known among inner city populations? And why were we unable to detect acute disease? Is it possible that subacute infections could actually lead to chronic renal disease? These observations may also rekindle the debate whether hypertension leads to chronic renal disease, or as we might suspect here, that the renal insult due to hantaviral infection may actually be the precursor of subsequent hypertension. Clearly there is much more to be done before any of these questions can be answered definitively. But at least we are now in a position to develop some testable hypotheses.

Subsequently, 3 patients at the Johns Hopkins Hospital have been identified who have seroconverted to the local Seoul-like hantavirus (Baltimore rat virus, BRV). Each of the patients resided in areas where infected rats had been collected. In all 3 cases the illness was characterized by acute onset of nausea, vomiting, fever, epigastric pain, proteinuria, and the development of hypotension, and variable renal and liver involvement. The course of illness for 2 of the patients was well characterized. The acute onset of illness with a febrile phase, followed by 1-2 days of hypotension, and renal failure with liver enzyme derangements is similar to rat-associated HFRS in other parts of the world. Two of the patients later developed chronic renal disease.

These data indicate the HFRS does occur in the United States at low levels but goes unrecognized. The development of chronic disease in 2 of the patients is consistent with our earlier observation that exposed individuals were more likely to suffer hypertensive renal disease than uninfected controls, and suggests hantaviral infection may be responsible for some portion of hypertensive renal disease, in endemic areas. This interpretation is supported by a case-control study of end-stage renal disease patients using hemodialysis clinics in inner-city Baltimore. Exposure to BRV was found only among patients with a primary diagnosis of hypertensive renal disease. Seroprevalence in this group was 7.0%.

I have purposefully concentrated on the epidemiologic aspects of the hantaviruses, but I would be remiss not to at least mention the significant advances that have been made in understanding the basic virology of this group of viruses. Very impressive strides have been made in taking a group of viruses, which only a decade ago could barely be grown in cell culture, to the point today where we recognize these as a complex of distinct viruses that form a new genus within the family Bunyaviridae (Schmaljohn et al., 1985). We have a firm grasp on their molecular characteristics and the prospects of a modern vaccine are well in sight.

In summary, although hemorrhagic fever with renal syndrome was well known for many years in Asia and parts of northern Europe, it was not until the isolation of Hantaan virus that a specific virus could be associated with the disease. The availability of Hantaan virus for use in diagnostic testing, and the fact that this virus is especially cross-reactive in the IFA test, led to the recognition and subsequent isolation of several other rodent-borne hantaviruses that appear to also be associated with human disease. Of these, one of the most intriguing is the Seoul-like viruses that are associated with domestic rats. Studies in Asia have clearly associated this virus with human HFRS. Very preliminary results suggest that prior infection with strains found here in the United States may be associated with an increased risk of chronic renal disease, hypertension, or cerebral vascular accidents. Our most recent data, mentioned above, provide additional evidence for both acute and chronic effects of infection in the United States.

ACKNOWLEDGMENT

The views of the authors do not purport to reflect the positions of the Department of the Army or the Department of Defense.

REFERENCES

Antoniadis, A., D. Grekas, C.A. Rossi, and J.W. LeDuc (1987). Isolation of a hantavirus from a severely ill patient with hemorrhagic fever with renal syndrome in Greece. J. Infect. Dis. **156**:1010-1013.

Childs, J.E., G.W. Korch, G.A. Smith, A.D. Terry, and J.W. LeDuc (1985). Geographic distribution and age related prevalence of antibody to Hantaan-like virus in rat populations of Baltimore. Am. J. Trop. Med. Hyg. **34**:385-387.

Childs, J.E., G.W. Korch, G.E. Glass, J.W. LeDuc, and K.V. Shah (1987). Epizootiology of Hantavirus infections in Baltimore: isolation of a virus from Norway rats and characteristics of infected rat populations. Am. J. Epidemiol. **126**:55-68.

Childs, J.E., G.E. Glass, G.W. Korch, R.R. Arthur, K.V. Shah, D. Glasser, C. Rossi, and J.W. LeDuc (1988). Evidence of human infection with a rat-associated Hantavirus in Baltimore, Maryland. Am. J. Epidemiol. **127**:875-878.

Earle, D.P. (1954). Symposium on epidemic hemorrhagic fever. Am. J. Med. **16**:617-709.

French, G.R., R.S. Foulke, and O.A. Brand (1981). Korean hemorrhagic fever. Propagation of the etiologic agent in a cell line of human origin. Science **211**:1046-1048.

Gajdusek, D.C. (1962). Virus hemorrhagic fevers. Special reference to hemorrhagic fever with renal syndrome (epidemic hemorrhagic fever). J. Pediatr. **60**:841-857.

Glass, G.E., J.E. Childs, A.J. Watson, and J.W. LeDuc (1990). Association of chronic renal disease, hypertension and infection with a rat-borne Hantavirus. Arch. Virol., Suppl. **1**:69-80.

LeDuc, J.W., A. Antoniadis, and K. Siamopoulus (1986a). Epidemiological investigations following an outbreak-of hemorrhagic fever with renal syndrome in Greece. Am. J. Trop. Med. Hyg. **35**:654-659.

LeDuc, J.W., G.A. Smith, J.E. Childs, F.P. Pinheiro, J.I. Maiztegui, B. Niklasson, A. Antoniadis, D.M. Robinson, M. Khin, K.F. Shortridge, M.T. Wooster, M.R. Elwell, P.L.T. Ilbery, D. Koech, E. Rosa, T. Salbe, and L. Rosen (1986b). Global survey of antibody to Hantaan related viruses among peridomestic rodents. Bull. WHO **64**:139-144.

Lee, H.W., P.W. Lee, and K.M. Johnson (1978). Isolation of the etiologic agent of Korean hemorrhagic fever. J. Infect. Dis. **137**:298-308.

Lee, H.W., P.W. Lee, and L.H. Baek (1981). Intraspecific transmission of Hantaan virus, etiologic agent of Korean hemorrhagic fever, in the rodent *Apodemus agrarius*. Am. J. Trop. Med. Hyg. **30**:1106-1112.

Lee, H.W., L.J. Baek, and K.M. Johnson (1982). Isolation of Hantaan virus, the etiologic agent of Korean hemorrhagic fever, from wild urban rats. J. Infect. Dis. **146**:638-644.

Schmaljohn, C.S., S.E. Hasty, J.M. Dalrymple, J.W. LeDuc, H.W. Lee, C.H. von Bonsdorff, M. Brummer-Korvenkontio, A. Vaheri, T.F. Tsai, H.L. Regnery, D. Goldgaber, and P.W. Lee (1985). Antigenic and genetic properties of viruses linked to hemorrhagic fever with renal syndrome. Science 227:1041-1044.

Xiang, C.M., M.Y. Guan, Z.M. Zheng, Z.A. Wu, X.Q. Ge, T.M. Zhang, G.H. Yuan, X.A. Gui, J.W. Huggins, T.M. Cosgriff, J. Smith, J.W. LeDuc, and J.M. Meegan (1988). Study of antiviral specific therapy of epidemic hemorrhagic fever with ribavirin. J. Exp. Clin. Virol. (China) 2:47-51.

15

Filoviruses

C.J. PETERS, E.D. JOHNSON, P.B. JAHRLING, T.G.
KSIAZEK, P.E. ROLLIN, J. WHITE, W. HALL, R. TROTTER,
AND N. JAAX

The viral family known as the Filoviridae is unique among animal virus families: we understand virtually nothing about the natural history and maintenance strategies of any member of the family, yet Marburg and Ebola viruses are highly pathogenic for man and are capable of epidemic transmission (Table 15.1). Surely they are a fitting subject for a book on emerging viruses.

DISCOVERY OF MARBURG VIRUS

Filoviruses first came to medical attention in 1967 when a lethal epidemic of viral hemorrhagic fever occurring in Marburg, Federal Republic of Germany (FRG); Frankfurt, FRG; and Belgrade, Yugoslavia (Serbia), was traced to a shipment of vervet or African green monkeys imported from Uganda (Martini and Siegert, 1971; Siegert, 1972). The causative agent was cultivated from the blood of sick humans and, as customary for arboviruses and other zoonotic viruses, was named *Marburg virus* after the site where the viral samples were obtained. The bizarre morphology of the virion, as well as its virulence and potential for human to human transmission, caught the imagination of virologists. Although there was some superficial similarity to rhabdoviruses (particularly plant rhabdoviruses), most scientists remained unconvinced that Marburg virus was just another rhabdovirus. Eventually, Marburg virus became the first member of the filovirus family (Kiley et al., 1982).

The impact of the 1967 Marburg virus epidemic went far beyond that of a rare disease, dangerous to a few people. Nonhuman primates are a vital resource to the biomedical community. They are, even today, essential to the development, safety testing, and production of viral vaccines. The fundamental biological similarities between these animals and man has made them an essential element of biomedical research programs in many areas, including simian lentiviruses that produce syndromes strikingly resembling human AIDS. Those concerned with the importation and use of nonhuman primates realized the potential disaster that could result from an introduction of Marburg virus into the primate user community and quarantine procedures were recommended for imported animals to prevent the dissemination of Marburg virus to vaccine facilities and biomedical research institutions. These precautions seemed particularly important, since ecological investigations failed to clarify any African fount of infection.

Marburg virus remained an obscure medical curiosity until 1975, when a naturally acquired human infection was recognized in South Africa. A young man traveling through Zimbabwe arrived in Johannesburg and was hospitalized with a viral hemorrhagic fever syndrome due to Marburg virus infection (Gear, 1989). After his death, two people who had cared for him during his illness, a traveling companion and a nurse, developed severe but nonfatal disease from Marburg virus. Epidemiologists retraced the travels of this young couple in an attempt to identify the source of infection. As with the original Marburg incident, these attempts failed. Interestingly, the publicity surrounding this episode in South Africa had important secondary consequences. Clinicians were alerted to the hemorrhagic fever syndrome and their interest led to the viral studies that first implicated Rift Valley fever virus as a cause of this same syndrome. Further studies in South Africa centered around the clinical complex also resulted in the recognition of Crimean Congo hemorrhagic fever virus as a significant public health problem in southern Africa.

AFRICAN EBOLA EPIDEMICS

The next indication of the existence of filoviruses came from an extraordinary pair of epidemics in 1976. Foci of disease appeared in southern Sudan and 600-700 km away in northern Zaire (Pattyn, 1978). Both epidemics were in clusters of small African communities situated in similar ecologic zones and lying along rural communication routes. The Zaire epidemic was clearly dependent on unsterilized needles and syringes for its major dissemination between villages, although multiple later generations of cases occurred among family contacts without any defined parenteral exposure. In the Sudan the initial focus was a cotton factory in Nzara, and several of the earliest recognized cases worked there in a single room. Travel to nearby Maridi introduced the virus into the medical care system, with subsequent iatrogenic dissemination that devastated the Maridi hospital.

Table 15.1   Filovirus Isolates

Year	Virus*	Number of cases (Percent mortality)		Comments
1967	MBG	25 (28)	from monkeys	Imported African green monkeys presumed to have been
		6 (0)	from man	infected in Uganda transmitted virus to European laboratory workers, particularly those exposed to blood and tissues. Secondary cases in medical personnel and family members.
1975	MBG	1 (100)	primary	Traveler infected in Zimbabwe transmitted disease to
		2 (0)	secondary	companion and nurse.
1976	EBO-Z	85 (100)	injection	Index case apparently introduced disease into Yambuku
		43 (91)	injection/contact	Hospital in Zaire. Secondary transmission occurred by
		149 (89)	contact	injection from unsterilized equipment and contact with sick people.
1976	EBO-S	280 (53)		An independent epidemic from that in Zaire arose in Nzara, Sudan, with a distinct EBO strain. Earliest cases were traced to cotton factory in Nzara. Transmission was both nosocomial and by contact in homes. Spread to adjacent towns, including Maridi, Sudan.
1977	EBO-Z	1 (100)		Child in Tandala, Zaire, died with hemorrhagic fever.
1979	EBO-S	34 (65)		Recurrent disease in Nzara, Sudan; the index case worked in same room in textile factory identified in 1976 epidemic.
1980	MBG	1 (100)	primary	French engineer in Nzoia, Kenya; he infected physician
		1 (0)	secondary	caring for him in ICU.
1987	MBG	1 (100)		Danish man visited parents living in Kisumu and traveled in western Kenya.
1989	EBO-R	4 (0)		Reston, Virginia: infected cynomolgus macaques imported from Philippines. Subsequent studies established Asian origin of virus. All 4 documented infections of man were subclinical. (Also identified in monkeys of same origin in Siena, Italy, 1992, and in Alice, Texas, 1990 and 1996.)
1994	EBO	1 (0)		Côte d'Ivoire, November: researcher became infected after necropsy on chimpanzee following a chimpanzee dieoff in Tai Forest; distinct EBO strain.
1995	EBO-Z	315 (77)		Epidemic in Kikwit, Zaire, January-July; index case identified as a charcoal vendor who lived in Kikwit but regularly collected wood in rainforest. As in the 1976 epidemics, most cases were nosocomial, also family contacts (caregivers).
1995	EBO	1 (0)		Liberia; 25 year old male, in area of Liberia near Côte d'Ivoire.
1996	EBO-Z	37 (57)		Gabon, January-March; initial cases had contact with a chimpanzee carcass. Cases included a 7 month old child.

*MBG = Marburg virus
EBO-Z = Ebola virus, Zaire strain
EBO-S = Ebola virus, Sudan strain
EBO-R = Ebola virus strain isolated in Reston, Virginia

Isolation of apparently identical viruses from the two epidemics led to the christening of "Ebola virus," named for a local river. Subsequently it has become apparent that the two viruses are not identical, but that they have significant antigenic, RNA sequence, and biologic differences (Buchmeier et al., 1983; Cox et al., 1983; Richman et al., 1983). Nevertheless, there were important similarities in the natural history of the two epidemics: needle/syringe transmission played a catalytic role in dissemination; person-to-person contagion occurred in 5-10% of household members, but generally only after close contact with desperately ill patients under conditions of primitive hygiene; and mortality was high. Human disease declined as hospitals were depopulated, less intimate association with sick persons was practiced, and increased use of modern barrier nursing practices was instituted by international assistance teams. Notable biosocial correlates included (1) the altruistic and effective international response to define the nature of these frightening threats to human health, and (2) the role of unsterilized injection equipment in disseminating disease. The introduction of sterile disposable needles and syringes has been of enormous benefit to the developed world, but these articles are by their nature not adaptable to preparation for safe reuse. Plastic syringes do not withstand even boiling and other simple methods applied in many third-world settings that might provide some measure of protection. This also has enormous implications for diseases with extraordinarily long viremic incubation periods, such as observed with AIDS.

The clinical disease observed in these Ebola epidemics resembled that described for Marburg (Pattyn, 1978; Peters et al., 1991). After an incubation period lasting 3 to 16 days, sudden fever and malaise developed followed by prostration, sore throat, chest pain, abdominal pain, skin rash, and diarrhea. Within a week to 10 days those destined to survive began to improve, even though recovery from the severe debilitating effects of the disease often required weeks. Patients with severe infections often experience diffuse or extensive hemorrhage, coma, and convulsions before death. The exact mechanisms by which filoviruses cause such serious disease are not known, but there is extensive viral involvement of liver, lymphoid organs, and kidneys. In experimental monkey Ebola infections, virus has been identified in vascular endothelial cells, suggesting at least one mechanism for the coagulopathy that occurs in a diffuse fashion in these animals as well as many filovirus-infected patients (Baskerville et al., 1985). Humans convalescent from Marburg or Ebola infection have had virus isolated up to 3 to 4 months later in semen or, in a uveitis patient, anterior chamber fluid. No evidence of long-term persistence, latency, or late degenerative disease has been adduced from the small number of patients under continued medical observation.

FURTHER VIRAL AND EPIDEMIOLOGICAL STUDIES

Both Marburg and Ebola viruses once again largely disappeared from mainstream medical interest. Isolated human cases were confirmed by virus isolation (Table 15.1), and occasional patients were presumptively diagnosed by serological means. A small outbreak occurred again in Nzara, Sudan, and the index case worked in the same small factory where the 1976 epidemic apparently originated. Retrospective epidemiologic investigations failed to find a source for either Marburg or Ebola virus in spite of attempts that included collection of ecologic samples for virologic tests. Bats, monkeys, spiders, and ticks were among the species suspected to be animal reservoirs of filoviruses on circumstantial evidence, but no definitive data were obtained. Some common factors emerged. The source of these viruses was embedded deep in rural African life. Casual visitors to cities were not at risk; expatriate cases had traveled in the countryside, had close contact with local people, and often had interests in local ecology. One particularly fertile area was recognized in the Mt. Elgon region on the Kenya-Uganda border. The 1980 and 1987 Marburg virus isolates came from Europeans traveling in nearby Kenya and visiting the Kitum cave atop Mt. Elgon. The 1967 shipment of African green monkeys, which resulted in recognition of the virus family, originated in Uganda within 100 km of Mt. Elgon. Facts surrounding the 1967 monkey collections were suppressed in the repressive political atmosphere of the time, but it now appears that there may have been monkey disease in the Ugandan exporting area (Johnson et al., 1982).

A major impediment to Ebola virus research has been the lack of a neutralizing antibody response in convalescent sera from patients or experimental animals surviving infection with filoviruses. This has worked in two ways, neither of which is necessarily obvious to the general scientific reader. First of all, to the virologist concerned with the biology of hemorrhagic fever viruses, virus neutralization is the basic tool for classifying related viruses, and the lack of access to this comfortable modality of established relevance makes it extraordinarily difficult to decide such questions as whether the Zaire and Sudan strains of "Ebola" are two different viruses. Second, the extent of in vitro virus neutralization often correlates with the ability of convalescent sera to protect against or treat disease from hemorrhagic fever virus infections. The lack of in vitro virus neutralization from filovirus antisera, not unexpectedly, is accompanied by a lack of protective capacity on passive transfer to infected experimental animals. This rather arcane point becomes particularly relevant to researchers who, in spite of the best containment technology, may be accidentally exposed to Ebola or Marburg viruses. Neither the antibodies in convalescent plasma nor other antiviral modalities such as drugs or alpha interferon have been shown to exert a protective effect in experimental animals (Peters et al., 1991).

The lack of a sensitive, specific neutralization test has also hampered researchers in their attempts to unravel the natural history of filoviruses. This test has served as the "gold standard" for seroepidemiological studies of most viruses until recent introduction of more sophisticated approaches. Large numbers of residents in central Africa have been found to have antibodies to Ebola virus by the widely used indirect fluorescent antibody (IFA) test. These tests are not simple false positives. Many IFA positive sera also react with Ebola virus by Western blot or radioimmunoprecipitation tests. The reactivity is reproducible on serial sampling and varies from village to village. Yet, based on the experience in Sudan and Zaire in 1976, the number of antibody positives observed should be reflected in the common occurrence of severe viral hemorrhagic fever. Even in the remote regions studied, these patients should have come to the attention of the medical profession and be remembered by local people; however, there are no recollections of such vivid and severe clinical syndromes. We have speculated that there may be other strains of Ebola-like filoviruses of lesser pathogenicity for man circulating in these regions.

It does seem that filoviruses are not common causes of serious human disease in Africa. Several attempts to isolate Ebola and Marburg viruses from putative viral hemorrhagic fever cases in West Africa (Liberia), East Africa (Kenya), central Africa (Central African Republic), and southern Africa (South Africa) have been largely unsuccessful. This does not exclude the possibilities that filoviruses kill a significant number of humans by their sporadic activity in Africa, that they may be more important in rural areas not yet tested, or that lethal epidemic disease may occur from time to time and not be recognized and reported.

In spite of dead ends in the epidemiology and therapy of filoviruses, progress was made in the molecular biology of these agents. Painstaking studies by Kiley, Regnery, Sanchez, and others at the Centers for Disease Control (CDC) led to our understanding of the filoviruses as a group of enveloped viruses with a single negative-polarity RNA strand, which is transcribed into monocistronic mRNA coding for the virion proteins (Kiley et al., 1988; Sanchez et al., 1989). The detailed findings and the lack of sequence homology with other virus families when combined with the detailed ultrastructural observations of Almeida, Peters, Muller, Murphy, and other workers led to the acceptance of the filovirus family (Kiley et al., 1982).

Thus, our attitude toward filoviruses in 1989 was highly ambivalent. These agents were capable of causing human disease with high mortality and with person-to-person spread, yet they seemed to be sufficiently uncommon that they presented no major health threat to

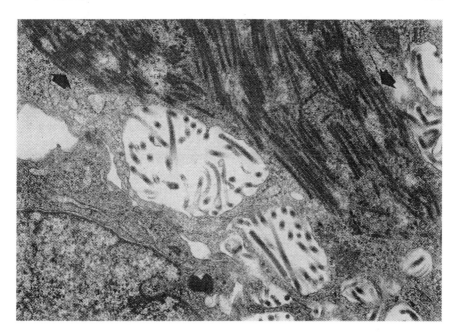

Figure 15.1 "Reston" strain of Ebola virus. Cultured MA-104 cells 2 days after inoculation with serum from an imported cynomolgus monkey dying of hemorrhagic fever. Arrows indicate array of viral nucleocapsids, which would appear as magenta inclusions on routine histopathological stains. Mature virions seen in vacuoles. Magnification, X 28,000. Courtesy of Mr. Tom Geisbert, USAMRIID.

residents or travelers in Africa. Indeed, disease from these viruses was so infrequent we had difficulty finding cases to study. Clearly there were other viral hemorrhagic fevers causing obvious health problems, either endemically, such as Lassa fever in West Africa, or epidemically, such as Rift Valley fever throughout sub-Saharan Africa, which seemed to call for a shift in resources away from Ebola virus. Yet it seemed unwise not to pursue more understanding of such a lethal viral disease when we had no real knowledge of its natural history or of the ways in which its activity was controlled. These considerations were preempted by an unusual series of events.

MONKEY EPIDEMICS IN THE U.S., 1989

In November 1989 we received samples for viral studies from cynomolgus macaques (*Macaca fascicularis*) recently imported from the Philippines. The veterinary clinician was aware that we had studied an epidemic of simian hemorrhagic fever (SHF) among imported *M. fascicularis* in April 1989 and suspected that this virus was causing an epidemic among a cohort of 100 monkeys housed in one room (Room F) in a quarantine facility in Reston, Virginia. Tissues taken from dead or moribund euthanized monkeys were inoculated into a cell line derived from rhesus monkey kidney (MA-104), and three animals were readily confirmed as having SHF viral infection; fluorescent antibody (FA) tests detected SHF antigens, and typical particles could be found by electron microscopy to confirm the infecting virus. Tissues from a fourth monkey, however, induced a different cytopathic effect in MA-104 cells and did not result in expression of SHF viral antigens. To our surprise, examination of these cell cultures with the electron microscope showed abundant filovirus particles (Fig. 15.1). Working into the evening and the next morning, we identified the filovirus to be not Marburg as suspected, but rather Ebola virus or a relative by its reaction with human and animal polyclonal Ebola viral antisera and several Ebola-specific monoclonal antibodies (Jahrling et al., 1990). By that evening the management of the quarantine facility, as well as state and national health authorities, had been notified of these findings. Because of spreading disease within the room all monkeys had already been euthanized, but more stringent precautions were instituted among the animals in other rooms and exposed personnel were placed under surveillance by the Virginia State Health Department and the CDC.

Two laboratory techniques developed for use in experimental infections of monkeys proved to be invaluable in reconstructing past events and monitoring ongoing animal disease: (1) Immunoperoxidase staining of formalin-fixed tissues had been valuable for studying the distribution of virus in animals inoculated with the Zaire strain of Ebola, and proved equally adaptable to retrospective examination of earlier monkey deaths within the building (Zaire strain antigen can be detected in paraffin-embedded tissue blocks from monkey necropsies performed more than 7 years previously); and (2) A rapid ELISA was also developed and applied to detect antigen in serum or tissues from infected animals, allowing a diagnosis of Ebola infection to be made within 4 hours (Ksiazek et al., 1992).

Events unfolded rapidly. A second room began to experience an unusually high mortality with ELISA antigen positivity in most dying animals, and at least one other room had Ebola involvement. One of the animal technicians then developed a febrile illness with digestive symptoms; he later proved *not* to have Ebola, but the event certainly helped crystallize thinking on potential lines of action. Because of the probability that the infection was spreading within the building, the remaining primates were euthanized. Since the monkeys were potentially infected with a lethal human pathogen, veterinarians, animal technicians, and other scientists with experience in working with dangerous organisms under high containment conditions were organized into teams to provide safe, humane euthanasia. Nursing personnel, specially trained in the use of self-contained protective gear to provide medical care to hemorrhagic fever patients, provided the training and support to utilize flexible plastic hoods with battery-powered blowers providing filtered sterile air. These head coverings interdigitate with impermeable overalls to give a high degree of protection against fomites, droplets, and aerosols. To assure that the building was safe for reuse, critical contents were surface decontaminated with hypochlorite or incinerated, followed by treatment of the entire structure with paraformaldehyde vapor. Tissues from animals outside the two heavily involved rooms, when tested by antigen ELISA, showed a very low prevalence of infection. Fortunately, clinical and serological surveillance by public health authorities of quarantine facility workers, veterinary personnel, and clinical laboratory technicians handling blood from infected animals revealed no signs of infection.

The mode of transmission within the quarantine facility could not be confidently established from an analysis of the initially collected data (Centers for Disease Control, 1990a). Disease first appeared in Room F and was probably introduced with that shipment. The second involved room could have become infected from Room F or have been infected before arrival. Because of the high susceptibility of *Macaca* to tuberculosis, arriving animals are tuberculin tested, with repeats at 2-week intervals. Many animals develop illness after shipment and receive injections of antibiotics and vitamins. Syringes (but not needles) were used for multiple animals, raising the possibility that parenteral transmission was largely responsible for spread. In any case, the quarantine procedures that had been put in place as a consequence of the 1967 Marburg episode had served to limit infected monkeys to the involved facility. Other factors also favored containment of the infection. Concern for herpes B virus (a natural infection in *Macaca* species, but potentially lethal for humans who may contract it from the monkeys) in the veterinary and HIV-1 in the medical communities has led to improved practices among those working with nonhuman primates and clinical laboratory samples. An alert veterinary clinician seeking laboratory confirmation of the monkey deaths brought samples to the microbiology laboratory where classical virology was critically important in identifying Ebola virus in the material (Jahrling et al., 1990).

The role of SHF virus was also unclear. This spherical, positive-stranded RNA virus has no antigenic or genetic relationship to the filovirus family (Gravell et al., 1986; Trousdale et al., 1975). It was first discovered as a lethal epidemic disease of captive *Macaca*, an Asian genus (Tauraso et al., 1970). However, SHF strains have been recovered from apparently healthy but chronically viremic patas monkeys (*Erythrocebus patas*, an African species). After some of the rare macaque epidemics of SHF were traced to cross-contamination from patas monkeys by unsterilized tatoo needles or injection equipment, it was hypothesized that patas monkeys were the true reservoir of SHF virus and that the macaques were only incidentally infected during captivity (London, 1977). Because no human disease has been observed in laboratory workers or animal handlers exposed to SHF, and because it is a relatively difficult virus to manipulate in the laboratory, the research effort on it has been modest.

Most animals tested from the first room, and some from the second room, had SHF in addition to Ebola virus detectable in serum or organs. Classical strains of SHF virus are virtually 100% lethal for macaques, as are previous Ebola isolates. Which was the primary pathogen and what was the interaction between the two viruses? We have begun to answer these questions in the laboratory. One of the Ebola isolates (H28) from Reston has been plaque-cloned and tested exhaustively to assure its freedom from SHF virus. This virus killed two of three cynomolgus macaques inoculated intramuscularly with 500 plaque forming units. Ebola antigen was present in the serum of all three infected monkeys; antibodies developed in all three as well. The simultaneous presence of Ebola antigen and antibody in serum from the two dying monkeys probably represents an ineffectual immune response occurring too late to mediate recovery from critical organ damage. It does contrast to most laboratory inoculations of macaques with Marburg, or with Sudan or Zaire strains of Ebola virus; antibody rarely appears in these animals, and they usually die.

FURTHER U.S. EPIDEMICS AND THE LINK TO ASIA

Of course the potential scientific payoff in this epidemic was the tracing of the source of filovirus infection in the monkeys and the opportunity to identify the elusive reservoir of Ebola virus. Collaborative international studies examined the ports of call of the cargo airplanes bringing the crucial shipment to the U.S. The first hypothesis was that these two known African viruses (SHF and Ebola) had been introduced into the Asian macaques during shipment. Careful shoe-leather epidemiological studies failed to find a direct link to monkeys or other animals from Africa during shipment. Of course, viruses can persist in injection apparatus, multidose medicine vials, or in dried material in the environment long after an infected animal has departed. However, this was not the explanation in this case; it appears that both Ebola and SHF strains also are present in Asia. The CDC had requested tissues from cynomolgus monkeys dying in quarantine facilities as part of a comprehensive effort to protect importers from Ebola virus. They succeeded in isolating another strain of Ebola virus from a cynomolgus monkey succumbing in Pennsylvania and the circumstances suggested an independent introduction of virus. Emerging serological data using the IFA test also pointed to widespread previous infection of macaques arriving from Indonesia and the Philippines, and indeed in several Old World species including rhesus macaques, *Cercopithecus* species (African green monkeys and their relatives), and *Papio* species (baboons).

Collaborative investigations in the Philippines (Dr. Betsy Miranda, the Philippine Department of Health; Dr. Mark White, the CDC Field Epidemiology Training Program consultant assigned to Manila; and Dr. Curt Hayes and LCDR James Burans, the U.S. Naval Medical Research Unit No. 2) confirmed the presence of antibodies in Asian macaques, found seropositives among monkey handlers,

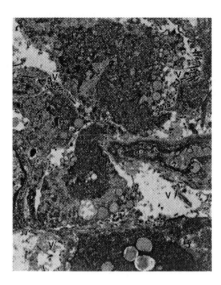 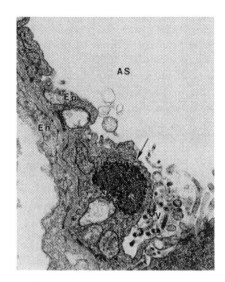

Figure 15.2 Lung from a rhesus monkey infected with the Zaire strain of Ebola virus by the aerosol route. Courtesy of Dr. John White, USAMRIID. **a.** A large number of virions (V) and some macrophages are shown in an alveolar space. Magnification, X 7,200;   **b.** A large cytoplasmic inclusion in an epithelial cell (Ep) contains viral nucleocapsids (I). Note the extracellular virions (V) in the adjacent alveolar space (AS). Magnification, X30,000.

and also identified Ebola-related deaths among monkeys held in an export compound near Manila on Luzon Island. IFA test suggested past infection among humans and monkeys on Mindanao, the island where wild cynomolgus monkeys were trapped for later export.

While data on infection in the Philippines were being developed, interesting findings were once again emerging from Reston, Virginia. Importation of macaques resumed in January 1990 and the first two shipments entered without apparent health problems. The few monkeys that died were tested by antigen capture ELISA and no positives were found. However, the next three shipments, arriving in February and March, yielded animals dying with Ebola virus infection. These deaths occurred in the first few days of arrival, were clinically and pathologically typical of the spectrum of primate Ebola infection previously seen at Reston and in the experimentally infected monkeys, and were associated with exuberant expression of Ebola virus (electron micrographs of tissues, immunohistochemical staining of antigens in fixed tissue, high-titered antigen present by ELISA, virus isolation). These data left little doubt that monkey infection occurred in the Philippines before or at the time of shipment and was highly suggestive that Ebola virus infection was the major factor in the monkey deaths. Furthermore, spread to additional monkeys in each of the involved rooms was progressive, with most inhabitants dying or being sacrificed when ill. More than 90% of the sick or dead animals tested during these room epidemics were positive by ELISA for Ebola antigen. The mortality in involved rooms was approximately 80%.

During this period of massive spread, disturbing clinical and pathological observations were made. Monkeys were noted to have extensive clinical evidence of respiratory involvement often with copious nasal discharge. High concentrations of viral antigen were detected by antigen ELISA and staining of smears from nasal and oropharyngeal swabs. The presence of virus in these samples was confirmed by electron microscopic visualization (Fig. 15.2) and by culture. Viral antigen was found in both upper and lower respiratory tracts and pneumonia was evident, both grossly and microscopically, in many animals.

The continuing spread of infection within the quarantine facility may be explained by these pathogenetic findings. The two shipments admitted in January had remained apparently healthy until, during March 1990, Ebola-specific deaths were found in the first arrivals and eventually deaths reached a level that required sacrifice of the entire room. By April 1990, virus was circulating in still another previously uninvolved room, this time involving the second January shipment and leading to elimination of the room's inhabitants.

The mechanism of cross-contamination between rooms is unknown. Infectious secretions may have been carried from one of the heavily involved rooms by animal caretakers in spite of quarantine precautions, but it is also possible that small particle aerosols may have circulated through the ventilation system. The most alarming finding was the development of serological evidence of infection in four of the five regular workers in the quarantine facility (Centers for Disease Control, 1990b). One was probably infected when he cut himself while performing a necropsy on an infected monkey; however, the other three had no defined exposure to virus. Fortunately, none of the workers experienced significant symptoms during the period while antibodies were rising. The seriousness of the efficient spread of a filovirus by such mechanisms cannot be overestimated; however, the context of the exposure must be borne in mind: literally hundreds of monkeys had died from infection within the facility, providing an enormous potential source of infectious material. The high incidence of acute infections at Reston contrasts markedly to the findings from surveys of others involved in the transport chain of the infected shipments as well as workers exposed to nonhuman primates for years (Centers for Disease Control, 1990c). CDC has found no seroconversions, a seroprevalence of around 1%, and no history of classical hemorrhagic fever. These IFA results, although confirmed by Western blot, represent a very low incidence of infection and require comparison to background serological findings in the general population.

Laboratory evidence for the extensive presence of virus in pulmonary secretions and the relentless spread within involved rooms (even in the absence of needle or syringe use) clearly established the ability of this filovirus strain to spread from monkey to monkey and even from monkey to man by droplets and/or small particle aerosols. This should be contrasted to the Marburg and African Ebola epidemics in which sick humans appeared to transmit virus primarily to those in close contact with their blood or secretions. Furthermore, even in the original Marburg epidemic, human disease acquired from monkeys only occurred in those exposed to blood, organs, or tissue cultures. However, before rejecting the possibility of occasional spread of Marburg or Ebola (Zaire and Sudan strains) by droplet or aerosol mechanisms, one must also consider the field observations that indicate a minority of Ebola secondary infections did not have close contact with patients' blood or body fluids, the primate studies in which monkeys housed in the same room (but not necessarily in adjacent cages) occasionally become infected, and a formal aerosol experiment in which as little as 500 PFU of the Zaire strain of Ebola virus fatally infected rhesus monkeys.

While these and similar observations on the pathogenesis and epidemiology of primate filovirus epidemics were being made in the United States by concerned scientists from industry, state health departments, CDC, and the U.S. Army Medical Research Institute of Infectious Diseases, new data on the geographic distribution of filoviruses in nonhuman primates were rapidly accreting. Cynomolgus macaques from the Philippines, Indonesia, and Thailand were found by IFA to have antibodies to filoviruses. As a matter of fact, monkey sera from numerous species, including *Macaca mulatta* (rhesus macaques) and several *Cercopithecus* species (particularly *C. aethiops*, also called African green or vervet monkey), have been positive by IFA. Thus, nonhuman primates seemed to be an important indicator species for filovirus infection. The findings of antibodies in monkey populations transplanted to different geographic areas suggested the possibility that Ebola virus might have a broad geographic distribution or perhaps an even closer relationship with the monkeys. The size of the populations that apparently sustained virus circulation is too small to imagine simple monkey to monkey transmission as the sole mechanism unless prolonged virus shedding occurred. Alternatively, one could envisage a mechanism of long-term infection with reactivation, similar to varicella and zoster or typhus and the Brill-Zinsser phenomenon. Another speculative possibility would invoke long-lived arthropods as mediators of infection. Some species of mites or lice could easily accompany monkeys on their journeys and be quite difficult to detect.

SOME CONCLUSIONS AND SPECULATIONS

What then have we learned about filoviruses from this episode? It now seems likely, based on serological information from the IFA test, that filoviruses circulate in Asia. Furthermore, an epidemic in a monkey facility in the Philippines led to multiple subsequent introductions into U.S. quarantine facilities. Available data do not permit a conclusion as to whether the monkeys are only incidentally infected or may play a more integral role in virus maintenance. Interestingly, antibodies that react with the Reston isolate imported from the Philippines are not the only ones found. Many Asian monkey sera react only with the Sudan or Zaire Ebola strains, and positive FA tests with Marburg virus antigen also occurs. The significance of this is unknown, but the findings certainly complicate simple hypotheses about strain antigenicity and geographical distribution. They also emphasize the need for additional serological tests for confirmation of seroepidemiological studies of filoviruses. The potential of filoviruses for droplet/aerosol transmission in appropriate circumstances has also been well established.

Are the Asian monkey isolates "Ebola virus?" The answer to the question as posed is clearly "yes." Morphology, cross-reactions with polyclonal and monoclonal antibodies, and the early biochemical data developed by A. Sanchez at the CDC support this classification. The Reston isolate does differ from the two African isolates in some significant ways: (1) Some polyclonal antisera react solely or significantly better with individual strains and one monoclonal antibody that reacts with Sudan and Zaire viruses fails to stain Reston virus-infected cells, (2) There appears to be less endothelial cell involvement in Reston virus-infected monkeys, and (3) Pathogenicity for man seems to be less than observed in the African epidemics. However, one could also ask, "What is Ebola virus?" For example, the IFA tests such as those applied to the Ebola strains might not clearly separate the highly pathogenic arenavirus, Lassa, from its much less dangerous relative, lymphocytic choriomeningitis virus. In fact, one must await additional serological and molecular data to understand the degree of taxonomic relatedness among the three isolates from Sudan, Zaire, and Reston, Virginia, called "Ebola virus."

What was the origin of the multiple introductions of this strain of Ebola virus in 1989-1990? The proximate cause seems to be an increased circulation of virus in holding facilities overseas, and the emerging evidence suggests that acutely infected animals were concentrated at a single exporter. It is possible that ordinary secular variations in filovirus transmission in nature may have led to introduction of active virus transmission into the exporter's facility, possibly with subsequent amplification by animal husbandry and injection practices. More speculatively, a variant virus with increased transmissibility may have arisen in nature or in the primate population destined for export. We are also pursuing the possibility that some interaction with SHF virus may have been responsible for the emergence of this Ebola strain as an epidemic pathogen; SHF has been coisolated from at least some sick animals in all the epizootics from which we have received samples. Other intercurrent infections with viruses such as hepatitis A, simian lentiviruses, or type D retroviruses, could also be involved. Regardless of the root causes of the epidemics, we now have knowledge and tools that did not exist in November 1989 and which permit a reasoned response to the threat. The high degree of transmissibility among monkeys housed in a single room dictates early identification of infected animals, both to protect the monkeys and to minimize risk of human infection. The antigen-detection ELISA appears to be a test that can accomplish this reliably in sick or dead animals and be readily applied to large numbers of samples. Testing serum samples for Ebola antigenemia or ribonucleic acid (A. Sanchez at the CDC has a sensitive polymerase chain reaction assay) will also identify many infected monkeys before they become ill. Although it seems likely that elimination of animals early in the infectious process should prevent continuing spread within monkey cohorts housed in the same room, this critical point remains to be established. The potential threat from imported antibody-positive animals also deserves further exploration. In our experience, IFA antibody titers in recently convalescent monkeys are considerably higher than those in most survey sera from healthy animals and animals with exceptional titers may form a special category. In general, however, there is no evidence that latent or chronic infection has played any role in the 1967 Marburg incident or in the last years' cynomolgus monkey epizootics, and the past record of safety in use of monkeys (many of which were IFA positive) and their tissues argues against any serious danger. However, a systematic exploration of latency seems particularly relevant in light of our ignorance of the mechanisms of filovirus maintenance in nature (Peters et al., 1992).

How dangerous are filoviruses from primates for man? Considering the experience since 1967, it would seem that the probability of significant disease is small, but that if an epidemic occurred it could be nasty. We were fortunate that the high infectivity of the Reston Ebola strain was not combined with the human pathogenicity of the 1967 Marburg virus. The only two recognized episodes have been in imported wild-caught monkeys and improved quarantine procedures are being implemented in the U.S. to further protect against this eventuality. An important aspect of any quarantine should be etiologic diagnosis of deaths. Improved use of pathological and microbiological diagnostic modalities in this country should minimize both primate loss and human risk. Increased concern for wildlife conservation and foreign licensing of exporters will further decrease the risk of filovirus spread to man.

What are the lessons for an "emerging virus" book? The obvious

answer is that we must have some flexibility in our research programs to explore some of the enigmas that may only give hints
regarding their possible future importance. Any "realistic" administrative review in 1989 could have established that filoviruses were
of little significance for human health and that scarce research funds
should not be allocated to expensive BL4 laboratories and overseas
field programs to study them. I imagine similar opinions would
have been proffered if a lentivirus had been isolated from a handful
of immunosuppressed people in Zaire in the mid-1970s.

ACKNOWLEDGMENTS

We would like to thank our colleagues in industry, State Health Departments, the
Centers for Disease Control, and in other Department of Defense laboratories who
have shared data and in some cases participated in evolving studies alluded to
above. The views of the authors do not purport to reflect the positions of the
Department of the Army or the Department of Defense.

In conducting the research described in this report, the investigators adhered
to the Guide for the Care and Use of Laboratory Animals, as prepared by the Committee
on Care and Use of Laboratory Animals of the Institute of Laboratory Animal
Resources, Commission on Life Sciences, National Research Council. The facilities
are fully accredited by the American Association for the Accreditation of Laboratory Animal Care.

REFERENCES

Baskerville, A., S.P. Fisher-Hoch, G.H. Neild, and A.B. Dowsett (1985).
    Ultrastructural pathology of experimental Ebola haemorrhagic fever
    virus infection. J. Pathol. **147**:199-209.
Buchmeier, M.J., R.U. DeFries, J.B. McCormick, and M.P. Kiley (1983).
    Comparative analysis of the structural polypeptides of Ebola viruses
    from Sudan and Zaire. J. Infect. Dis. **147**:276-281.
Centers for Disease Control (1990a). Update: Ebola-related filovirus infec-
    tion in nonhuman primates and interim guidelines for handling nonhu-
    man primates during transit and quarantine. Morbidity and Mortality
    Weekly Reports **39**:22-24, 29.
Centers for Disease Control (1990b). Update: Filovirus infection in animal
    handlers. Morbidity and Mortality Weekly Reports **39**:221.
Centers for Disease Control (1990c). Update: Filovirus infections among
    persons with occupational exposure to nonhuman primates. Morbidity
    and Mortality Weekly Reports **39**:266-267, 273.
Cox, N.J., J.B. McCormick, K.M. Johnson, and M.P. Kiley (1983). Evidence
    for two subtypes of Ebola virus based on oligonucleotide mapping of
    RNA. J. Infect. Dis. **147**:272-275.
Gear, J.H.S. (1989). Clinical aspects of African viral hemorrhagic fevers.

Rev. Infect. Dis. **11**: Suppl. 4, S777-S782.

Gravell, M., W.T. London, M.E. Leon, A.E. Palmer, and R.S. Hamilton (1986). Differences among isolates of simian hemorrhagic fever (SHF) virus (42231). Proc. Soc. Exp. Biol. Med. **181**:112-119.

Jahrling, P.B., T.W. Geisbert, D.W. Dalgard, E.D. Johnson, T.G. Ksiazek, W.C. Hall, and C.J. Peters (1990). Preliminary report: Isolation of Ebola virus from monkeys imported to USA. Lancet **335**:502-505.

Johnson, B.K., L.G. Gitau, A. Gichogo, et al. (1982). Marburg, Ebola and Rift Valley fever virus antibodies in East African primates. Trans. R. Soc. Trop. Med. Hyg. **76**:307-310.

Kiley, M.P., E.T. Bowen, G.A. Eddy, M. Isaacson, K.M. Johnson, J.B. McCormick, F.A. Murphy, S.R. Pattyn, D. Peters, O.W. Prozesky, R.L. Regnery, D.I.H. Simpson, W. Slenczka, P. Sureau, G. van der Groen, P.A. Webb, and H. Wulff (1982). Filoviridae: taxonomic home for Marburg and Ebola viruses? Intervirology **18**:24-32.

Kiley, M.P., N.J. Cox, L.H. Elliott, A. Sanchez, R. DeFries, M.J. Buchmeier, D.D. Richman, and J.B. McCormick (1988). Physicochemical properties of Marburg virus: evidence for three distinct virus strains and their relationship to Ebola virus. J. Gen. Virol. **69**:1957-1967.

Ksiazek, T.G., P.E. Rollin, P.B. Jahrling, E. Johnson, D.W. Dalgard, and C.J. Peters (1992). Enzyme immunosorbent assay for Ebola virus antigens in tissues of infected primates. J. Clin. Microbiol. **30**:947-950.

London, W.T. (1977). Epizootiology, transmission and approach to prevention of fatal simian haemorrhagic fever in rhesus monkeys. Nature **268**:344-345.

Martini, G.A., and R. Siegert (eds.) (1971). *Marburg Virus Disease.* Berlin and New York: Springer-Verlag.

Pattyn, S.R. (ed.) (1978). *Ebola Virus Haemorrhagic Fever.* Amsterdam: Elsevier/North-Holland Biomedical Press.

Peters, C.J., E.D. Johnson, and K.T. McKee Jr. (1991). Filoviruses and management of viral hemorrhagic fevers. In *Textbook of Human Virology* (R.B. Belshe, ed.), second ed., Chap. 26 (pp. 699-712). St. Louis: Mosby-Year Book.

Peters, C.J., P.B. Jahrling, T.G. Ksiazek, E.D. Johnson, and H.W. Lupton (1992). Filovirus contamination of cell cultures. Devel. Biol. Stand., in press.

Richman, D.D., P.H. Cleveland, J.B. McCormick and K.M. Johnson (1983). Antigenic analysis of strains of Ebola virus: Identification of two Ebola virus serotypes. J. Infect. Dis. **147**:268-271.

Sanchez, A., M.P. Kiley, B.P. Holloway, J.B. McCormick, and D.D. Auperin (1989). The nucleoprotein gene of Ebola virus: Cloning, sequencing, and in vitro expression. Virology **170**:81-91.

Siegert, R. (1972). *Marburg Virus* [Virology Monograph 11, pp. 97-153]. Berlin and New York: Springer-Verlag.

Tauraso, N.M., M.G. Myers, K. McCarthy, and G.W. Tribe (1970). Simian hemorrhagic fever. In *Infections and Immunosuppression in Subhuman Primates* (H. Balner and W.I.B. Beveridge, eds.), pp. 101-109. Copenhagen: Munksgaard.

Trousdale, M.D., D.W. Trent, and A. Shelokov (1975). Simian hemorrhagic fever virus: a new togavirus (39111). Proc. Soc. Exp. Biol. Med. **150**:707-711.

16

Human Monkeypox, A Newly Discovered Human Virus Disease

FRANK FENNER

MONKEYPOX IN CAPTIVE MONKEYS

In 1958, Dr. P. von Magnus and his colleagues at the State Serum Institute in Copenhagen recovered an orthopoxvirus from the skin lesions of a cynomolgus monkey during an outbreak of a pox disease in their laboratory monkeys. They noted that the pocks it produced on the chorioallantoic membrane were very similar to those produced by variola virus (although subsequently differences were found), but unlike variola virus, the new virus produced large lesions in rabbit skin. It was a new orthopoxvirus, which they called "monkeypox virus". Over the next 10 years nine more outbreaks were recognized in captive primates in North America and Europe, all in monkeys shipped from Asia, except for a case in a chimpanzee very recently imported from Sierra Leone and a large outbreak in the Rotterdam Zoo in 1964-1965 which was introduced by two South American anteaters. No cases occurred in animal handlers, and no cases were reported in captive monkeys after 1968.

Retrospectively, the occurrence of these outbreaks, except the case in a chimpanzee from Sierra Leone, which was incubating the disease when captured, must have been due to infection of susceptible Asian monkeys, and the South American anteater, in transit. During the period 1958-1968, large numbers of monkeys were being imported into laboratories in Europe and North America for polio vaccine production and testing. Initially the conditions for shipping and handling in transit were deplorable, all kinds of animals from different places being crowded together. Presumably during this period Asian monkeys were in close enough contact with infectious African monkeys to contract the disease from them.

THE DISCOVERY OF HUMAN CASES OF MONKEYPOX

When the Intensified Smallpox Eradication Programme of the World

Health Organization was launched in 1967, the Chief of the Smallpox Eradication Unit, Dr. D. A. Henderson, recognized that it was essential to establish whether there was an animal reservoir of variola virus. Since primates were the most likely reservoir host, special attention was given to the only known orthopoxvirus of monkeys, monkeypox virus. A committee of poxvirologists was established and first met in Moscow in 1969. The meeting focused on monkeypox virus, and the committee agreed that it was definitely a species distinct from variola virus.

By 1970 smallpox was well on the way to eradication from West and Central Africa, but in August 1970 a "sporadic" case of "smallpox" was reported from a village in the tropical rain forests of Zaire, in a district where the last outbreak of smallpox had occurred in 1968. Scabs were collected and sent through WHO Headquarters to the WHO Collaborating Laboratory in Moscow, where Dr. S. S. Marennikova recognized that this case of "smallpox" was caused by monkeypox virus, and informed Henderson by telephone. Henderson immediately got in touch with colleagues in the other WHO Collaborating Laboratory in Atlanta, and told them of Marennikova's finding, for they had received some puzzling specimens from Liberia. The virus from Liberian specimens, and from specimens received shortly afterwards from Sierra Leone and Nigeria, also turned out to be monkeypox virus.

THE ORGANIZATION OF FIELD RESEARCH

In the early 1970s the eradication of smallpox remained the highest priority of the World Health Organization, but by 1976 global eradication was sufficiently well advanced for the Smallpox Eradication Unit to try to determine the public health importance of this newly discovered disease. A Coordination Meeting was held in the WHO Regional Office in Brazzaville, at which it became clear that the best surveillance program for human monkeypox was that operating in Zaire. Four years later, when the General Assembly of WHO declared smallpox to have been eradicated, it endorsed a proposal for further research on monkeypox, and a WHO-supported program was set up in Zaire. This program, planned by Dr. I. Arita and carried out under the direction of Dr. Z. Jezek of WHO Headquarters and Dr. Kalisa Ruti of the Zaire health services, operated until 1986. With laboratory assistance supplied by the WHO Collaborating Centers in Atlanta (chief, Dr. J. H. Nakano) and Moscow (chief, Dr. S. S. Marennikova), this program obtained a wealth of information that has been assembled in a monograph (Jezek and Fenner, 1988), in which a detailed account of the disease and all relevant references can be found.

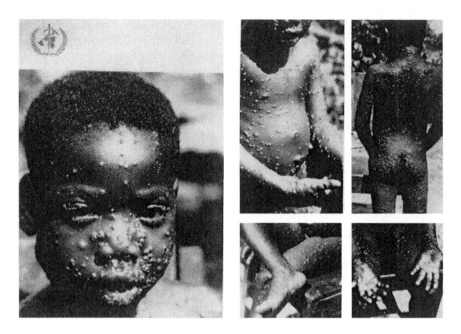

Figure 16.1 Monkeypox recognition card. Adapted from the smallpox recognition card used for surveillance during the Intensified Smallpox Eradication Programme of the World Health Organization, this card, in color, illustrates the clinical features of a typical case. It helped greatly in surveillance for cases of human monkeypox in Zaire. Courtesy of the World Health Organization.

THE INCIDENCE OF HUMAN MONKEYPOX

Table 16.1 sets out the geographic and annual incidence of human monkeypox over the period 1970-1986. Although occurring in several countries in West Africa, by far the highest incidence was in Zaire. This was partly due to the better surveillance in Zaire, which was based in health institutions and supported by experts from WHO, but is also a reflection of the much more extensive rain forests in Zaire, and the fact that such rain forest areas as are present in West Africa have been extensively cleared in the last 20 years.

CLINICAL FEATURES OF HUMAN MONKEYPOX

Clinically human monkeypox is very like smallpox (Fig. 16.1), and because of the importance of ensuring that smallpox cases were not still occurring after 1976, all suspected cases were subjected to laboratory confirmation. One clinical feature that occurred in most cases of human monkeypox but not in smallpox was gross

Table 16.1
Human Monkeypox Cases Reported in Western and Central Africa, 1970-1986*

Countries Reporting Cases of Human Monkeypox

	Cameroon	Central African Republic	Côte d'Ivoire	Liberia	Nigeria	Sierra Leone	Zaire	Total
Population in thousands (1980)*	8,554	2,290	8,247	1,871	80,555	3,296	28,532	124,791
Rain forest area (1980) (thousands of hectares)	17,920	3,590	4,458	2,000	5,950	740	105,650	140,308
Number of monkeypox cases								
1970	-	-	-	4	-	1	1	6
1971	-	-	1	-	2	-	-	3
1972	-	-	-	-	-	-	5	5
1973	-	-	-	-	-	-	3	3
1974	-	-	-	-	-	-	1	1
1975	-	-	-	-	-	-	3	3
1976	-	-	-	-	-	-	5	5
1977	-	-	-	-	-	-	6	6
1978	-	-	-	-	1	-	12	13
1979	2	-	-	-	-	-	8	10
1980	-	-	-	-	-	-	4	4
1981	-	-	1	-	-	-	7	8
1982	-	-	-	-	-	-	40	40
1983	-	-	-	-	-	-	84	84
1984	-	6	-	-	-	-	86	92
1985	-	-	-	-	-	-	62	62
1986	-	-	-	-	-	-	59	59
Total no. of cases	2	6	2	4	3	1	386	404

*From Jezek and Fenner, 1988.

lymphadenopathy, sometimes localized but often generalized. In the 404 cases that were carefully observed, no cases were seen that resembled flat or hemorrhagic smallpox. The case-fatality rate was about 10%, all in unvaccinated children between 3 months and 8 years of age. Epidemiologic and serologic studies indicated that a few subclinical cases occurred; some 5% of unvaccinated close household contacts of clinical cases showed serologic evidence of infection but no evidence of disease or pockmarks.

EPIDEMIOLOGIC FEATURES OF HUMAN MONKEYPOX

The vast majority of cases of human monkeypox occurred in children living in small villages in the tropical rain forests. There was no clearcut seasonal incidence, but more cases occurred in June through August, the period of maximum agricultural activity and hunting. The most interesting and important epidemiologic feature, however, was the pattern of transmission. The sporadic nature of most cases and the pattern of distribution of the disease indicated that human monkeypox was a zoonosis. However, among 338 cases that were intensively investigated in Zaire, there were 203 isolated cases (i.e., primary cases infected from an animal source), and 135 cases that occurred in clusters of two or more cases (Table 16.2). The incubation period in three cases where exact data were available was 12-14 days—that is, the same as in smallpox. Extrapolating from evidence that the extremes of the incubation period in smallpox were 7 and 19 days, it was found that the rash-to-rash intervals in the 135 cases that occurred in clusters gave a bimodal distribution. Forty-two cases occurring with an interval of 7 days or less were classified as coprimary cases, possibly infected from the same animal source. The rest, with intervals of up to 22 days, were classified as secondary cases—that is, cases infected from a human source. There was evidence of serial transmission from one case to another in 24 of the 103 secondary cases, but never was a chain of transmission main-

Table 16.2
Monkeypox Patients by Year, Origin of Infection, and Generation Rank*

	Number of Cases Infected by Presumed Source						
Year	Animal		Human In Generation				Total cases
	Primary	Co-primary	First	Second	Third	Fourth	
1981	6	-	1	-	-	-	7
1982	22	2	13	3	-	-	40
1983	47	11	19	3	3	1	84
1984	52	10	18	6	-	-	86
1985	40	7	11	4	-	-	62
1986	36	12	7	3	1	-	59
Total	203	42	69	19	4	1	338

*From Jezek and Fenner, 1988.

tained for more than 4 generations.

Vaccination, which protects against monkeypox as well as it protected against smallpox, had been continued in Zaire until 1980. However, although the proportion of unvaccinated children steadily increased from 1980, the maximum incidence of infection occurred in 1984, and the incidence fell in 1985 and 1986, in spite of continued intensive surveillance. Based on available data on transmission and taking a "worst case" scenario, the probable rate of case-to-case transmission in the total absence of vaccination was modeled. Although in the model an occasional large outbreak occurred, and some chains lasted for as long as 14 generations, the basic reproductive rate was less than one. This agrees with the intuitive extrapolation from what is known of the history of the people of the affected regions. It is reasonable to speculate that monkeypox has been occurring as a zoonosis, with occasional secondary cases, for as long as humans have been living in the tropical rain forests, but it has never been recognized as an infectious disease like smallpox, which caused epidemics whenever it entered a village.

THE ECOLOGY OF MONKEYPOX VIRUS

Laboratory studies showed that monkeypox virus had a wide host range. Over a period of some 7 years, sera were collected from a wide range of wild and domestic animals in the Zaire rain forests, in the vicinity of villages where cases of human monkeypox had occurred. As a result primates of 10 species, belonging to five genera, have been shown to be infected with monkeypox virus under natural conditions. Most of these are rain forest species; one that is not, and may be significant as the probable source of infection of Asian monkeys in transit to the laboratory, is *Cercopithecus aethiops*, the species of African monkey most widely used in the laboratory. It was difficult to see how primates, animals that moved in small self-contained groups and had a relatively long life span, could be the reservoir hosts of a virus that caused acute nonpersistent infections. A large number of several species of commensal rats were tested, but were all negative. However, positive results were obtained with a high proportion of sera from four species of squirrel of the genera *Funisciurus* and *Heliosciurus* (up to 49% of one collection of sera from *Funisciurus lemniscatus*). Further, in 1986 monkeypox virus was recovered from the tissues of a sick *Funisciurus anerythrus* that had been captured in an oil palm plantation near a village. Studies of the ecology of these squirrels shows that they occur in considerable numbers in the agricultural areas close to villages in the rain forest. They are often captured for food, especially by boys making their first ventures in hunting.

CONDITIONS RELEVANT TO HUMAN INFECTION WITH MONKEYPOX VIRUS

Based on experience gained from the ecologic surveys carried out in Zaire, a number of conclusions can be drawn concerning the natural history of monkeypox virus. (1) Monkeypox virus circulates among mammals inhabiting arboreal levels of the forest; terrestrial rodents and domestic animals do not participate in the cycle. (2) Squirrels, especially those of the genus *Funisciurus*, are important hosts and circumstantial evidence indicates that they are the reservoir host in the secondary forests surrounding human settlements. (3) Monkeypox virus-specific antibodies were found in primates that dwell in forest strata also occupied by squirrels. However, comparison of their lifespan and antibody prevalence rates with those of squirrels suggested that monkeys were infected with monkeypox virus by at least an order of magnitude less frequently than *Funisciurus*. (4) There is no evidence that arthropods participate in the circulation of monkeypox virus. (5) The absence of cases of human monkeypox does not necessarily mean that the virus does not circulate in wildlife in that area, since customs or nutritional habits may restrict contact between infected animals and humans.

Conditions that facilitate the occurrence of human infections with monkeypox virus include the enzootic circulation of the virus in wild animals in the agricultural areas and forest surrounding human settlements, the use of meat of wild animals as an important source of animal protein, and close contact of humans with wild animals, including such activities as trapping, killing, skinning, playing with carcasses, and the consumption of raw or partially cooked meat.

PREVENTION OF HUMAN MONKEYPOX

Vaccination with smallpox vaccine would undoubtedly be protective, but the disease is so rare (average annual incidence 0.63 cases per 10,000 population per year in the highest incidence area in Africa), and occurs among a population so much in need of other forms of medical intervention (malaria 32.1, helminthiasis 27.6 per 10,000 per year), that the benefits of vaccination do not warrant its expense. Control therefore depends on health education aimed at changing habitual eating customs of the populations at risk (without prejudicing the adequacy of their diet), so that they do not come into contact with infected animals.

THE FUTURE OF HUMAN MONKEYPOX

A striking feature of the incidence of human monkeypox since its discovery in 1970 is that only one case has been reported from countries of western Africa since 1978 and only two others since eight cases were reported from four different countries in 1970-1971 (see Table 16.1). To some extent this may reflect the absence of adequate surveillance in all countries except Zaire, but it is difficult to believe that this is the complete explanation. There has been great destruction of the forests in most countries in West Africa since 1970, and it is possible that this has greatly diminished the wildlife source of the virus, or the contact between man and infected animals.

Conversion of forest into agricultural land is less advanced in Zaire, and the changes observed there so far may, if anything, have increased contact between man and infected animals. Conversion of the primary forest into secondary forest creates a favorable habitat for various species of *Funisciurus* that appear to be reservoir hosts of monkeypox virus.

On the other hand, intensified agricultural development turns hunters into agricultural laborers and farmers and increases the concentration of population on the newly exploited areas to the extent that the surrounding forest no longer serves as an useful source of animal protein. In these circumstances animal husbandry is expanded, thus decreasing the chances of contracting monkeypox from infected wild animals. In this sense human monkeypox may become a "disappearing" disease.

REFERENCE

Jezek, Z., and F. Fenner (1988). *Human Monkeypox* [Monographs in Virology, 17]. Basel: S. Karger.

17

Seal Plague Virus

BRIAN W.J. MAHY

In 1988, beginning about April and reaching a peak in August, several thousand dead seals were washed up on the shores of Europe. In the U.K. alone, 2,800 seals were found dead on the coast. Most were concentrated in East Anglia, where more than half of the seal population was affected. Towards the end of the epidemic, seals also began to be washed up around the Irish Sea, and there were considerable numbers found up in the Hebrides, the Orkney Islands, and the north of Scotland. Deaths also occurred in the Netherlands, Germany, and in various areas around the North Sea. The animals that actually washed up probably represented a third of the total numbers of dead seals. All the dead animals belonged to the species known as common, or harbor seals (*Phoca vitulina*). Relatively few deaths have been reported among seals in the United Kingdom since the end of 1989 and it may well be that, like many of these plagues, this particular episode has ended. A similar disease in seals in Lake Baikal, Siberia, was seen somewhat earlier than the European epizootic, in December 1987 (Grachev et al., 1989; Likhoshway et al., 1989; Osterhaus et al., 1989a, 1989b). The disease was also found in porpoises (*Phocoena phocoena*) (Kennedy et al., 1988) and more recently evidence was obtained of a similar infection in Mediterranean dolphins (*Stenella coeruleoalba*) (Domingo et al., 1990).

The clinical signs that were found in the seals included respiratory distress and nasal discharge. On necropsy, there was severe pneumonia, with evidence of bronchiolar damage and intracytoplasmic inclusions in bronchiolar cells. The symptoms resembled those of canine distemper; in addition, there were signs of central nervous system involvement and damage.

In the past, the best known virus causing disease in seals was influenza A (H7N7), a strain of which caused severe disease outbreaks in early 1980 (Geraci et al., 1982). However, in 1988 the disease was not due to influenza virus, and the first virus to be isolated from the diseased seals was a picornavirus. This led to my being telephoned and asked whether Pirbright Laboratory, the high-security animal virus facility in England, could have a look at this picornavirus from seals to see whether it was related to foot and mouth disease virus, a notorious picornavirus of livestock. Subsequently, a herpesvirus was also isolated from the seals, but the disease symptoms suggested the possibility that a morbillivirus could be involved (Osterhaus and Vedder, 1988). This proved to be the case, as I shall describe.

Morbilliviruses are RNA viruses that form a genus within the family Paramyxoviridae, which includes many viruses that cause respiratory disease. The morbilliviruses include the viruses of measles, canine distemper, and two diseases of livestock: rinderpest, in bovine species, and peste des petit ruminants, in sheep and goats. The virus I will discuss was called seal plague by Gordon Scott, of the Centre for Tropical Veterinary Medicine in Edinburgh. He recently delivered an interesting lecture about plagues over the centuries and noted that there have been 32 plagues between 1977 and 1987 alone, including a large number of animal plagues. An alternative name that has been suggested for the disease is phocid distemper (Table 17.1).

If we do not confine ourselves to human disease, probably the greatest plague of all time was rinderpest, or cattle plague (Scott, 1985). In South Africa during the 1920s, this virus was killing roughly two million cattle every year. Rinderpest was so serious that it led to the formation of the State Veterinary Service in the United Kingdom in 1867, as well as the State Veterinary Services in several other European countries. These actions eventually resulted in the elimination of the disease from Europe by slaughter. Now rinderpest is controlled by an excellent tissue culture vaccine developed by Plowright and Ferris (1962). So although rinderpest, or cattle plague, was a very serious disease, it is now under control in most parts of the world. It still causes occasional very threatening epidemic waves in Africa and India, however. The cause of rinderpest, of course, was the subject of a tremendous amount of scrutiny. I am always rather amused by a contemporary picture of the famous nineteenth-century microbiologist Robert Koch looking for the causative agent of rinderpest under his light microscope (Fig. 17.1). We now know that he would not have been able to see it that way, because rinderpest is caused by a virus which, as I mentioned, belongs to an antigenically related genus of paramyxoviruses known

Table 17.1   Morbilliviruses

Virus	Principal Host
Measles	Man, monkey
Canine Distemper	Dog
Rinderpest	Cattle, other ruminants
Peste des petits ruminants	Sheep, goats
Phocid distemper/seal plague	Seals

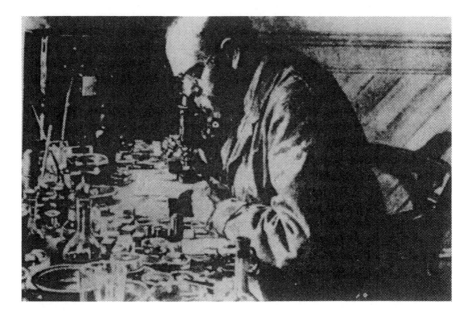

Figure 17.1   Koch looking for rinderpest (cattle plague) microbe

as the morbilliviruses. At present, this genus consists of four members, but I am now suggesting, and will discuss evidence to show, that there is at least a fifth virus, namely seal plague. There may also be others out in the sea mammal population.

The morbilliviruses, measles of man, distemper of dogs (CDV), rinderpest (RPV) in bovine species, and peste des petit ruminants (PPR) of sheep and goats, form a very closely linked group, both genetically and antigenically. Cross reactions occur in many of the antigenic sites so that vaccines against one of these viruses frequently protect against another.

Peste des petit ruminants is the least familiar of the group. It was described as the fourth member of the group by Paul Gibbs and others (Gibbs et al., 1979), we now know from genetic analysis that it is distinct from the other viruses. PPR virus is found to cause economically important diseases in sheep and goats in Africa and in India (Shaila et al., 1989). In Africa, when one sees rinderpest virus in sheep and goats, it seems to be an inapparent infection without disease. Cattle can be infected by rinderpest virus from sheep, and the cattle develop a serious disease. PPR virus does not infect cattle, but appears to cause disease in the local species of sheep and goats.

The organization of the genomes of all the morbilliviruses is similar (Barrett et al., 1991). These (as all paramyxoviruses) are negative strand RNA viruses. In the conventions of virology, positive strand RNA is the kind that can code directly for proteins (in

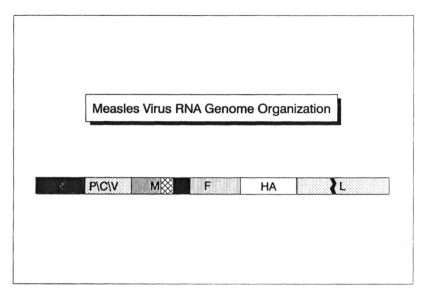

Figure 17.2   Measles virus RNA genome organization

other words, it can serve as a messenger RNA). The negative strand is therefore the RNA strand with a sequence complementary to the positive strand (imagining the positive and negative RNA as if they were the two strands of a hypothetical double helix). As the cell has no mechanism for copying negative strand RNA into a positive strand, this function is carried out by a viral RNA polymerase, which is contained in the virion. Paramyxoviruses differ from the similar-looking orthomyxoviruses (such as influenza), which are also negative strand viruses, by having their genome in a single long piece of RNA rather than in segments. The genome of morbilliviruses, typified by measles, consists of 15,000 bases which encode six structural proteins, and at least two nonstructural proteins (Fig. 17.2). The most prominent protein produced is the nucleocapsid (N) protein; a phosphoprotein (P) and two nonstructural proteins called C and V are made from overlapping reading frames in the same gene (Cattaneo et al., 1989). There are also a matrix (M) protein, involved in viral assembly in the host cell; a fusion (F) protein, which is important in viral interactions with cells, including transport and release; a hemagglutinin (H), important in attachment to host cells; and a large polymerase (L) protein. The only grossly noticeable protein difference between the four morbilliviruses is that the N protein of rinderpest migrates more slowly on polyacrylamide gels than that of the other viruses; this seems to be true of all the strains we have seen.

When we came to analyze samples from the seals, we began with serum samples collected from sick or dead seals. Material like this is often poor, and it is very difficult to know what the condition of the animals was at the time the samples were collected. The sera were analyzed using two types of tests to detect antibodies, a virus neutralization test and an ELISA test, both using rinderpest antigen which was grown in cell culture. Antibodies to canine distemper virus were tested in parallel by Osterhaus' group in Holland.

A striking observation was that a number of gray seal populations (*Halichoerus grypus*, a different species from the harbor seal), which apparently had no disease, typically showed positive reactions against morbilliviruses. This was not true of the harbor seals, where we found both disease and antibodies. We obtained over 1,000 different seal sera from animals that had been found dead in different areas around the coast of Europe. Selecting 180 representative sera from these, we found that 50 percent of the sera showed positive neutralization tests against both canine distemper and rinderpest viruses, so they appeared to have antibodies that would inhibit either of these two viruses. Ten percent of the sera were negative to both viruses. Some additional sera were positive for either rinderpest or canine distemper, but not both. Although not definitive, this suggested that the seal virus had antigenic determinants which were shared with both canine distemper and rinderpest.

When we tested sera taken from harbor seals before the epidemic began, we found no antibodies reacting with morbilliviruses. We assume that these are examples of animals without exposure to virus. There were also negative sera from sick or dead animals during the epidemic; there, we assume, the animals probably died in the early stages of infection before an antibody response developed. Finally, there were healthy animals with low titers of antibody, and sick or dead animals with high ELISA titers.

Using a different type of test, indirect ELISA (Bostock et al., 1990), we could differentiate the other morbilliviruses from one another. Relative reactivity of each antigen for the antibodies in the seal serum could be determined by comparing dilutions of each antigen. Antibodies to a goat PPR vaccine from Nigeria react very strongly against PPR antigen, but show very little reaction against rinderpest virus and only a small reaction against canine distemper. By contrast, with a bovine rinderpest vaccine strain, there is considerable cross-reaction against PPR, and a much stronger reaction against rinderpest, but little reaction against canine distemper. The seal serum, on the other hand, showed considerable cross-reaction against all three of these morbilliviruses, again suggesting that the seal virus is related to these viruses but is not one of the three.

Subsequently, sera collected from seals from other parts of Northern Europe were examined for the presence of antibodies using both CDV and RPV indirect ELISA with protein A and anti-seal conjugates as well as virus neutralization tests for both viruses (Osterhaus et al., 1989c). This study confirmed that the virus that infected

European seals induced antibodies that cross-neutralized both CDV and RPV. It also confirmed the specificity of the CDV and RPV ELISAs for detecting the presence of antibodies to the seal virus and, for sera collected after the onset of the epizootic, the correlation between positive ELISA and virus neutralization tests was high (Osterhaus et al., 1989c).

We went on to look more specifically by genetic hybridization using cloned DNA for the nucleoprotein (N) genes from rinderpest and PPR. This readily discriminates between the different morbilliviruses (Diallo et al., 1989). We had already used this method to advantage in studying a disease outbreak in Sri Lanka which occurred in 1987 (Anderson et al., 1990). In that outbreak, we were able to show that the virus causing a disease in goats there was rinderpest, rather than PPR that had been introduced from India probably by soldiers. This success made us confident that the test could distinguish the viruses.

We took a series of morbillivirus probes, including cloned F and N genes from the three animal morbilliviruses, and reacted them with RNA extracted from spleen tissue of diseased seals. Controls of known morbilliviruses gave the expected results, with specificity for each virus. The seal tissue gave a slight reaction against the F gene probe of canine distemper and rinderpest, but strong reactions against the N genes of both rinderpest and PPR, which we would never see if the seal virus were actually one of these two viruses. There was some reaction against rinderpest F gene. These data supported the hypothesis that we had a novel morbillivirus (Mahy et al., 1988). More specific genetic probes that we prepared later seem to bear this out. A virus was isolated in Hannover from tissues of a diseased seal (Liess et al., 1989) and a specific cDNA clone representing the P gene was prepared from this virus (Haas et al., 1991). The nucleotide sequence of this clone was found to share only about 80 percent homology with a similar clone derived from canine distemper virus. Whereas the seal virus P gene clone hybridized strongly with tissues from many different diseased seals from various parts of Europe, a P gene clone from canine distemper virus showed no hybridization (Barrett et al., 1991a). Sequencing studies in other laboratories confirmed the distinction between seal plague virus and canine distemper virus (Curran et al., 1990).

We then tested a specific radioimmunoprecipitation assay. The idea was to see whether the seal sera contained antibodies that would specifically react with and precipitate the F proteins of canine distemper virus or rinderpest, produced by introducing these viral genes into cells. We did this because it appears, from a number of studies, that neutralizing antibodies are directed primarily against the F protein, and evidence from Norrby's group suggests that anti-F protein antibodies alone will protect against canine distemper

(Norrby et al., 1986). We found a lot of variation in the seal sera, but, with some exceptions, most of the sera were able to immunoprecipitate F proteins from one or more of the morbilliviruses.

Overall, there is a good correlation between antibody titers in the rinderpest virus ELISA, and radioimmunoprecipitation assay using the cloned rinderpest F gene. Neutralization titers against rinderpest virus are also fairly well correlated with radioimmunoprecipitation assay against the N gene. The specifics are not clarified because only recently have we been able to grow the virus in cell culture. Now that the virus is finally cultivated in vitro, more precise studies are underway to define its relationship to the other viruses (Harder et al., 1991). All of this only goes to show the difficulties of studying viruses in the process of emergence.

What is unusual is that we can see instances where sera from gray seals, particularly, will be strongly positive against morbilliviruses, but the seal, although presumably infected, is completely healthy and shows no evidence of disease. We suspect that gray seals may not be significantly affected by this infection. One possible scenario is that the virus has been present for some time in the gray seal population, and its moving into the common, or harbor seal, caused this particular epidemic (Osterhaus et al., 1989c).

Another possibility, which has been raised by Goodhart (1988), is that neither species is the primary source of the virus. He noted that another seal species, the harp seal (*Pagophilus groenlandicus*), which is normally confined to the much colder waters up in the north, for some reason in 1988 came down in large numbers to the North Sea. Studies of harp seals collected in Greenland in 1985 and 1986 revealed antibodies to a morbillivirus in 12 out of 40 animals tested (Dietz et al., 1989), which supports the Goodhart hypothesis. The only other species that has been implicated and is known to have been diseased is the porpoise. At least two or three porpoises have been found with similar sorts of symptoms as were seen in the harbor seals (Kennedy et al., 1988).

This is an example of a virus in the process of emergence. It is also likely that this virus was a notable example of interspecies transfer, perhaps originating in another species of marine mammal (Likhoshway et al., 1989; Osterhaus et al., 1989a,c). There is every evidence that the seal plague morbillivirus is present in the sea mammal population, and there could well be other morbilliviruses in these populations. For example, the disease in seals (*Phoca sibirica*) in Lake Baikal, Siberia, was originally thought to be caused by the same virus as is responsible for seal disease in other parts of Northern Europe. Using a panel of monoclonal antibodies against canine distemper virus, however, the Siberian virus was clearly closely related to canine distemper virus, unlike the European seal plague virus (Osterhaus et al., 1989a). Once the seal plague virus was isolated in cell culture (Liess et al., 1989), monoclonal antibodies were prepared against the virus. These gave a similar pattern of reaction against sixteen different seal virus isolates (Harder et al., 1991), but the Siberian isolate was different, reacted like canine distemper virus, and could be easily distinguished (Barrett et al., 1991), Visser et al., 1990). Molecular genetic studies also confirm that the Siberian virus is more closely related to canine distemper virus than to other seal plague viruses from Northern Europe (Barrett et al., 1991). Indeed, it has been suggested that the Lake Baikal seals may have been infected by land animals infected with canine distemper virus (Grachev et al., 1989). The number of viruses recently found in dolphins and seals suggests that the sea mammal population might contain a number of poorly characterized viruses that are in many cases closely related to known mammalian viruses. This population, therefore, may be a viral reservoir of considerable potential significance. The patterns of interspecies transfer of these viruses in marine populations are still largely unknown.

ACKNOWLEDGMENTS

There was considerable collaboration in the early stages of this study with John Harwood and Sheila Anderson of the Sea Mammal Research Unit in Cambridge and Dr. Ab Osterhaus in Utrecht, Holland. In Pirbright, I thank John McCauley, John Crowther, Chris Bostock, Euan Anderson, John Anderson, Paul Thomas, Sharon Evans, Shaila Subbarao, and especially Tom Barrett, who were all involved in these studies. In Atlanta, I thank Bill Bellini and Joann House.

REFERENCES

Anderson, E.C., A. Hassan, T. Barrett, and J. Anderson (1990). Observation on the pathogenicity and transmissibility for sheep and goats of the strain of virus isolated during the rinderpest outbreak in Sri Lanka in 1987. Vet. Microbiol. 21:309-318.

Barrett, T., S.M. Subbarao, G.J. Belsham, and B.W.J. Mahy (1991). The molecular biology of the morbilliviruses. In The Paramyxoviruses (D. Kingsbury, ed.), pp. 82-103. New York: Plenum.

Barrett, T., J. Crowther, A.D.M.E. Osterhaus, S.M. Subbarao, J. Groen, L. Haas, L.V. Mamaev, A.M. Titenko, I.K.G. Visser, and C.J. Bostock (1992). Molecular and serological studies on the recent seal virus epizootics in Europe and Siberia. Sci. Total Environ., in press.

Bostock, C.J., T. Barrett, and J.R. Crowther (1990). Characterisation of the European seal morbillivirus [Advances in Veterinary Virology: Proceedings of the 1st Congress of the European Society for Veterinary Virology, Liege, 5-7 April 1989]. Vet. Microbiol. 23:351-360.

Cattaneo, R., K. Kaelin, K. Baczko, and M.A. Billeter (1989). Measles virus editing provides an additional cysteine rich protein. Cell 56:759-764.

Curran, M.D., D. O'Loan, and B.K. Rima (1990). Nucleotide sequence analysis of phocine distemper virus reveals its distinctions from CDV. Vet. Rec. **127**:430-431.

Diallo, A., T. Barrett, S.M. Subbarao, and W.P. Taylor (1989). Differentiation of rinderpest and peste des petits ruminants viruses using specific cDNA clones. J. Virol. Meth. **23**:127-137.

Dietz, R., C.T. Ansen, P. Have, and M.-P. Heide-Jørgensen (1989). Clue to seal epizootic? Nature **338**:627.

Domingo, M., L. Ferrer, M. Pumarola, A. Marco, J. Plana, S. Kennedy, M. McAlisky, and B.K. Rima (1990). Morbillivirus in dolphins. Nature **348**:21.

Geraci, J.R., D.J. St. Aubin, I.K. Barker, R.G. Webster, V.S. Hinshaw, W.J. Bean, H.L. Ruhnke, J.H. Prescott, G. Early, A.S. Baker, S. Madoff, and R.T. Schooley (1982). Mass mortality of harbor seals: pneumonia associated with influenza A virus. Science **215**:129-1131.

Gibbs, E.J.P., W.P. Taylor, M.J.P. Lawman, and J. Bryant (1979). Classification of peste des petits ruminants as the fourth member of the genus morbillivirus. Intervirology **11**:268-274.

Goodhart, C.B. (1988). Did virus transfer from harp seals to common seals? Nature **336**:21.

Grachev, M.A., V.P. Kumarev, L.V. Mamaev, V.L. Zorin, L.V. Baranova, N.N. Denikina, S.I. Belikov, E.A. Petrov, V.S. Kolesnik, R.S. Kolesnik, V.M. Dorofeev, A.M. Beim, V.N. Kudelin, F.G. Nagieva, and V.N. Sidorov (1989). Distemper virus in Baikal seals. Nature **338**:209.

Haas, L., S.M. Subbarao, T. Harder, B. Liess, and T. Barrett (1991). Detection of phocid distemper virus RNA in seal tissues using slot hybridisation and the polymerase chain reaction amplification assay: genetic evidence that the virus is distinct from canine distemper virus. J. Gen. Virol. **72**:825-832.

Harder, T.C., V. Moennig, I. Greiser-Wilke, T. Barrett, and B. Liess (1991). Analysis of antigenic differences between sixteen phocine distemper virus isolates and other morbilliviruses. Arch. Virol. **118**:261-268.

Kennedy, S., J.A. Smyth, P.F. Cush, S.J. McCullough, G.M. Allan, and S. McQuaid (1988). Viral distemper now found in porpoises. Nature **336**:21.

Liess, B., H.R. Frey, and A. Zaghawa (1989). Morbillivirus in seals: isolation and some growth characteristics in cell cultures. Deut. Tierarztl. Wchschr. **96**:180-182.

Likhoshway, Ye.V., M.A. Grachev, V.P. Kumarev, Yu.V. Solodun, O.A. Goldberg, O.I. Belykh, F.G. Nagieva, V.G. Nikulina, and B.S. Kolesnik (1989). Baikal seal virus. Nature **339**:266.

Mahy, B.W.J., T. Barrett, S. Evans, E.C. Anderson, and C.J. Bostock (1988). Characterization of a seal morbillivirus. Nature **336**:115.

Norrby, E., G. Utter, C. Orvell, and M.J.G. Appel (1986). Protection against canine distemper virus in dogs after immunisation with isolated fusion protein. J. Virol. **58**:536-541.

Osterhaus, A.D.M.E., J. Groen, P. De Vries, F.G.C.M. Uytdehaag, B. Klingeborn, and R. Zarnke (1988). Canine distemper virus in seals. Nature **335**:403-404.

Osterhaus, A.D.M.E., and E.J. Vedder (1988). Identification of virus causing recent seal deaths. Nature **335**:20.

Osterhaus, A.D.M.E., H.W.J. Broeders, J. Groen, F.G.C.M. Uytdehaag, I.K.G. Visser, M.W.G. Bildt, C. Van De Orvell, V.P. Kumarev, and V.L. Zorin (1989a). Different morbilliviruses in European and Siberian seals. Vet. Rec. **125**:647-648.

Osterhaus, A.D.M.E., J. Groen, F.G.C.M. Uytdehaag, I.K.G. Visser, M.W.G. v.d. Bildt, A. Bergman, and B. Klingeborn (1989b). Distemper virus in Baikal seals. Nature **338**:209-210.

Osterhaus, A.D.M.E., J. Groen, F.G.C.M. Uytdehaag, I.K.G. Visser, E.J. Vedder, J. Crowther, and C.J. Bostock (1989c). Morbillivirus infections in European seals before 1988. Vet. Rec. **125**:326.

Plowright, W., and R.D. Ferris (1962). Studies with rinderpest virus in tissue culture. The use of attenuated culture virus as a vaccine for cattle. Res. Vet. Sci. **3**:172-182.

Rima, B.K., S.L. Cosby, N. Duffy, C. Lyons, D. O'Loan, S. Kennedy, S.J. McCullough, J.A. Smyth, and F. McNeilly (1990). Humoral immune responses in seals infected by phocine distemper virus. Res. Vet. Sci. **49**:114-116.

Scott, G.R. (1985). Rinderpest in the 1980s. Progr. Vet. Microbiol. Immun. **1**:145-174.

Shaila, M.S., V. Purushothaman, D. Bhavasar, K. Venugopal, and R.A. Venkatesan (1989). Peste des petits ruminants of sheep in India. Vet. Rec. **125**:602.

Visser, I.K.G., V.P. Kumarev, C. Van De Orvell, P. De Vries, H.W.J. Broeders, M.W.G. Van De Bildt, J. Groen, and J.S. Teppema (1990). Comparison of two morbilliviruses isolated from seals during outbreaks of distemper in North West Europe and Siberia. Arch. Virol. **111**:149-164.

18

Canine Parvovirus 2: A Probable Example of Interspecies Transfer

COLIN R. PARRISH

The virus now known as canine parvovirus type 2 (CPV-2) first emerged around 1978 as an epidemic disease of dogs. The attention and concern it aroused when it first appeared was reflected by a flurry of press stories in a variety of media. Even the *National Enquirer* ran headlines of the sort "killer virus turns dog's heart to sponges".

After this understandable initial reaction, the interest has waned. There are reasonably good vaccines that control the disease under most circumstances, and the virus itself is now accepted as an endemic canine pathogen in most countries in the world. I will take the opportunity here to describe this virus and what we know of its origins.

The parvoviruses are a large group of very small viruses, found in a wide variety of hosts. Among human parvoviruses are B19 virus, associated with erythema contagiosum (Fifth Disease of childhood), and human adeno-associated virus (AAV), but other mammals also have a wide range of parvoviruses. There are two canine parvoviruses; in addition to CPV-2, there is another parvovirus of dogs, described around 1970 and now usually called minute virus of canines (MVC), or CPV-1. It is not closely related to CPV-2. Other naturally occurring parvoviruses of carnivores include feline panleukopenia virus (FPV), which causes a disease of cats sometimes known as feline distemper, as well as raccoon parvovirus and mink enteritis virus.

Canids, the members of the family Canidae, include foxes, dogs, and jackals. Cats and their relatives, constituting the family known as the Felidae, are classified in a separate family from the dogs and their relatives (Canidae). Felids all appear susceptible to FPV, as are the Procyonidae (the carnivore family that includes raccoons and relatives). A parvovirus of raccoons has been known for many years, and may be the same as FPV. It is not known whether pandas can become infected with FPV, but I suspect not, which is interesting because some classifications place at least the lesser panda with raccoons in the Procyonidae. There may be a poorly characterized parvovirus of civets, another carnivore that is sometimes called a cat but which is more closely related to the mongoose, and is in a separate family from the Felidae. Not all carnivores have known parvoviruses, although many species have not been tested. At present, however, there is no known parvovirus that affects bears or seals.

Both European and American mink are infected by a parvovirus called mink enteritis virus (MEV), which was first observed in Ontario, Canada in 1947 as a cause of severe, often fatal, diarrhea in ranch mink. Subsequently, the disease caused by MEV was seen in farmed mink in many countries of the world, including Scandinavia. Whether MEV was a new virus in 1947 (i.e., newly emerged in mink), or whether its appearance was due to some change in a preexisting virus of mink, was not known at that time.

I mentioned earlier that canine parvoviruses can infect various members of the Canidae, including domestic dogs and their South American relatives, as well as an animal called the raccoon dog (*Nyctereutes procyonoides*), a primitive canine from Asia and eastern Russia. At least one parvovirus infects foxes. Its identification is not definite, but present evidence suggests that it is very similar to the feline virus. This may seem surprising, because foxes are also members of the Canidae. It therefore appears that the canine parvoviruses infect the wolflike canids and the South American canids, whereas the foxes are affected by the FPV-like virus.

EMERGENCE OF CANINE PARVOVIRUS (CPV-2)

Canine parvovirus type 2 appears to have emerged as a totally new virus of dogs around 1976 to 1978 (Parrish, 1990). There is no evidence for the existence of the virus before the early 1970s. A paper that reports serological evidence for infection of dogs in Greece around 1974 is the earliest report of the virus, and there is no evidence for infection of dogs before that time (Parrish et al., 1988b; reviewed in Parrish, 1990). Based on retrospective serological surveys, which tested for antibody to CPV in stored sera from dogs, the next confirmed positive we know of comes from Belgium and dates from October 1976. Other similar studies have identified the virus in sera from the Netherlands from 1977, in Australia from May 1978, and in Japan from about July 1978. In the United States, the first positive sera in domestic dogs dated from July 1978, and positives were first found in sera collected in 1979 and 1980 from wild populations of coyotes and wolves, respectively. The rapid spread of the virus in the coyote population after 1979 suggests that it was a recent introduction in late 1978.

CPV-2 spread globally within a year or two of its first emergence in the dog population (Parrish et al., 1988b). Most of this spread occurred during 1978. CPV-2 is now endemic in every country where it has been tested for. More recently, slight variants, which I have designated CPV-2a and CPV-2b, appear to have subsequently displaced the original CPV-2 in the dog population (Parrish et al., 1985; Parrish et al., 1988b; Parrish et al., 1991). Work on this virus in my own laboratory began with a comparison of CPV-2 with the previously known feline and mink viruses. The three viruses are very similar. Initially, specific monoclonal antibodies were prepared that could be used to distinguish CPV from the feline, mink, and raccoon parvoviruses. This was possible since CPV has an antigenic determinant that is not present on the other viruses. Conversely, another antigenic site is present on most feline, mink, and raccoon viruses, but not on CPV.

DISPLACEMENT OF CPV-2 BY VARIANT STRAINS

Encouraged by these results with antigenic analysis, we decided to analyze field isolates of CPV-2. As my laboratory became established in research on this virus, people would send various tissue or fecal samples to be tested for virus. The virus is present in feces of infected animals, and it is probably through infected feces that the virus is usually transmitted from infected to uninfected dogs.

As we began to characterize these field isolates using our monoclonal antibodies, something surprising turned up. The viruses isolated from samples collected after 1980 all appeared to be antigenically different from the viruses that were collected before that year. Additional monoclonal antibodies prepared against one of these post-1980 isolates revealed the presence of a new antigenic determinant in the later virus isolates, which was not present in the pre-1980 isolates. This was not due to a geographic difference, as these isolates had all been collected in the United States. Apparently there was some sort of change in the virus type going on during this period. Along with the antigenic change, there was also a corresponding change in the DNA sequence, which is revealed by digestion with the *Hph*I restriction enzyme and by DNA sequence analysis. I designated the new virus CPV-2a (Parrish et al., 1985).

A collaborative study involving our laboratory and other scientists in the United States, Denmark, France, Belgium, Japan, and Australia showed that CPV-2a did not appear before 1979. Most viruses that were collected in 1978 and 1979 were CPV-2, the original type. By 1979 and 1980, a change of the virus type was beginning; after that, the balance shifted rapidly. In Japanese isolates from 1980, CPV-2 outnumbered CPV-2a by 5 to 1. However, in Denmark,

CPV-2a had already displaced the original strain by 1980, the earliest year for which isolates are available. Only 4 out of 125 Danish CPV isolates from that year that were tested with the monoclonal antibodies were of the original type; the rest were type 2a. By the mid-1980s, the shift was complete worldwide, with an apparently complete replacement of the original virus type by CPV-2a.

More recently a further strain of CPV-2 has been recognized as first being present around 1984. Provisionally designated CPV type 2b, that virus has largely replaced the CPV-2a strain amongst dogs in the United States. The CPV-2b isolates differ in only a single antigenic epitope from CPV-2a strains, and genetically those viruses differ by only two coding changes in the VP-1/VP-2 (coat protein) genes (Parrish et al., 1991).

The reasons for the apparent global displacement of CPV-2 by CPV-2a and CPV-2b in the dog population are poorly understood. What were the selective forces that gave CPV-2a an advantage? One possible mechanism might be antigenic selection, but there seems to be efficient cross-protection between all strains. Dogs that have recovered from infection by one virus appear to be completely protected against infection by the other strain. It is possible that dogs with a low level of immunity, such as puppies with declining levels of maternally acquired antibodies, might be more susceptible to the second strain, and perhaps this was able to drive the displacement.

Another possible selective factor might be the stability of the virus. CPV-2a or CPV-2b might be more stable than CPV-2, allowing it to spread more efficiently. But, again, data are lacking. In addition, most parvoviruses are very stable and very difficult to inactivate under most circumstances, and CPV-2 seems to be no exception.

CPV-2a and CPV-2b might also represent better adapted viruses, and might have supplanted the original virus by replicating more rapidly after infection and achieving higher levels in feces shed from infected dogs. However, although natural infections could be different, preliminary experimental studies have showed that all these viruses replicate to similar levels and are shed in the feces in similar amounts.

DOGS AND CATS:
FACTORS INVOLVED IN HOST RANGE OF CPV-2

CPV-2 can be distinguished from the other parvoviruses by additional criteria besides its antigenic type (Parrish, 1990). Under suitable conditions, each of these viruses will hemagglutinate, or clump red blood cells, with the range of conditions for the hemagglutination (HA) reaction varying with the virus. Canine parvovirus can hemagglutinate in solutions as alkaline as pH 8, while feline and mink viruses do not hemagglutinate in buffers above pH 6.8. Another property, of course, is host range. Canine parvovirus is so named because it was first isolated from domestic dogs. CPV clearly infects dogs, but grows poorly in cats. Conversely, feline panleukopenia virus grows well in cats but replicates only to low titers in dogs. It is not entirely negative, however, and it appears that FPV isolates can replicate in the dog at a low level of efficiency. The virus produced in the dog is insufficient to initiate a second cycle of infection when tissues from the first passage in dogs are inoculated into further dogs. Unlike the situation in animals, CPV-2 replicates very well in cat cells in tissue culture. On the other hand, FPV replicates very poorly, or not at all, in dog cells in culture.

To determine what accounted for these differences in host range, my laboratory performed genetic studies with the feline and canine viruses. In order to understand these studies, it is first necessary to describe parvoviruses in a little more detail. At about 20-22 nanometers in diameter, parvoviruses are among the smallest viruses. In fact, the name *parvo* is from the Latin word for small. The viral DNA genome is about 5,000 bases long (about 5,130 bases for CPV-2), encoding nonstructural proteins and capsid (coat) proteins. The capsid protein comes in two forms, called VP-1 and VP-2; the genes coding for each are partly separate but a considerable portion overlaps. The nonstructural proteins are encoded at what by convention is the left hand end of the genome, while the VP-1 and VP-2 are both encoded in the right hand end. The viral DNA is protected by a capsid, or coat, made up of a total of 60 copies of the VP-1 or VP-2 capsid proteins. As with most viruses, the capsid gives the virus particle its shape, which has icosahedral symmetry in the case of these viruses.

Using standard recombinant DNA technologies, we made recombinants in vitro between FPV (the feline virus) and CPV, with different portions of the DNA derived from each virus. The most informative recombinant virus consisted almost entirely of the FPV genome, but a short segment (730 bases) of the capsid protein gene was replaced with a segment from CPV that is common to both the VP-1 and VP-2 genes of CPV. The resulting recombinant virus gained the antigenic type of canine parvovirus, being recognized by the CPV-specific monoclonal antibodies. The same recombinant virus also gained the HA and host range properties of canine parvovirus for tissue culture cells and for dogs (Parrish et al., 1988a). This demonstrated that most of the host range properties of the virus are encoded by a short region within the capsid protein gene.

The three-dimensional structure of CPV has recently been solved by X-ray crystallography (Tsao et al., 1991), clarifying some of the basis for these differences. The viral capsid is comprised of 60 copies of VP-1 or VP-2. Most of the differences between CPV and FPV are on the surface of the capsid, and many of these differences are found in one area, a raised region of the structure surrounding the three-fold axis of symmetry of the virus. One of the structural differences located on this axis determines the CPV-specific antigenic epitope, while one or more differences in this region determine the FPV-specific epitope. The pH dependence of hemagglutination appears to be determined by a difference in amino acid residue 375. That amino acid residue is not on the surface of the virus, but is directly below a surface residue which is on the side of a dimple at the twofold axis of symmetry. This suggests that the dimple might be a receptor binding site.

RELATIONSHIPS AMONG THE PARVOVIRUSES OF CARNIVORES

Tabulating all the differences in the capsid protein gene sequence, those differences that distinguish the canine and feline viruses fall in two or three major regions. The changes that are most significant in terms of biological properties appear to occur in the region of the capsid gene (VP-1/VP-2 common portion) represented by nucleotide positions 780 to 1,200. Of the four differences in that region, three are coding changes, which alter the protein product, and one is a noncoding change. My interpretation of the data from our recombination mapping is that these changes are sufficient to determine the antigenic site specific to canine parvovirus, as well as the HA pattern of canine parvovirus and at least part of the host range of canine parvovirus for dogs. In other words, only about four or five changes, all localized to the capsid gene, are sufficient to make FPV into a virus with biological properties like CPV. Changes at other positions in the capsid protein gene appear to be the primary determinant of the antigenic difference between CPV-2 and 2a. The antigenic difference between those two viruses may well be due to a combination of three or four nucleotide substitutions in the capsid protein gene.

Having found that the capsid gene appears to determine host range, we sequenced the capsid protein genes from a number of different parvoviruses, including mink enteritis virus, raccoon parvovirus, FPV, and the two CPV types, CPV-2 and CPV-2a, in order to further characterize the relationships of these viruses by the methods of molecular biology. A phylogenetic, or family, tree of the carnivore parvoviruses, based on differences in their DNA sequences, indicated that the mink, raccoon, and feline parvoviruses were not readily distinguishable from one another and formed a single cluster. In contrast, the canine parvoviruses formed a separate cluster, with the CPV-2 virus isolates being distinguishable from the CPV-2a strain. I will later summarize what has been speculated about the origin of CPV-2.

ORIGIN OF MINK ENTERITIS VIRUS (MEV)

Similar questions surround the origin of MEV. The first cases of disease caused by mink enteritis virus were identified in 1947. It is unknown whether MEV was then a new virus of mink or whether it was preexisting. There are no pre-1947 mink sera that could be used to resolve whether the virus existed in mink before 1947. Work in my own laboratory supports the suggestion that MEV is a preexisting virus that has been around for a long time but, for some reason, underwent changes in virulence (reviewed in Parrish, 1990). We found that mink could be experimentally infected with at least some strains of other parvoviruses. Feline panleukopenia virus and raccoon parvovirus replicate quite efficiently in mink, and they can be propagated serially in mink. Mink enteritis virus replicates to a slightly higher titer, but the differences are not statistically significant. However, the viruses show differences in their virulence for mink. In mink, only MEV consistently caused extensive damage to the intestinal villi, resulting in severe and often fatal disease. In contrast, FPV isolates do not cause significant clinical disease in mink.

There is an interesting parallel in the natural history of MEV. In the 1970s and early 1980s, it was recognized that MEV had been endemic for some time among farm mink in the United States and in Scandinavia without much disease being reported. In the past few years, there have been significant outbreaks of disease in both the United States and in Scandinavia. The viruses isolated from those outbreaks appear to be genetically distinct from the viruses that were collected during the late 1970s and early 1980s. This may be similar to the original emergence of MEV in 1947, where a low level of mild disease had previously been occurring unnoticed for a long time. It is possible that a change in the virus or in farming practices resulted in the propagation of a variant virus type causing a significant level of disease.

POSSIBLE ORIGINS OF CPV-2

It appears therefore that the emergence of MEV in the 1940s is a different story from the emergence of canine parvovirus in the 1970s. The mink virus probably already existed. Canine parvovirus appears to have emerged as a truly new virus type in the 1970s, and subsequently has become globally distributed so that it is now endemic in dogs around the world.

Although the genesis of CPV-2 is unknown, there are several possible hypotheses. One possible origin is a long existing virus of dogs that was maintained in an isolated population. At the moment there is no evidence for this, and, given the rapid spread of CPV during 1978, it seems unlikely that the virus would have stayed isolated for very long. There may have been a progenitor virus or an ancestor virus that was less able to spread, and that was contained for a longer period in an isolated population of dogs. If so, that virus has not yet been identified.

Another possibility is a virus of a closely related species becoming adapted to dogs. There are many wild carnivores that have been little studied virologically, and that could have been hosts to a progenitor of CPV-2. One intriguing candidate is the fox parvovirus, which appears to be endemic in many populations of Arctic and red foxes. The fox virus infects farmed fur foxes in Finland and several other countries. A second possibility is the Asiatic raccoon dog, already mentioned, which might have maintained a virus like CPV-2.

Another source of CPV could be chance natural variation of FPV under conditions that allowed transmission to a dog, but this seems unlikely. Another plausible version of this hypothesis that has been put forward, but which has not yet been either eliminated or confirmed, is the possibility of a tissue culture or vaccine strain of FPV mutating in tissue culture, and then spreading to dogs. In support of this, we do know that both the feline and canine viruses can replicate in feline cell lines in tissue culture. This suggests that if a virus like CPV-2 had arisen from FPV under those circumstances, it might have been propagated and later possibly spread into dogs by a presently unknown route.

At the moment, there is no evidence for this origin. None of the FPV vaccine strains studied to date has proved to be a direct ancestor of canine parvovirus. Suggestions that some of the vaccine strains of FPV had genetic similarities to CPV were not confirmed when we sequenced the DNA of those particular strains.

Just a few appropriate mutations in the capsid genes would probably have sufficed to convert FPV into CPV. Although its actual origin is unknown, the relationship of CPV-2 to FPV suggests that CPV-2 could have arisen from that virus, or another naturally occurring carnivore parvovirus, and that a mutation or series of mutations in the capsid gene conferred the ability to infect dogs. Whatever the exact origin of CPV, it seems likely that some sort of interspecies transfer then introduced the parvovirus into the dog population.

REFERENCES

Parrish, C.R. (1990). The emergence, natural history and variation of canine, mink and feline parvoviruses. In *Advances in Virus Research* (K. Maramorosch, F.A. Murphy, and A.J. Shatkin, eds.), vol. 38, pp. 404-450. San Diego: Academic Press.

Parrish, C.R., C.F. Aquadro, and L.E. Carmichael (1988a). Canine host range and a specific epitope map along with variant sequences in the capsid protein gene of canine parvovirus and related feline, mink, and raccoon parvoviruses. Virology **166**:293-307.

Parrish, C.R., C.F. Aquadro, M.L. Strassheim, J.F. Evermann, J.-Y. Sgro, and H.O. Mohammed (1991). Rapid antigenic-type replacement and DNA sequence evolution of canine parvovirus. J. Virol. **65**:6544-6552.

Parrish, C.R., P. Have, W.J. Foreyt, J.F. Evermann, M. Senda, and L.E. Carmichael (1988b). The global spread and replacement of canine parvovirus strains. J. Gen. Virol. **69**:1111-1116.

Parrish, C.R., P.H. O'Connell, J.F. Evermann, and L.E. Carmichael (1985). Natural variation of canine parvovirus. Science **230**:1046-1048.

Tsao, J., M.S. Chapman, M. Agbandje, W. Keller, K. Smith, H. Wu, M. Luo, T.J. Smith, M.G. Rossmann, R.W. Compans, and C.R. Parrish (1991). The three-dimensional structure of canine parvovirus and its functional implications. Science **251**:1456-1464.

19

Replication Error, Quasispecies Populations, and Extreme Evolution Rates of RNA Viruses

JOHN HOLLAND

INTRODUCTION

The purpose of this chapter is to introduce non-specialists to recent insights into the extreme genetic variability and great adaptability of RNA viruses (those which have RNA genomes, or which utilize RNA as an intermediate template to replicate their DNA genomes). This topic has been reviewed in considerable detail recently, so this chapter will present a summary and overview without excessive elaboration or references. Readers are referred to the many reviews in Domingo et al. (1988) and Holland (1992) for detailed references.

THE RNA BIOSPHERE

There is now support (see Cech, 1989 and Robertson, 1992) for the hypothesis that the first biosphere on earth consisted of primitive replicating RNA molecules, some of which had enzymatic functions. Catalytic RNA molecules (ribozymes) have been widely investigated recently and RNA self-replication appears increasingly feasible (Cech, 1989; Robertson, 1992). RNA self-replication at best would be an extremely error-prone process. But infidelity offers obvious advantages in generating the extreme RNA genome diversity necessary for the earliest stages of "life" on earth. Following the earliest evolution, the greater chemical and genetic stability of DNA would have allowed larger genome sizes and the regulatory sophistication necessary for cells and organisms as we presently know them. Thus, today's biosphere is DNA-based, and the only known RNA "life forms" are RNA viruses. These depend on DNA-based host cells for their existence. Whether any existing RNA virus genomes contain sequence vestiges of the earliest RNA life forms is unknown (and probably unknowable), but it is clear that RNA viruses are ubiquitous, extremely successful cellular parasites of considerable disease importance. The majority of all plant, animal and human viruses are RNA viruses. The reasons for this are not immediately evident given the capacity for DNA to integrate and recombine with host cell DNA, to utilize and modify host DNA regulatory pathways, and so on. It is the author's conviction that RNA virus genomes are successful because they are small, simple, rapidly-replicating and efficient, but most importantly because RNA genomes are genetically plastic and enormously adaptable to changing environmental challenges since they consist of extremely heterogeneous populations (quasispecies populations). This would explain the apparently bizarre genome replication strategies of retroviruses, which reverse transcribe RNA genomes to produce DNA proviruses, and of hepadnaviruses (such as hepatitis B virus). The latter have virion DNA genomes, but they replicate via RNA transcripts that are reverse-transcribed to produce DNA for viral genomes. Such convoluted replication schemes allow the advantages of both worlds; the genetic plasticity and adaptability of the RNA world and the stable integration capacity and recombinational and regulatory capacities of the DNA world. Thus, it is no surprise that nearly all viruses that replicate in both plants and insects, or in both animals and insects, are either RNA viruses, or else DNA viruses that replicate via reverse transcription of RNA genomic copies.

WHY CANNOT DNA VIRUSES ALSO BE GENETICALLY PLASTIC AND ADAPTABLE?

Some DNA viruses may have high mutation frequencies and great adaptability (Smith and Inglis, 1987). Drake (1969) pointed out that the spontaneous mutation rates of all living organisms tend to be inversely proportional to the sizes of their DNA genomes. The obvious reason for this is the need to increase fidelity of DNA replication as the number of targets (genes) susceptible to lethal or damaging mutations increases with the increasing complexity of higher organisms. Thus, errors during DNA replication are usually corrected by "proofreading" exonucleases associated with DNA polymerases (these excise terminal mismatched bases) and by "mismatch excision-repair" systems. Excision-repair, recombination repair systems, and other repair systems also function for DNA damaged by such means as oxygen-derived free radicals, by UV light, by mutagenic chemicals, and so on. Therefore, DNA has a variety of mechanisms for maintaining or restoring informational integrity

(Radman and Wagner, 1986; Lahue and Modrich, 1989). In contrast, RNA proofreading and RNA mismatch-repair systems have not been confirmed to date. RNA synthesis appears to be inherently error-prone and not corrected, whereas the products of DNA polymerases (which are also intrinsically error-prone) are generally corrected. Adelman et al. (1988) estimated the average DNA damage rate in humans to be thousands of oxidative DNA "hits" per cell per day! The long life span of humans attests to the efficiency with which such damaged bases are correctly replaced by repair systems.

Despite the presence of host cell DNA proofreading/repair systems, some DNA viruses could have high mutation frequencies (Smith and Inglis, 1987). This could be achieved in a number of ways (e.g., absence or suppression of proofreading, sequestering of viral DNA away from mismatch repair systems, replication of DNA as single strands which cannot be subjected to mismatch repair, etc.). The advantages to DNA (or RNA) viruses of high mutation frequencies (and of high adaptability) are obvious. Hall et al. (1984) selected "antimutator" strains of herpes simplex virus exhibiting mutation frequencies orders of magnitude lower than those of wild-type strains. The fact that wild-type herpes viruses had maintained quite high mutation rates strongly suggests that much lower rates are neither generally advantageous, nor selected in nature. This review will focus on RNA viruses (and viruses replicating their genomes via RNA templates), but similar principles may apply to some DNA viruses as well (Smith and Inglis, 1987).

AVERAGE MISINCORPORATION FREQUENCIES OF DNA AND RNA POLYMERASES

Quantum mechanics and quantum electrodynamics tell us that we live in a probabilistic, rather than deterministic universe. There are few completely-predictable processes even at the macroscopic level, and polymerases copying DNA or RNA templates are subject to inevitable probabilistic misincorporation errors. Mutations occur for many reasons (e.g., mispairing due to rare (transient) tautomeric forms of bases in the template or substrate; syn-anti rotation of the substrate; depurination, deamination, protonation-deprotonation of bases; polymerase slippage or "jumping" or "stuttering", oxidative damage to bases, etc.). These events can vary with different polymerases, with varying nucleotide pool ratios or pool sizes, pH, temperature, pressure, oxygen levels, and other factors. The sum of individual probabilities of all mutagenic effects must set upper limits on the average fidelity level of any DNA or RNA replication. We do not yet know the dimension of this limit, but studies of DNA polymerases in vitro suggest minimal average error levels of the order of 10^{-4} to 10^{-5} misincorporations per site prior to proofreading/repair (reviewed in Loeb and Cheng, 1990). Proofreading and mismatch repair systems can greatly increase fidelity, but the energy cost is high (Radman and Wagner, 1986; Lahue et al., 1989; Fersht et al., 1982). Likewise, in vivo and in vitro estimates of the average error frequencies of virus RNA replicases and reverse transcriptases also suggest misincorporation frequencies of the order of 10^{-3} to 10^{-5} (see reviews in Domingo et al., 1988; Holland, 1992). There is as yet no evidence for efficient RNA proofreading. Thus, RNA synthesis may generally be error prone, thereby assuring great diversity (and adaptability) for all viruses that replicate RNA genomes (or RNA copies of DNA genomes). However, some studies (Smith and Palese, 1988; Sedivy et al., 1987; Durbin and Stollar, 1986; Hahn et al., 1989a,b) suggest much lower error rates at some sites (or regions) of certain RNA virus genomes. However, even if some sites have low mutation frequencies, high mutation frequencies at average sites still produce quasispecies populations. Much more work is required before it will be possible to provide firm data regarding minimum, maximum, and average error rates of viral RNA replicases. Furthermore, we cannot yet eliminate the possibility of RNA proofreading mechanisms capable of correcting basic RNA replicase error levels. In any case, there is no RNA virus for which consistently low RNA mutation frequencies have been reported, whereas very high frequencies have been observed at many sites in a wide variety of RNA viruses studied. It is important to note that DNA and RNA polymerases have mutational biases and these can differ. That is, certain specific base substitutions are made with much lower probabilities than others. For example, *E. coli* DNA polymerase I exhibits a C·A mispairing frequency of 2×10^{-5}, but the C·T mispairing frequency is 100-fold lower (2×10^{-7}) (Fersht et al., 1982). So specific mutation frequencies will often differ from **average** frequencies. It will be assumed in discussions below that a reasonable approximation of the average RNA virus replicase error frequency is of the order of 10^{-4} to 10^{-5} base substitutions per site, even though certain sites or regions may have much higher fidelity while others may be mutational hot spots.

EXTREMELY HIGH MUTATION FREQUENCIES OF RNA VIRUSES

Average error frequencies of the order of 10^{-4} to 10^{-5} per site in RNA virus genomes exceed by a millionfold or more the average (corrected) error frequencies of their animal, plant, and human hosts. This discrepancy is frequently reflected in rates of evolution, which can also proceed up to millionsfold faster than that of their hosts.

Obviously rapid evolution is facilitated if populations contain diverse arrays of mutants, and this is a characteristic of RNA viruses. RNA genomes are always quite limited in size (and therefore in information content). The average RNA virus genome is about 10,000 bases (10 kb) or less in size, so the number of genes (and their protein products) averages less than 10. It is, of course, this size limitation which makes possible very high mutation frequencies. For example, a replicating virus genome of 10 kb size will produce an average of 1 mutation per 10 replications if the replicase error frequency averages 10^{-5} per nucleotide site per replication; it will average 1 mutation per replication if the error frequency is 10^{-4}, and 10 mutations per replication if the mean error frequency is 10^{-3}. As discussed above, RNA genome mutation frequencies measured to date have varied, but the average is so high that enormous diversity of RNA virus populations is the norm.

WHEN IS A VIRUS CLONE NOT REALLY A CLONE?

When it is an RNA virus clone. With error frequencies per site averaging 10^{-5} or greater, we cannot envision an RNA virus as "a virus" nor an RNA clone as "a clone" (i.e., a collection of identical virus genomes). This is true even when nucleic acid sequencing provides an unequivocal sequence for the entire virus genome. The sequence obtained at each base position must necessarily be viewed as an average or consensus sequence for that site. Many individual genomes in an RNA virus clone may have different nucleotides at that site (and other sites), so sequencing the mixed genome population provides information only about the nucleotides most frequently present at each site. Thus, RNA virus clones must be viewed as quasispecies populations (i.e., as swarms of related mutants rather than fixed entities). The quasispecies concept is reviewed in Eigen and Biebricher (1988) and is discussed below.

CAN WE DETERMINE THE EXACT GENOME SEQUENCE OF AN INDIVIDUAL RNA VIRUS GENOME?

No, there is an uncertainty principle working against virologists seeking exact sequence information about an individual RNA virus genome, particularly if it is desired later to study the biological behavior of the sequenced virus genome and its progeny.

The most obvious way to attempt exact sequencing of an individual RNA virus genome is via molecular cloning of cDNA copies. Since DNA replication can be much less error-prone (due to proofreading and repair), DNA copies of an RNA genome can be amplified with fidelity. However, all known reverse transcriptases are error-prone so there will necessarily be uncertainty regarding the fidelity of the cDNA copy that is cloned, amplified and sequenced. It is unlikely that a high fidelity viral reverse transcriptase will be found (i.e., one with proofreading/mismatch repair) since this would lessen the adaptability of any retrovirus encoding it. Perhaps in future years such a reverse transcriptase might be engineered. For the same reasons, exact sequencing of one RNA genome cannot be achieved by the powerful polymerase chain reaction (PCR) approach, even if a high fidelity DNA polymerase were used for DNA amplification in vitro. Once again the investigator must begin with the uncertainty inherent in reverse transcriptase copies of the viral RNA.

One might anticipate eventual employment of direct physical methods for sequencing a single RNA genome (e.g., direct use of scanning tunneling microscopy or atomic force microscopy), but these may never provide sufficient resolution of biological materials. Even if they do, exact, full-length sequence accuracy is unlikely, and precise location and recovery of a single RNA molecule would be daunting. Even if a single RNA molecule could be sequenced and replicated with complete fidelity, uncertainty would still exist because the recovered genome came from a quasispecies swarm of related variants (see below).

Finally, use of cDNA clones to generate infectious, replicating RNA viruses (including retroviruses) has the obvious advantage of starting with a defined DNA sequence, which can be specifically modified for genetic studies. However, this does not eliminate the RNA sequence uncertainties in transcribed RNAs. Obviously, numerous mutations will be introduced into the RNA virus population during RNA polymerase transcription of the cDNA, and during subsequent replication (by viral RNA replicase or reverse transcriptase) of the transcribed RNA. Therefore, it must be understood that some uncertainty always accompanies studies of genome sequences of RNA viruses whether from diseased tissue or from laboratory clones.

MANFRED EIGEN'S QUASISPECIES MODEL FOR RNA VIRUS POPULATIONS

Eigen, Schuster, and their colleagues have elaborated a "quasispecies" model to describe distributions of related replicating RNA molecules that contain a wide variety of different mutations (see Eigen and Biebricher, 1988). This model was originally developed to explain the early evolution of life on earth among self-replicating RNA molecules, but it has application to present day RNA virus populations and perhaps to many DNA-based populations as well. The essence of the quasispecies concept lies in the fact that RNA virus populations (even populations derived from clones) are usually very large populations comprised of many millions to many billions of genomes, each of which has a high probability of being a mutant with regard to the average genome sequence. In very large and diverse quasispecies populations, every possible single-base change is represented, and every possible two-base mutant combination and many higher order combinations are represented. This is true even when the population is recently expanded from a single virus particle (a clone), and even when RNA sequencing of the population provides a definitive average (consensus) sequence for the entire genome. This concept is counterintuitive to some and is not accepted by all virologists. Another major tenet of the quasispecies model is that the target of biological selection is not the single most fit genome sequence present (i.e., the master sequence) nor any single RNA molecules in the population. Rather, it is the entire mutant swarm that is acted upon by selective forces, as well as being the product of selection. There may be only one master sequence that exhibits maximum fitness in any defined environment, or there may be a number of equally fit master sequences. However, it is the master sequences together with their inevitable (and unavoidable) mutant swarms that are selected. When environmental conditions change so that new master sequences are required, diverse quasispecies swarms increase the probability that appropriate new master sequences will be available to evolve away from the swarm in which it originated. Master sequences and consensus sequences may exhibit relative stability in some environments, or they may change extremely rapidly, with some being present only for very short time periods, as discussed below.

VIRUS RNA GENOMES CAN EVOLVE EXTREMELY RAPIDLY

As might be expected, as a result of high mutation frequencies, RNA viruses can exhibit extreme rates of evolution. Remarkably, rates of evolution of RNA viruses can exceed average rates of evolution of their DNA-based hosts by factors of millions. Base substitution rates of higher eukaryotes vary, but the average is apparently less than 10^{-9} base substitutions per site per year. In contrast, RNA viruses such as poliovirus, influenza virus, HIV (AIDS) viruses, enterovirus, Moloney retrovirus, foot-and-mouth disease virus, and others can evolve at rates in excess of 10^{-3} base substitutions per site per year (reviewed in Domingo and Holland, 1988; Holland, 1992). Thus, the "molecular clocks" of RNA viruses can spin at blinding speeds as compared to those of their hosts. This was clearly demonstrated in an outbreak of poliomyelitis (Kew et al., 1981) caused by a Sabin poliovirus vaccine strain (which was cloned by Sabin). During this

1-year outbreak of polio, the viral genome underwent mutational change approximating $1\text{-}2 \times 10^{-2}$ base substitutions per site per year in infected humans (see also Kinnunen et al., 1990). Clearly the high mutation frequencies of RNA genomes often allow very rapid evolution. It is not surprising that the host immune system has also evolved mechanisms to allow extremely high mutation frequencies in immunoglobulin variable region genes of pre B cells (Wabl et al., 1985). These frequencies are of the same order of magnitude as those of RNA virus genomes and the basis for this extremely low fidelity of DNA synthesis at selected genetic sites is not yet known. Perhaps proofreading and repair are suppressed during replication at these sites, or post-replicative modification may be promoted. Regardless of mechanisms, the advantages for immune system adaptability are obvious.

DO HIGH MUTATION RATES NECESSITATE CONTINUOUS RAPID EVOLUTION OF RNA VIRUS GENOMES?

No, RNA virus populations can frequently maintain quite stable master sequences and consensus sequences. This is true in nature and in controlled laboratory experiments (see reviews in Holland, 1992). These "equilibrium populations" are still diverse quasispecies swarms, but if the selective environment is not greatly altered, and if the genome RNA master sequences are highly fit (as compared to all other genomes in the mutant spectrum) then the consensus sequence can be maintained for long periods. We have observed remarkable equilibrium stability of VSV genomes for hundreds of passages in cell culture at low multiplicities of infection (Steinhauer et al., 1989). However, changes in the selective environment can quickly upset stable equilibrium populations and promote very rapid viral evolution. For example, VSV passaged repeatedly at high multiplicities is selected for resistance to the interfering effects of defective interfering (DI) particles. However, these variants generate new DI particles and must then mutate to escape from these in successive cycles. This "cycling" leads to recurring rapid changes in viral replicase specificity and in genome RNA sequences at virus (and DI) replicase recognition sites (O'Hara et al., 1984a,b). Thus, the same virus population may exhibit either great consensus sequence stability or rapid evolution depending upon conditions. So the evolutionary clocks of RNA genomes clearly can run very rapidly, or more slowly, or not at all for long periods. This can be observed in nature also. For example, eastern equine encephalitis virus in North America has undergone remarkably little sequence divergence (0.7%) since 1933 (Weaver et al., 1991). At the other end of the spectrum is the rapid, continuous evolution of HIV (Coffin, 1986; Temin, 1989).

ARE THE NUMBERS OF DIFFERENT VIABLE GENOME SEQUENCES RATHER LIMITED FOR A PARTICULAR TYPE OF RNA VIRUS?

No, but it is obvious that there must be strict constraints on virus genome size, replication strategy, genome organization, host range, and so on, and this in turn constrains viral genome evolution during any given interval of time. However, the number of all possible viable mutants can never be tested in nature. Sequence comparisons of some evolving related RNA virus genomes have shown that well over half of all genome sites can accommodate mutations. This means that for a 10 kb viral RNA genome, more than 4^{5000} sequence permutations and combinations must be tested to find all possible viable mutants. (If possibilities for genome expansion and contraction by additions, deletions and recombinations, and reassortments, are included, the situation is worse.) This assures that not even a minuscule fraction of all possible viable RNA virus genomes has arisen, nor can ever appear (to be tested for fitness), in our universe. New virus sequences arise gradually and continuously, and are sooner or later displaced by yet newer ones, but the possibilities are limitless. The regular emergence of "new" viruses and "new" human, animal, and plant diseases should therefore come as no surprise. It is inevitable, and must occur at irregular intervals.

CAN DIRECTIONS OF VIRUS EVOLUTION AND THE TIMING OF NEW OUTBREAKS OF VIRUS DISEASE BE PREDICTED WITH ANY CONFIDENCE?

No, this is not possible because the evolution of quasispecies populations of viruses is not deterministic, but probabilistic. During any epoch of our biosphere, the numbers of possible new virus mutants are finite and limited by the genome structures and sequences, and the mutation rates and replication rates of all currently-existing viruses. But of course these involve extremely large numbers. Furthermore, "founder effects" in virus populations are often stochastic (e.g., the chance infection of an individual by a single virus particle that represents a rare mutant, or the early appearance of an uncommon mutant in a replicating virus clone). Even when a single VSV virus population was divided into aliquots and passaged in persistently infected cells in nude mice (Spindler et al., 1982), rapid sequence divergence occurred (up to 1% divergence in 12 to 15 weeks!). Clearly these in vivo passage conditions promoted extreme virus population disequilibrium and rapid evolution. Many specific environmental conditions can regularly select certain types of mutants (e.g., drug-resistant variants, antibody resistant variants, variants able to replicate in a certain cell type, etc.), but the overall directions and timing of major evolutionary changes in virus populations cannot be predicted with any certainty. It is obvious, however, that as virus host populations (or potential host populations) increase, there is a concomitant increase in the probability of major evolutionary changes in virus populations due to increased opportunities for replication, mutation, recombination, and selection. As the world population of humans (and of their domestic animals and plants) increase, the probability for new viral disease outbreaks must inevitably increase as well. AIDS is not the first "new" virus disease of humans, and it will not be the last. However, it is unrealistic to hope to predict the time, place, or nature of future outbreaks. Nobody could have predicted the AIDS epidemic, for example.

CAN THE AVERAGE MUTATION FREQUENCIES OF RNA VIRUSES BE GREATLY INCREASED BY MUTAGENESIS?

Apparently not. Eigen and Biebricher (1988) pointed out a threshold relationship correlating the mean error rate in replication, $1-\hat{q}$ (where $\hat{q}$ is the replicase fidelity rate) with the maximum length of a defined genome sequence, V_{max}, that can be maintained reproducibly during replication. This is not a fixed value; rather, it can vary with the function σ_0 which represents the selectivity or efficiency of the master sequence's reproductive advantage relative to the mean competitive abilities of the mutant spectrum in a quasispecies population. They suggest that maximum genome size, V_{max}, is determined by σ_0 and mean replicase fidelity, $\hat{q}$:

$$V_{max} \leq \frac{\log_e \sigma_0}{1-\hat{q}} \qquad \text{(Eqn. 19.1)}$$

Selectivity functions are not known for any virus, and of course will vary with different viruses and mutants, different host environments, and so on. But in the range of σ_0 between 2 and 10, the natural log of σ_0 is not far from 1; σ_0 for most RNA viruses may be in this range, since this would limit mean replicase error rates to approximately the reciprocal of the genome size. Since the high mutation frequencies (of the order of 10^{-4}) often observed for RNA viruses are in fact approximately equal to the reciprocal of the genome length, this suggests that RNA viruses may often have an average error frequency that is near maximal. That is, they may be near the threshold for error catastrophe, beyond which loss of information content will result from increased errors in replication. This can be tested using

RNA mutagens. We have recently examined the quantitative effects of various chemical mutagens on RNA virus survival and mutational adaptability. Surprisingly, large increases in mutation frequency at single genome sites were never obtained with any mutagen tested. Severalfold increases were the maximum observed at any level of virus survival after mutagenesis (Holland et al., 1990). This suggests that RNA virus replicase mean error levels are generally adjusted to provide near-maximal genetic adaptability (quasispecies mutant distributions) without loss of information content. This does not mean that mutagens cannot increase the relative abundance of mutants nor increase the rate of virus evolution. In fact, they do (Pringle, 1970), but they do so at the cost of reduced virus yields and reduced mutant yields. Reduced virus yields after mutagenesis increase the probability of emergence to dominance of induced mutants. They can do this by promoting genetic bottlenecks, followed by frequent "founder effects" for mutants in the surviving populations. Mutagen treatment clearly increases rates of evolution of RNA virus populations (Clewley and Bishop, 1979; Steinhauer et al., 1989), even though it usually reduces the total number (but not the percentage) of mutants.

It should be stressed that such experiments necessarily deal with **average** error levels and **average** effects of mutagens. Even in clonal quasispecies populations of RNA viruses (with or without mutagens), there may be a quasispecies distribution of viruses having different replicase error frequencies. For example, the majority of temperature-sensitive (*ts*) mutants of vesicular stomatitis virus (VSV) map to the large polymerase (L) gene whether they were spontaneous or mutagen-induced *ts* mutants. Pringle et al. (1981) have characterized one *ts* mutant clone of VSV that apparently exhibits an increased average mutation frequency. It seems possible that replicase fidelities of RNA viruses might undergo frequent deterioration and improvement with the end result generally being the adjustment of average error rates to an optimal level (above, but close to, the error threshold). This might vary somewhat with different virus strains, but most RNA viruses are probably near the edge of error catastrophe because this maximizes adaptability and competitive ability.

WILL HIGH RATES OF MUTATION AND EVOLUTION OF RNA VIRUSES PREVENT DEVELOPMENT OF EFFECTIVE VACCINES AND ANTIVIRAL DRUGS?

No, but they may often complicate such efforts. Some of the most successful virus vaccines are for RNA viruses, such as poliovirus, measles, mumps, and rubella. Even the vaccines for rabies and influenza A viruses are effective in the majority of vaccinees, and it is still too early to be pessimistic regarding the possibility of effective AIDS vaccines. How can vaccines be effective over many decades for highly-mutable RNA viruses? First, if there are numerous neutralization epitopes, the frequency of variants resistant at all epitopes should be so low that long time periods will be requested for their stepwise generation. At any interval in their evolution all virus genomes are constrained in the numbers and positions of base and amino acid substitutions they can sustain within a given time period because a large fraction of mutations will be lethal or debilitating. There are many amino acid sites which are, for long time periods, either invariant or capable of providing only debilitated mutants (until compensatory mutations restore fitness). An effective vaccine will generally exploit such sites and epitopes. Even highly variable epitopes can be immunogenic if they are numerous and/or if the immune response against them is able to abort or slow natural infections so that large numbers of virus particles (and resistant mutants) are never produced. The same is true for an antiviral drug used for prophylaxis (or even for treatment if given early enough). Even though drug-resistant mutants can be produced at high frequency (Domingo, 1989), a ten thousandfold or greater early reduction in production of (sensitive) virus may often allow an effective immune response to develop before significant numbers of resistant mutants accumulate. In any case, it is clear that vaccines against quite variable viruses have been very effective. It is conceivable that optimal deployment of these might be able to eliminate certain RNA disease agents (such as measles and the polioviruses) from the human population. Even if resistant virus strains were to arise and begin to circulate widely, they might lose much (or all) of their disease potential due to vaccine-selected mutations. Finally, if vaccine failures became common due to resistant strains, the newer strains can then be incorporated into a polyvalent vaccine. Regular updating of vaccine antigens is already routine for influenza A vaccines and may eventually become necessary for some of the less-rapidly-evolving RNA disease agents. In general, drug-resistant and immune-resistant mutants of RNA viruses may cause frequent problems for prophylaxis and therapy, but these should not be insurmountable. Obviously, these problems become much more difficult for viruses (such as AIDS viruses) in which the nature of the infection regularly leads to immune suppression coupled with persistent virus replication. But even here, combined drug therapies together with polyvalent vaccines may ultimately prove effective. In general, antiviral drugs and vaccines should not select resistant virus mutants in the general circulating virus population as long as the major reservoirs of infection are not treated or immunized. For example, the antigenicity of yellow fever virus in a rain forest canopy or of "wild-type" measles virus in unimmunized third world human populations should not be affected significantly by vaccine programs deployed elsewhere. On the other hand, a successful effort to treat nearly all HIV-infected persons in the United States with AZT would be expected to lead to wide circulation of AZT-resistant HIV strains (Richman, 1990). At present, most sources of infection are untreated so most circulating "wild-type" virus strains remain AZT-sensitive and resistance develops in most infected persons only after AZT treatment of that individual.

IN A WORLD OF RAPIDLY-EVOLVING (AND RAPIDLY-INCREASING) POPULATIONS OF HUMAN VIRUSES, WHAT CAN BE DONE TO IMPROVE CAPABILITIES FOR EARLY DETECTION AND RESPONSE TO "NEW" VIRUS DISEASES?

Of course many (mostly costly) measures can be taken to increase rapid response capabilities for serious outbreaks of "new" virus diseases of humans that certainly will occur in future years. However, stochastically-spaced virus disease outbreaks represent only a fraction of the problems faced by the burgeoning human population, so early detection-response approaches must be kept relatively inexpensive, yet potentially effective in an emergency.

There is an existing excellent model for a worldwide virus surveillance laboratory, the Yale World Reference Center for Arboviruses at the Yale Arbovirus Research Unit. With additional responsibilities and capabilities, and with modest additional support, this Center (or one modeled after it) could serve a vital function in future outbreaks. The following approach is suggested as one possibility for a World Reference Center for emerging viruses:

1. This Center should be a single worldwide "Emerging Virus Surveillance Laboratory" (under WHO auspices), which would be independent of all national governments, regardless of (multiple) funding sources, and regardless of geographic location.

2. Its accomplished scientists—physicians, epidemiologists, toxicologists, and other suitably trained persons—would pursue individual research interests in the absence of outbreaks, but would have prior worldwide passport clearances to help with investigations of new or unusual outbreaks of infectious diseases, to provide information, and to transport tissue specimens, sera, and other needed materials. Prior clearances pose obvious (but surmountable) political difficulties.

3. Such a laboratory could provide worldwide information, tissues, sera, virus isolates, DNA clones, and similar materials to all qualified research laboratories, vaccine and pharmaceutical firms, and others. They in turn would agree to provide the

laboratory (and through it the world scientific community) with all new data, clones, drugs, reagents, vaccine strains, and other useful products as they become available during a new virus outbreak of serious proportions.

4. This approach would supplement, not supplant, the roles of existing governmental agencies (such as CDC). It could maximize early involvement of all laboratories with requisite expertise, and might, in a rapidly spreading outbreak, reduce the effective response time below a critical level. Highly qualified governmental agencies (such as CDC in the United States) might frequently have problems gaining access in certain countries.

5. A single Center is preferable to multiple centers to reduce costs, to eliminate competition-driven delays, and to provide a single coordination and communication center. Support would be augmented during a serious outbreak.

6. Finally, to promote international trust and cooperation, such a Center should be available at all times for visits by qualified scientists from all countries. Such a Center would not supplant field stations or medical intelligence offices, but would cooperate with them and provide advanced isolation and identification and communication capabilities.

It is impossible to predict whether serious emerging virus disease outbreaks during the next century will be slowly transmissible, chronic disease outbreaks (like AIDS) or rapidly transmitted (like influenza). It is equally impossible to know whether an "Emerging Virus Surveillance Laboratory" would really be needed or effective in near-future outbreaks. However, such preparedness at modest cost seems a prudent precaution.

ARE RNA VIRUSES GOOD MODELS FOR EVOLUTION GENERALLY?

Perhaps. They certainly can provide insights into basic principles of evolution. Viruses lack many important features of higher organisms (e.g., sensory and behavioral adaptations, chromosome segregation, meiotic crossing over, sexual competition, etc.). Nevertheless, their vast populations, rapid growth, and extreme rates of evolution offer opportunities for well-controlled studies that are not feasible with other organisms. Powerful new techniques for rapid sequence analysis of variants should help provide some definitive evolutionary insights using RNA viruses as model systems.

ACKNOWLEDGMENTS

The author thanks Drs. Esteban Domingo, Juan Carlos de La Torre, and David Steinhauer for their many helpful discussions of these topics. Our work was supported by NIH grant AI 14627 from the National Institute of Allergy and Infectious Diseases.

REFERENCES

Adelman, R., R.L. Saul, and B.N. Ames (1988). Oxidative damage to DNA: Relation to species metabolic rate and life span. Proc. Natl. Acad. Sci. USA 85:2706-2708.

Cech, T.R. (1989). RNA enzymes. Adv. Enzymol. 62:1-36.

Clewley, J.P., and D.H.L. Bishop (1979). Assignment of the large oligonucleotides of vesicular stomatitis virus to the N, NS, M, G and L genes and oligonucleotide ordering within the L gene. J. Virol. 30:116-123.

Coffin, J.M. (1986). Genetic variation in AIDS viruses. Cell 46:1-4.

Domingo, E. (1989). RNA virus evolution and the control of viral disease. Prog. Drug Res. 33:93-133.

Domingo, E., and J.J. Holland (1988). High error rates, population equilibrium and evolution of RNA replication systems. In RNA Genetics, vol. 3 (E. Domingo, J.J. Holland, and P. Ahlquist, eds.), pp. 3-36. Boca Raton, Fla.: CRC Press, Inc.

Drake, J.W., E.F. Allen, S.A. Forsberg, R.M. Preparata, and E.O. Greening (1969). Spontaneous mutation. Nature 221:1128-1132.

Durbin, R.K., and V. Stollar (1986). Sequence analysis of the E1 gene of a hyperglycosylated, host restricted mutant of Sindbis virus and estimation of mutation rate from frequency of revertants. Virology 154:135-143.

Eigen, M., and C.K. Biebricher (1988). Sequence space and quasispecies distribution. In RNA Genetics, vol. 3 (E. Domingo, J.J. Holland, and P. Ahlquist, eds.), pp. 211-245. Boca Raton: CRC Press, Inc.

Fersht, A.R., J.W. Knill-Jones, and W.-C. Tsui (1982). Kinetic basis of spontaneous mutation. J. Mol. Biol. 156:37-51.

Hahn, C.S., C.M. Rice, E.G. Strauss, E.M. Lenches, and J.H. Strauss (1989a). Sindbis virus ts103 has a mutation in glycoprotein E2 that leads to defective assembly of virions. J. Virol. 63:3459-3465.

Hahn, Y.S., E.G. Strauss, and J.H. Strauss (1989b). Mapping of RNA temperature sensitive mutants of Sindbis virus: assignment of complementation groups A, B and G to nonstructural proteins. J. Virol. 63:3142-3150.

Hall, J.D., D.M. Coen, B.L. Fisher, M. Weisslitz, S. Randall, R.E. Almy, P.T. Gelep, and P.A. Schaffer (1984). Generation of genetic diversity in herpes simplex virus: an antimutator phenotype maps to the DNA polymerase locus. Virology 132:26-37.

Holland, J., E. Domingo, J.C. de la Torre, and D.A. Steinhauer (1990). Mutation frequencies at defined single codon sites in vesicular stomatitis virus can be increased only slightly by chemical mutagenesis. J. Virol. 64:3960-3962.

Holland, J.J. (ed.) (1992). *Genetic Diversity of RNA Viruses* [Current Topics in Microbiology and Immunology, 176]. Berlin and New York: Springer-Verlag.

Kew, O., M.B.K. Nottay, M.H. Hatch, J.H. Nakano, and J.F. Obijeski (1981). Multiple genetic changes can occur in the oral poliovaccines upon replication in humans. J. Gen. Virol. **56**:337-347.

Kinnunen, L., A. Huovilainen, T. Püyry, and T. Hovi (1990). Rapid molecular evolution of wild type 3 poliovirus during infection in individual hosts. J. Gen. Virol. **71**:317-324.

Lahue, R.S., K.G. Au, and P. Modrich (1989). DNA mismatch correction in a defined system. Science **245**:160-164.

Loeb, L.A., and K.C. Cheng (1990). Errors in DNA synthesis: a source of spontaneous mutations. Mutation Res. **238**:297-304.

O'Hara, P.J., F.M. Horodyski, S.T. Nichol, and J.J. Holland (1984a). Vesicular stomatitis virus mutants resistant to defective-interfering particles accumulate stable 5'-terminal and fewer 3'-terminal mutations in a stepwise manner. J. Virol. **49**:793-798.

O'Hara, P.J., S.T. Nichol, F.M. Horodyski, and J.J. Holland (1984b). Vesicular stomatitis virus defective interfering particles can contain extensive genomic sequence rearrangements and base substitutions. Cell **36**:915-924.

Pringle, C.R. (1970). Genetic characteristics of conditional lethal mutants of vesicular stomatitis virus induced by 5-fluorouracil, 5-azacytidine, and ethyl methanesulfonate. J. Virol. **5**:559-567.

Pringle, C.R., V. Devine, M. Wilkie, C.M. Preston, A. Dohn, and D.J. McGeoch (1981). Enhanced mutability associated with a temperature-sensitive mutant of vesicular stomatitis virus. J. Virol. **39**:377-389.

Radman, M., and R. Wagner (1986). Mismatch repair in *Escherichia coli*. Ann. Rev. Genet. **20**:523-538.

Richman, D.D. (1990). Viral drug resistance. Curr. Opin. Infect. Dis. **3**:819-823.

Robertson, H.D. (1992). Replication and evolution of viroid-like pathogens. In *Genetic Diversity of RNA Viruses* (J.J. Holland, ed.) [Curr. Top. Microbiol. Immunol. 176]. Berlin and New York: Springer-Verlag.

Sedivy, J.M., J.P. Capone, U.L. RajBhandary, and P.A. Sharp (1987). An inducible mammalian amber suppressor: Propagation of a poliovirus mutant. Cell **50**:379-389.

Smith, D.B., and S.C. Inglis (1987). The mutation rate and variability of eukaryotic viruses: an analytical review. J. Gen. Virol. **68**:2729-2740.

Smith, F.I., and P. Palese (1988). Influenza virus: high rates of mutation and evolution. In *RNA Genetics*, vol. 3 (E. Domingo, J.J. Holland, and P. Ahlquist, eds.), pp. 123-135. Boca Raton, Fla.: CRC Press, Inc.

Spindler, K.R., F.M. Horodyski, and J.J. Holland (1982). High multiplicities of infection favor rapid and random evolution of vesicular stomatitis virus. Virology **119**:96-108.

Steinhauer, D.A., J.C. de la Torre, E. Meier, and J.J. Holland (1989). Extreme heterogeneity in populations of vesicular stomatitis virus. J. Virol. **63**:2072-2080.

Temin, H.M. (1989). Is HIV unique or merely different? J. AIDS **2**:1-9.

Wabl, M., P.D. Burrows, A. von Gabain, and C. Steinberg (1985). Hypermutation at the immunoglobulin heavy chain locus in a pre-B-cell line. Proc. Natl. Acad. Sci. USA **82**:479-482.

Weaver, S.C., T.W. Scott, and R. Rico-Hesse (1991). Molecular evolution of eastern equine encephalitis virus in North America. Virology **182**:774-784.

20

The High Rate of Retrovirus Variation Results in Rapid Evolution

HOWARD M. TEMIN

The AIDS pandemic can be viewed as a paradigm of the emergence of new diseases and of apparently new pathogens. In discussing this pandemic, I first consider if the AIDS pandemic is unique, and then I describe what properties of viruses, especially retroviruses, give them the potential to give rise to apparently novel agents.

IS THE AIDS PANDEMIC UNIQUE?

I do not think that the AIDS pandemic is unique relative to other epidemics when those epidemics are considered from the perspective of their time rather than in hindsight. In the past, major epidemics frequently occurred when there were new patterns of communication and transportation among separate populated areas and/or new patterns of settlement. William McNeill, in his impressive book *Plagues and Peoples* (1976), describes the occurrence of major epidemics throughout history in terms of this hypothesis.

One of the first examples of urbanization in the ancient world was in Athens during the Peloponnesian war. For defensive purposes, all of the Athenian population was pulled behind walls, and the city was supplied by ship. This congestion resulted in a great epidemic in 430-429 B.C.E., described by Thucydides.

In the middle of the sixth century, when extensive sailing ship traffic between India and the Mediterranean was established, there was a great outbreak of bubonic plague in the Mediterranean countries. In the thirteenth century, Mongol horsemen roamed from Burma and Yunnan all the way to Europe. McNeill believes that as a result bubonic plague reached Northern Europe. As a consequence, in 1346-1350, one-third of the population of Northern Europe died from bubonic plague, the Black Death.

In the sixteenth century, after Europeans reached America, there were devastating epidemics among the native peoples, resulting in a 90% population loss among American Indians in 120 years.

In the seventeenth and eighteenth centuries, regular trade by sailing ships between Africa and the Americas brought yellow fever to the Americas resulting in regular recurring epidemics. In 1793 in Philadelphia, then the nation's capital, social order broke down entirely. Of a population of approximately 45,000, half the people fled the city altogether (including all city officials except the mayor and most federal officials), and over 4,500 of those remaining perished.

In the early nineteenth century, with steamship travel becoming regular between India and Europe, both bubonic plague and cholera became worldwide. For example, in 1831, 13% of the population of Cairo died from cholera; and in 1832, more than 3,500 New Yorkers died of cholera within a few months.

Accompanying the disruptions of World War I, twenty million persons world-wide died in the 1918-1919 influenza pandemic.

Thus, it is not surprising that after World War II, with the changes in urbanization, enormous population increases in Africa, freer life styles in North America, and jet travel, a major new pandemic occurred. If anything, the surprise might be that there has been only one new pandemic (Temin, 1989).

HOW DOES A NOVEL PATHOGENIC AGENT SUDDENLY APPEAR?

The answer to this question can be a historical description; that is, for a new pathogenic virus, the answer could be "a precursor virus infected members of species *a* and then as a result of altered or special conditions *xyz*, the virus spreads in a particular locale to members of species *b*, and causes disease in *b*". In some cases discussed in this book, this description is available. However, it is not yet clear what was the immediate precursor virus for HIV-1, although HIV-2 appears to be directly descended from an SIV (Dietrich et al., 1989; Allan et al., 1991; see also Chapter 12 in this volume).

We do know, however, that viruses, especially RNA viruses, can evolve very rapidly (Eigen and Biebricher, 1988; Domingo and Holland, 1988; Domingo et al., 1985; Doolittle et al., 1989; Pathak et al., 1990). I shall discuss, using retroviruses as an example, the molecular basis for that rapid evolution and how the high rate of virus genetic variation allows mutation-driven evolution.

TYPES AND RATES OF RETROVIRUS VARIATION

There are two types of data relating to this question. One is nucle-otide sequence data from virus isolates. The most extensive data is from HIV-1 (Goodenow et al., 1989; Meyerhans et al., 1989; Vartanian et al., 1991; Balfe et al., 1990; Simmonds et al., 1990). The polymerase chain reaction was used to sequence repeatedly 350 base pairs (bp) of DNA from several clones of HIV-1 amplified directly from patient material. The data indicate that in any one AIDS patient, at any one time, there are many different virus genomes. (Eigen has called this distribution a quasispecies, although I think "population" or "swarm" is clearer. A quasispecies is a population with particular properties [Eigen and Biebricher, 1988].)

The other kind of data is direct measurements of the retroviral mutation and recombination rates. Early quantitative experiments involved a reversion assay at a single site in an oncoretrovirus vector (Dougherty and Temin, 1988). A figure of 2×10^{-5} substitutions per base pair per replication was found. Other experiments used a forward mutation assay involving a change in electrophoretic mo-bility of RNA from certain regions of another oncoretrovirus (Leider et al., 1988). A similar rate of base pair substitution was found.

More recently a modification of the oncoretrovirus vector sys-tem was developed to measure the rate of forward mutations in a single cycle of retrovirus replication (Pathak and Temin, 1990a,b). Briefly, a retrovirus shuttle vector containing a selectable marker for mammalian and bacterial cells and sequences for replication as both a retrovirus and a bacterial plasmid was constructed (shuttle vec-tor); the vector also contained the lacZα peptide gene as a reporter gene. This vector was used in a single cycle of replication as a retrovirus, the proviral DNA was recovered as plasmids, and mu-tants were selected and sequenced.

The results indicated rates (per replication cycle per base pair) for base pair substitution of 7×10^{-6}, for frame shifting of 1×10^{-6}, for deletion of 2×10^{-6}, and for deletions with insertions of 2×10^{-6}. A high rate of deletion was also found previously (Dougherty and Temin, 1986). However, recent work (Pulsinelli and Temin, 1991) shows that these deletions are the result of mistakes in plus strand strong stop DNA synthesis and transfer.

Additional sequencing indicated that in about 1 per 10^4 provi-ruses, there was a 2% substitution rate over a 600 bp stretch. This high rate of mutation is called hypermutation and apparently results from an error-prone reverse transcriptase (see also Vartanian, et al., 1991). An error in transcription or translation could yield such a reverse transcriptase, which could then give rise to the hypermutated provirus. (Other experiments showed that the rate of transcription-

ALTERNATIVE MODES
OF RETROVIRUS REPLICATION
As virus

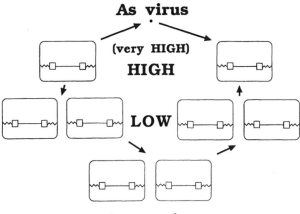

As provirus

Figure 20.1 Alternative modes of retrovirus replication. Cells containing proviruses (small boxes connected by straight line) integrated with cell DNA (zig-zag lines) are shown replicating and producing viruses (small filled circle). The rate of variation is shown as very high for hypermutation, high for usual retrovirus replication as virus, and low for retrovirus replication as provirus.

translation base substitution errors is about 10^{-4} per RNA molecule [Yang and Temin, unpublished observations].)

A modification of this single cycle protocol was used to measure the rate of recombination during retrovirus replication (Hu and Temin, 1990a). The rate of recombination between two markers separated by 1 kbp was about 2%. Calculation shows that this result indicates a rate for a full-sized retrovirus of 0.4 recombinations per replication cycle. However, restriction enzyme analysis of recombinants using six additional nonselected markers indicated that genomes with a recombination between the selected markers were likely to contain additional recombinations (Hu and Temin, 1990b). Thus, recombination will rapidly scramble the genomes of related retroviruses infecting the same cell.

These data indicate that retroviruses have a high probability of undergoing a mutation or recombination during every viral replication cycle. In addition, in about 1 per 10^4 viral replications a retrovirus will undergo hypermutation over part of its genome. Finally, retroviruses can persist as proviruses and only change at the rate of cell DNA. The figure (Fig. 20.1) shows these three modes of replication. A further consequence of the existence of a proviral step in retrovirus replication is the opportunity thereby given for recombination with cellular genes to introduce new sequences into the retrovirus genome (Bishop and Varmus, 1985; Temin, 1988).

CONSEQUENCES OF HIGH RATE OF MUTATION AND RECOMBINATION

A consequence of the high rate of mutation and recombination in retrovirus replication is that many variant viruses will be present in any retrovirus population. Any variant with a selective advantage will increase, and successful variants can become "frozen" as proviruses. In addition, retroviruses have a very high frequency of phenotypic mixing. This phenomenon allows retroviruses to undergo multiple mutations and recombinations before they are subject to selection (analogous to the effect of recessive mutations in diploid organisms). Thus, at any one time there will be in a retrovirus population a pool of variants that may be less than optimal for the present environment, but that will be more fit in a different environment.

Returning to our discussion of the origin of epidemics, we see that when the human population changes, which results in a new environment for viruses, a novel virus variant could easily spread and cause an epidemic, for example, HIV-1 and AIDS.

It is important to realize that retroviruses are not the only viruses with a high rate of mutation. All single-stranded RNA viruses mutate at the same high rates, and thus they exist in infected persons as populations of variants. However, single-stranded true RNA viruses (not retroviruses) have neither the high rate of recombination characteristic of retroviruses nor the ability to "freeze" good variants as proviruses. (It is not known if these RNA viruses undergo hypermutation, but analogous mechanisms might exist.)

The ability of viruses to evolve rapidly and thus take advantage of new environmental niches is inherently unpredictable. Since these mutational and recombinational processes are random, novel combinations of characteristics insure that new viral pathogens will appear when they have new opportunities to replicate.

ACKNOWLEDGMENTS

I thank G. Pulsinelli for helpful comments on this manuscript. The research in my laboratory is supported by Public Health Service grants CA 22443 and CA 07175 from the National Cancer Institute. I am an American Cancer Society Research Professor.

REFERENCES

Allan, J. S., M. Short, M.E. Taylor, S. Su, V.M. Hirsch, P.R. Johnson, G.M. Shaw, and B.H. Hahn (1991). Species-specific diversity among simian immunodeficiency viruses from African green monkeys. J. Virol. **65**:2816-2828.

Balfe, P., P. Simmonds, C.A. Ludlam, J.O. Bishop, and A.J.L. Brown (1990). Concurrent evolution of human immunodeficiency virus type 1 in patients infected from the same source: Rate of sequence change and low frequency of inactivating mutations. J. Virol. **64**:6221-6233.

Bishop, J. M., and H. Varmus (1985). Function and origins of retroviral transforming genes. In *RNA Tumor Viruses: Molecular Biology of Tumor Viruses* (R. Weiss, N. Teich, H. Varmus, and J. Coffin, eds.), 2nd ed., vol. 2 [Supplements and Appendixes], pp. 249-356. Cold Spring Harbor, N.Y.: Cold Spring Harbor Laboratory.

Delassus, S., R. Cheynier, and S. Wain-Hobson (1991). Evolution of human immunodeficiency virus type 1 *nef* and long terminal repeat sequences over 4 years in vivo and in vitro. J. Virol. **65**:225-231.

Dietrich, U., M. Adamski, R. Kreutz, A. Seipp, H. Kuhnel, and H. Rubsamen-Waigmann (1989). A highly divergent HIV-2-related isolate. Nature **342**:948-950.

Domingo, E., and J.J. Holland (1988). High error rates, population equilibrium, and evolution of RNA regulatory systems. In *RNA Genetics*, vol. 3 (E. Domingo, J. J. Holland, and P. Ahlquist, eds.), pp. 3-36. Boca Raton, Fla.: CRC Press, Inc.

Domingo, E., E. Martinez-Salas, F. Sobrino, J.C. de la Torre, A. Portela, J. Ortin, C. Lopez-Galindez, P. Perez-Brena, N. Villanueva, R. Najera, S. VandePol, D. Steinhauer, N. DePolo, and J. Holland (1985). The quasispecies (extremely heterogeneous) nature of viral RNA genome populations: biological relevance - a review. Gene **40**:1-8.

Doolittle, R. F., D.-F. Feng, M.S. Johnson, and M.A. McClure (1989). Origins and evolutionary relationships of retroviruses. Quart. Rev. Biol. **64**:1-30.

Dougherty, J. P., and H.M. Temin (1986). High mutation rate of a spleen necrosis virus-based retrovirus vector. Molec. Cell. Biol. **6**:4387-4395.

Dougherty, J. P., and H.M. Temin (1988). Determination of the rate of base-pair substitution and insertion mutations in retrovirus replication. J. Virol. **62**:2817-2822.

Eigen, M., and C.K. Biebricher (1988). Sequence space and quasispecies distribution. In *RNA Genetics*, vol. 3 (E. Domingo, J. J. Holland, and P. Ahlquist, eds.), pp. 211-245. Boca Raton: CRC Press, Inc.

Goodenow, M., T. Huet, W. Saurin, S. Kwok, J. Sninsky, and S. Wain-Hobson (1989). HIV-1 isolates are rapidly evolving quasispecies: Evidence for viral mixtures and preferred nucleotide substitutions. J. AIDS **2**:344-352.

Hu, W.-S., and H.M. Temin (1990a). Genetic consequences of packaging two RNA genomes in one retroviral particle: Pseudo-diploidy and high rate of genetic recombination. Proc. Natl. Acad. Sci. USA **87**:1556-1560.

Hu, W.-S., and H.M. Temin (1990b). Retrovirus recombination and reverse transcription. Science **250**:1227-1233.

Leider, J. M., Palese, P., and F.I. Smith (1988). Determination of the mutation rate of a retrovirus. J. Virol. **62**:3084-3091.

McNeill, W.H. (1976). *Plagues and Peoples.* Garden City, N.Y.: Anchor Press/Doubleday.

Meyerhans, A., R. Cheynier, J. Albert, M. Seth, S. Kwok, J. Sninsky, L. Morfeldt-Månson, B. Asjö, and S. Wain-Hobson (1989). Temporal fluctuations in HIV quasispecies in vivo are not reflected by sequential HIV isolations. Cell **58**:901-910.

Pathak, V., and H.M. Temin (1990a). Broad spectrum of in vivo forward mutations, hypermutations, and mutational hotspots in a retroviral shuttle vector after a single replication cycle: Substitutions, frameshifts, and hypermutations. Proc. Natl. Acad. Sci. USA **87**:6019-6023.

Pathak, V. K., and H.M. Temin (1990b). Broad spectrum of in vivo forward mutations, hypermutations, and mutational hotspots in a retroviral shuttle vector after a single replication cycle: Deletions and deletions with insertions. Proc. Natl. Acad. Sci. USA **87**:6024-6028.

Pathak, V., W.-H. Hu, and H.M. Temin (1991). Retrovirus variation and hypermutation. In *Somatic Hypermutation in V-region* (E. J. Steele, ed.), pp. 149-158. Boca Raton, Fla.: CRC Press, Inc.

Pulsinelli, G.A., and H.M. Temin (1991). Characterization of large deletions occurring during a single round of retrovirus replication: A novel deletion mechanism involving errors in strand transfer. J. Virol. **65**:4786-4797.

Simmonds, P., P. Balfe, C.A. Ludlam, J.O. Bishop, and A.J.L. Brown (1990). Analysis of sequence diversity in hypervariable regions of the external glycoprotein of human immunodeficiency virus type 1. J. Virol. **64**:5840-5850.

Temin, H.M. (1988). Evolution of cancer genes as a mutation-driven process. Cancer Res. **48**:1697-1701.

Temin, H.M. (1989). Is HIV unique or merely different? J. AIDS **2**:1-9.

Vartanian, J.-P., A. Meyerhans, B. Asjö, and S. Wain-Hobson (1991). Selection, recombination, and G-A hypermutation of human immunodeficiency virus type 1 genomes. J. Virol. **65**:1779-1788.

21

Evolution of Influenza and RNA Viruses

PETER PALESE

This chapter and the one following will deal with the evolutionary emergence in nature of human influenza viruses. There are three major types of influenza viruses, designated A, B, and C, all of which cause the disease we characteristically recognize as influenza, but only influenza A has been associated with pandemics. There is a uniquely rapid and uniform rate of evolution in influenza A virus genes. At the other end of the spectrum, influenza C viruses exhibit a much slower evolutionary rate, with coexistence in man of several evolutionary lineages. Influenza B viruses appear to be intermediate between influenza A and influenza C viruses in terms of their evolutionary rate.

For influenza A, viruses with the H1 hemagglutinin subtype predominated from 1918 all the way to 1957. The earliest human isolates available for analysis in the laboratory date from 1933, when the virus was first grown in an experimental host system. In 1957, a shift occurred from the H1 to the H2 subtype. This subtype was prevalent until 1968, when another shift occurred, to the H3 subtype; these viruses are still the predominant type today. Finally, in 1977 there was the apparent reemergence of H1 viruses. There is far less diversity in influenza types B and C. The earliest available influenza B isolate dates from 1940; unlike influenza A, there is only one major hemagglutinin type. The first influenza C virus was isolated in 1947, and distinct subtypes of the hemagglutinin have not been observed with this virus either.

Unlike these, influenza A virus changes readily. The work in my own laboratory, which I will discuss, uses the tools of molecular biology to analyze the mutation rates of various genes of influenza viruses. One can analyze changes in the hemagglutinin and neuraminidase, the surface proteins undergoing the shifts, but if one wishes to study long-term evolution of the human influenza A viruses, it is preferable to focus on a gene that, unlike the surface proteins, is not exchanged by reassortment. The NS gene, which is the gene coding for nonstructural proteins, meets these criteria. It has the added advantage of being

Figure 21.1 Most parsimonious evolutionary tree for influenza A virus NS genes. The length of the trunk and the side branches of the evolutionary tree are proportional to the minimal number of substitutions required to account for the differences in sequence. Nonintegral numbers arise from averaging over all possible minimal solutions. The broken line connects the 1950 and the 1977 H1N1 strains. (From Buonagurio et al., 1986a. Copyright 1986 by the American Association for the Advancement of Science.)

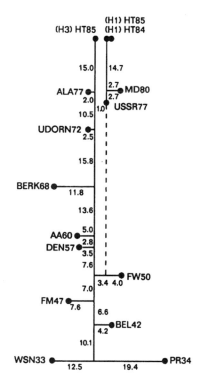

short, only 890 nucleotides long, simplifying complete analysis.

NS genes of 20 strains were sequenced and the nucleotide differences—mutations—in their NS genes were analyzed and arranged in a phylogenetic tree, using the procedure known technically as maximum parsimony tree analysis. The analysis itself was conducted in collaboration with Walter Fitch. The procedure basically involves using computer calculations to determine most probable evolutionary relationships of these sequenced genes by arranging the individuals in the order that gives the shortest pathways that will link them (Buonagurio et al., 1986a).

This phylogenetic, or family, tree of the human influenza A viruses possesses a main trunk with side branches (Fig. 21.1). The main trunk contains changes that are conserved over time. Side branches represent unique changes, leading to potential new lineages. As one might expect, the distance between viruses is proportional with time for influenza A viruses in humans. Examining strains isolated between 1933 and the present time, the most distantly related strains are those separated by the greatest amount of time. There is a very rapid evolution of the viruses as seen by just testing this one fairly well-conserved gene. The one exception is the reappearance of H1 viruses in 1977. These H1 viruses appear basically identical to the 1950 strains.

Figure 21.2 Linearity with time of number of substitutions in the NS genes of influenza A viruses. The abscissa represents the year of isolation of the influenza A viruses used in the analysis. The ordinate indicates the number of substitutions observed in their NS genes between the first branching point formed by the WSN/33 and PR/8/34 sequences in Figure 21.1 and the tips of all branches of the evolutionary tree. A line, generated by linear regression analysis, is drawn through the points. The slope of the line is 1.73 (0.08 substitutions per year). In addition to the sequences found on the trunk of the evolutionary tree (filled circles), the NS genes of the four new H1N1 viruses are also represented in this graph (filled squares). (From Buonagurio et al., 1986a. Copyright 1986 by the American Association for the Advancement of Science.)

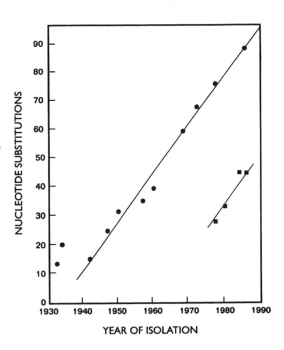

Another way of representing these data is to plot the year of isolation versus the number of nucleotide substitutions (Fig. 21.2). This gives two parallel lines. The first line represents all early H1 isolates and continues with the H2 and H3 isolates, to the present. The second line represents the H1 viruses isolated after 1977. This system makes it possible to determine the evolutionary rate of influenza viruses in nature. From the main trunk, since the number of mutations is approximately linear over time, one can readily calculate a rate of approximately 2×10^{-3} changes per RNA base site per year. The H1 viruses, in the second parallel line, change at approximately the same rate, despite having diverged. This emphasizes that two systems with similar mutation rates can proceed in different directions. These evolutionary rates are much higher than the rates for eukaryotic genes, which hover around 10^{-9} changes per nucleotide per year, about one million times slower.

EVOLUTIONARY PATTERNS OF OTHER INFLUENZA TYPES

Using the same approach, sequencing the genes of different influenza C viruses isolated between 1947 and 1984, we showed that influenza C viruses change at a much smaller rate (Fig. 21.3). There are 10 changes in the NS gene between the Taylor strain of 1947, and a strain isolated in 1954. However, Johannesburg 1966 virus, a virus that was isolated almost 20 years later than the Taylor strain, shows no NS gene sequence differences from the 1947 strain. This extreme conservation of sequences has never been seen with influenza A viruses (Bonagurio et al., 1986b).

In the HE gene (the influenza C equivalent of the hemagglutinin), the changes are similarly slow, and do not occur at a constant rate. There were a total of 110 nucleotide changes between the 1947 and the 1980 strain, but a 1981 strain differs from the 1947 strains by only 29 nucleotide changes.

There are two main conclusions of this study with influenza C viruses. First, situations occur in which there is little or no change for approximately 20 years or more. Second, the increases are not linear with time. From these data, we postulate a pattern for the evolution of influenza C viruses different from that of A viruses. Influenza A viruses exhibit rapid evolution, Darwinian style, in which a parent sheds off variants, only one of which may be successful (Fitch et al., 1991). The result is a slender evolutionary tree. In essence, with the exception of the H1 viruses, there is only one evolutionary lineage of influenza A. In contrast, influenza C viruses have several cocirculating evolutionary lineages and the genetic distances among isolates obtained in successive seasons may be small. In other words, the influenza C viruses evolve slowly, and several lineages can cocirculate in the population.

An analysis of influenza B viruses was also performed. The NS and hemagglutinin genes obtained from different viruses were sequenced and a phylogenetic tree was constructed. Here, again unlike influenza A, the branching order is not a function of time. For example, a 1984 strain turns out most closely related to a 1973 strain, but 1987 strains are much more distantly related. The interpretation of the data for influenza B viruses is that there is more change over time with influenza B than with influenza C virus and less than with influenza A. In addition, there appear to be cocirculating evolutionary lineages of influenza B viruses similar to what was observed for influenza C viruses.

Recently, the complete nucleotide sequence of an influenza C virus has been completed, allowing us to compare all the genes of the three influenza virus types (Yamashita et al., 1989). Comparing the amino acid identities among the proteins of influenza A, B, and C viruses, two points are notable. The protein that is most conserved among the three virus types is the polymerase basic protein, PB1, which shows a 60 percent sequence identity between influenza A and B, and a 40 percent identity between influenza C and the two other types. Second, in terms of divergence of these viruses, the receptor destroying enzyme, neuraminidase, is present only in influenza A and B viruses. In place of this protein, influenza C has a

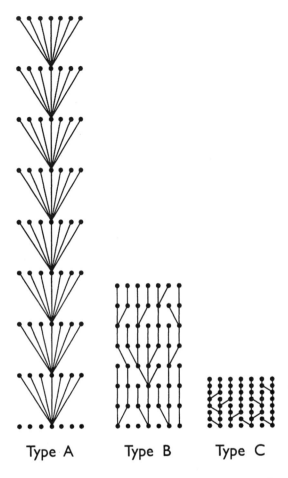

Type A   Type B   Type C

Figure 21.3 Evolutionary model for the propagation of influenza A, B, and C viruses in man. Dots lying on a horizontal plane represent influenza virus variants arising in the same season (year). The branch lengths indicate average relative change from the preceding season. The left part of the diagram shows influenza A virus. The variants arise from only one lineage because of the dominating effects of favorable variants. The middle and right of the diagram show, respectively, the cocirculation of multiple influenza B and C virus lineages. Variation of influenza B viruses appears to be slower than that of influenza A viruses and faster than that of C viruses. This is illustrated by the intermediate length of the evolutionary branches of the influenza B virus pattern. For all influenza A, B, and C viruses an arbitrary number of seven seasonal cycles is shown on the diagram. (From Yamashita et al., 1988. Reprinted by permission of Academic Press, Inc.)

domain in its glycoprotein, which is coded by a 300 nucleotide region and which has receptor destroying activity. This region is the influenza C equivalent of the neuraminidase. It should also be noted that a similar enzyme is also present in coronaviruses, a positive strand RNA virus (and hence an RNA virus quite different from influenza), which has interesting evolutionary implications (Vlasak et al., 1988). Finally, we recently determined (in collaboration with Frederick J. Fuller's group in Raleigh, North Carolina) that the P-alpha protein of the tick-borne Dhori virus shares between 27% and 31% sequence identity with the PB1 polypeptides of the influenza A, B, and C viruses (Lin et al., 1991).

MEASUREMENT OF VIRAL MUTATION RATE IN TISSUE CULTURE

These experiments were performed in order to better understand the factors which determine the evolutionary rate of viruses in nature. The evolutionary rate may depend on parameters such as mutation rate, number of replication cycles, constraints on protein and RNA structure, and on selective pressure. Clearly, it is a very complex system.

In order to define the effects of individual factors, a system was developed for measuring mutation rates in vitro (Parvin et al., 1986). A single infectious influenza virus particle is placed on a monolayer of susceptible cells in culture, giving a single plaque (a hole in the cell sheet) in the culture dish. A plaque is caused by the progeny of the original single viral particle. In a period of 40 hours, influenza A virus undergoes five cycles of replication. The number of mutations present in this plaque, representing the viral progeny of the original single particle, is determined. Analyzing the individual viruses is done by sequencing. Testing the NS gene, seven mutations were identified out of a total of 100,000 bases sequenced from 100 individual viruses. Assuming five replication cycles during this plaque formation, this yields a figure of 10^{-5} mutations per replication cycle (Parvin et al., 1986).

The same approach with polio virus gave a different result. Despite the sequencing of approximately 100,000 nucleotides, no mutations were found among 100 poliovirus isolates. This would translate into a mutation rate at least one-tenth than that of influenza A. Similar results were obtained by Philip Sharp's laboratory, with a figure of 10^{-6} mutations per nucleotide per infectious cycle, using a different method (Sedivy et al., 1987). John Holland and his colleagues have reported much higher mutation rates for polio virus, but the experimental system to measure the mutation rates is different from ours and from that of Sedivy and colleagues (de la Torre et al., 1990).

We also have recently analyzed the mutation rate of a retrovirus by the same approach, starting with a cloned DNA of the Rous sarcoma virus (RSV) genome (Leider et al., 1988). Retroviruses are more complex than influenza or polio viruses because the virus first makes a DNA form, the provirus, from the viral RNA. This requires the viral enzyme reverse transcriptase. Replication of progeny viral RNA from this DNA uses host RNA polymerase II. The involvement of two different polymerases, the

232 EMERGING VIRUSES

host RNA polymerase II, and the viral reverse transcriptase, complicates the estimates of the mutation rate. Rather than sequencing directly, it is possible to take a shortcut by making RNA probes with the "standard" sequence and then hybridizing them to the regions of interest in the viral RNA. The hybrids are analyzed by a biochemical technique, denaturing gradient gel electrophoresis. If there is a mismatch, indicating that one or more bases of the progeny virus differ from the probe sequence, the mismatched heteroduplex runs more slowly in this gel system.

For RSV, nine mutations were detected in 65,000 nucleotides screened. This translates into a mutation rate of about 10^{-4} changes per replication per nucleotide site, the highest rate of any of the viruses we have tested so far. Thus, influenza A virus is intermediate and polio virus has the lowest rate among the three viruses we tested in our laboratory.

In summary, human influenza A viruses show unique rapid evolution with a uniform rate over a 50-year period. We can say that the NS gene shows approximately 2×10^{-3} changes per site per year. Variation in influenza B virus appears to be slower than that of influenza A virus, but faster than that of influenza C viruses. Both influenza B and influenza C viruses exhibit multiple cocirculating lineages in man. Our studies on the genome structure of influenza viruses show that the PB1 (RNA polymerase) protein is the most highly conserved among influenza virus genes. Other viruses, such as coronaviruses, may have an evolutionary relationship with influenza C viruses; perhaps these viruses share a common ancestor at least for certain genes or domains of genes. An evolutionary relatedness was also observed between the tick-borne Dhori virus and the type A, B, and C influenza viruses. Finally, comparing the mutation rates of different RNA viruses, a retrovirus was found to possess the highest mutation rate, the overall rate being 10^{-4} mutations per nucleotide per replication cycle. In comparison, using similar analyses in tissue culture systems, influenza A virus had a mutation rate of only 10^{-5} mutations per nucleotide per cycle, and poliovirus was lower still.

REFERENCES

Buonagurio, D.A., S. Nakada, J.D. Parvin, M. Krystal, P. Palese, and W.M. Fitch (1986a). Evolution of human influenza A viruses over 50 years: Rapid, uniform rate of change in NS gene. Science 232:980-982.
Buonagurio, D.A., S. Nakada, W.M. Fitch, and P. Palese (1986b). Epidemiology of influenza C virus in man: Multiple evolutionary lineages and low rate of change. Virology 153:12-21.
Fitch, W.M., J.M.E. Leiter, X. Li, and P. Palese (1991). Positive Darwinian evolution in human influenza A viruses. Proc. Natl. Acad. Sci. USA 88:4270-4274.
Leider, J.M., P. Palese, and F.I. Smith (1988). Determination of the mutation rate of a retrovirus. J. Virol. 62:3084-3091.

Lin, D.A., S. Roychoudhury, P. Palese, W.C. Clay, and F.J. Fuller (1991). Evolutionary relatedness of the predicted gene product of RNA segment 2 of the tick-borne Dhori virus and the PB1 polymerase gene of influenza viruses. Virology **182**:1-8.

Parvin, J.D., A. Moscona, W.T. Pan, J.M. Leider, and P. Palese (1986). Measurement of the mutation rates of animal viruses: Influenza A virus and polio virus type 1. J. Virol. **59**:377-383.

Sedivy, J.M., J.P. Capone, U.L. RajBhandary, and P.A. Sharp (1987). An inducible mammalian amber suppressor: Propagation of a poliovirus mutant. Cell **50**:379-389.

de la Torre, J.C., E. Wimmer, and J. Holland (1990). Very high frequency of reversion to guanidine resistance in clonal pools of guanidine-dependent type 1 poliovirus. J. Virol. **64**:664-671.

Vlasak, R., W. Luytjes, W. Spaan, and P. Palese (1988). Human and bovine coronaviruses recognize sialic acid containing receptors similar to those of influenza C viruses. Proc. Natl. Acad. Sci. USA **85**:4526-4529.

Yamashita, M., M. Krystal, W.M. Fitch, and P. Palese (1988). Influenza B virus evolution: Co-circulating lineages and comparison of evolutionary pattern with those of influenza A and C viruses. Virology **163**:112-122.

Yamashita, M., M. Krystal, and P. Palese (1989). Comparison of the three large polymerase proteins of influenza A, B and C viruses. Virology **171**:458-466.

22

Factors Restraining Emergence of New Influenza Viruses

BRIAN MURPHY

The segmented genome of influenza virus can readily undergo reassortment, an exchange of genes between two virus strains coinfecting a cell at the same time. As Webster discusses in Chapter 4, the evolution of new pandemic influenza A strains appears to result from reassortment of genes of human and avian influenza A viruses. The emergence of new pandemic influenza strains is rare and has occurred most recently in 1918, 1957, and 1968. Avian influenza viruses are very common. It is likely that virtually every one of the enormous number of ducks in the world becomes infected. Human influenza is also common, with an estimated 100,000,000 infections in humans annually. Both ducks and primates can be hosts for coinfection by two influenza strains, both being susceptible, at least experimentally, to infection with a number of different influenza strains of either avian or mammalian origin. Avian influenza viruses normally replicate in both the respiratory tract and the gut of infected waterfowl, with prolonged virus shedding and little overt disease. Most human influenza virus strains do not replicate efficiently in the intestinal tract of ducks, but can infect their respiratory tract. Considering this enormous potential for gene exchange between avian and human viruses to occur, why do pandemic influenza viruses emerge only infrequently? The question is crucial because, given the many opportunities for new influenza reassortants to arise, the factors that prevent a new avian-human influenza A virus reassortant from efficiently infecting humans may well be the major determinants of whether a pandemic can occur. In this chapter, I will consider possible answers.

As Palese demonstrated, one can trace a linear evolution and conservation of influenza virus genes, beginning from the first human influenza virus isolated in 1933, which is the oldest human influenza strain that can be tested directly, down to the present. Most of the genes are the same in all these strains. However, a major exception is represented by the gene that codes for the hemagglutinin (H) protein. In each successive human pandemic influenza strain, a new hemagglutinin subtype has appeared, sometimes but not necessarily with a concomitant change in the neuraminidase protein. The pandemic of 1918-1919 was caused by an H1N1 virus, which was replaced by an H2N2 virus in 1957. In 1968, that virus was replaced, in turn, by an H3N2 virus that is still persisting in the population today.

In contrast to the situation with the H protein, the same NS (nonstructural proteins) gene has appeared in every human influenza A strain. This is also true of most other genes of pandemic influenza, subject to the occasional exception, such as the strain responsible for the 1957 pandemic. As demonstrated by Kawaoka and Webster, that strain arose from an exchange of three genes; in addition to the hemagglutinin and the neuraminidase, it also differed from previously circulating human strains in its gene for PB1, which is part of the viral RNA polymerase, or RNA copying enzyme. Thus the H2N2 pandemic virus had three genes presumably of avian origin, the H, N, and PB1 genes, and the other five genes were from the human virus. In 1968, only the H and PB1 genes were derived from the avian reservoir.

ABILITY OF AVIAN INFLUENZA STRAINS TO INFECT PRIMATES

Notwithstanding these minor exceptions, the variety of human influenza strains is extremely limited in comparison to the great diversity of avian influenza viruses. With all the genetic diversity in the avian reservoir from which to select, it is natural to ask why strains bearing a wider variety of avian influenza virus genes do not ever appear in the human population.

Confirming the epidemiologic finding of a limited range of influenza viruses in the human population, experimental studies also demonstrate that avian influenza viruses vary greatly in their ability to replicate in primates. An analysis of the factors responsible for this will constitute the major thrust of this chapter.

One serious limitation in answering these questions is the difficulty of designing suitable experimental systems. It is, of course, neither wise nor feasible to conduct experiments with new influenza viruses on human subjects, especially reassortant viruses containing H genes not presently circulating in the human population. As a result, most of what we know about influenza viruses in humans comes from natural disease. A considerable amount of work has been done in cell culture, with valuable information gained, but cell cultures do not offer the same challenge to a virus as does the whole organism. As a surrogate for human infection, we have concentrated on an animal model using a primate, the squirrel monkey (*Saimiri sciureus*), which is relatively easy to work with in the laboratory and responds much like humans after infection with various human influenza A viruses. Briefly, in this model, squirrel monkeys are exposed to specific influenza viruses by inhalation and are tested for virus in the lower respiratory tract a few days later. Quantities of virus produced in various parts of the respiratory tract and duration of infection can be determined, making it possible to define quantitatively as well as qualitatively the relative ability of specific influenza viruses to replicate in primates.

Comparing 10 avian influenza isolates for their ability to replicate in the lower respiratory tract of squirrel monkeys, we found that they varied in ability to replicate in the primate. While many strains grew, most did so more poorly than the human influenza viruses tested. Besides validating the model, this finding also further confirmed that not all avian influenza viruses were equal in their ability to infect primates.

RESTRICTION OF AVIAN INFLUENZA VIRUSES IN MONKEYS

What is responsible for these differences in influenza strains? One way to approach this question is by genetics, testing for viral genes that cause a virus to be restricted in its ability to replicate in primates.

Influenza makes a number of protein products that perform various functions. The information for all of these products is, of course, coded in the eight segments of the influenza virus genome, offering numerous possibilities for viral reassortment. The surface glycoproteins inserted into the viral envelope, H and N, are important in entry and exit from the host cell, and have been discussed elsewhere. Below the surface, the M (matrix) protein is the main structural component surrounding the core of the virus particle, and is also required for virus maturation. The major internal component of the virion is the nucleoprotein (NP), another structural protein which is bound to the viral RNA as well as to other proteins. The virus has its own RNA polymerase, with its three component proteins designated PB1, PB2, and PA. Finally, there are two nonstructural proteins of unknown function; both are encoded by the same RNA segment, NS.

KEY VIRAL GENES RESTRICTING AVIAN INFLUENZA VIRUSES

The genetic approach we have used has been to make reassortant influenza viruses containing specific combinations of genes from avian and human influenza strains (reviewed in Treanor and Murphy, 1990). These reassortants can then be tested in the squirrel monkey to determine the effects of specific viral genes on replication in primates. The first reassortants tested were single gene reassortant viruses, standard human influenza strains containing a single gene from a particular avian strain. Some of these replicated comparatively well. In these cases, the virus could be isolated from the monkeys, to confirm that it had not changed significantly during primate infection. Many other reassortants did not replicate well. One such reassortant we tested showed highly restricted replication in the monkey lower respiratory tract, yielding one ten-thousandth as much virus as its human virus parent. This reassortant replicated so poorly that it was not possible to isolate it from the exposed monkeys.

Several reassortants containing the avian virus NP or M genes were attenuated in squirrel monkeys, while the NS gene often seemed less critical. This indicated that at least two genes in the avian virus, NP and M, were capable of reducing replication of the avian-human influenza A reassortant virus in primates. For the NP gene in particular, every single reassortant that contained this particular avian NP gene, irrespective of any other genes it possessed, showed a restricted phenotype. Human influenza strains could be rendered highly attenuated for primates simply by substituting the new avian NP gene.

These results had all been obtained using one avian isolate, derived originally from a mallard duck, as the donor for the avian genes. In order to confirm whether these results were generally applicable, we made and tested additional single gene reassortants derived from a different avian donor virus, a strain isolated from the pintail duck. Many of these reassortants, including all possessing the avian NP gene, also showed restricted replication in primates. Consequently, for this avian isolate as well, the NP gene of the pintail virus conferred host restriction. Because these studies are very complicated and involve primates, the number of such studies is limited, but the results have been consistent. To generalize from these data, the NP gene, at least in many avian strains, appears to be attenuating for humans.

The M gene of this particular avian virus did not reduce viral replication in primates, unlike the M gene of the other avian strain we tested. To further clarify the role of the M gene, reassortant viruses were derived that contained either the mallard or the pintail M gene in a human influenza strain, using the same human parent virus throughout. As in previous experiments, only the reassortant with the mallard M gene was attenuated. The M protein genes of these two avian viruses differ by only three amino acids, representing minuscule genetic divergence between the two avian viruses.

But those few amino acid differences are sufficient to cause attenuation for primates.

ROLES OF OTHER GENES IN HOST RESTRICTION

A third type of restriction was also identified. Certain combinations of avian and human influenza A virus genes prevented replication in primates. One virus with a particular constellation of polymerase genes failed to replicate at all in the respiratory tract of the squirrel monkeys. This virus was also unable to replicate in mammalian cells in culture, indicating that for some presently unknown reason these polymerase genes were not functioning appropriately in the mammalian cell in culture or in the respiratory tract in the monkeys. However, the virus replicated efficiently in cells of avian origin, indicating a profound effect of the host on the replication of such a reassortant virus.

The NS gene may show a different subtlety. Recent work has demonstrated that the NS gene exists as two versions, or alleles, designated allele A and allele B. These two alleles differ in their amino acid sequences by about 30 percent. Each allele, of course, also exhibits some variation among different strains that possess it, but these differences are much smaller, on the order of 10 percent. Oddly, although avian influenza strains may possess either allele, only the A allele is found in human influenza A virus isolates. A possible explanation, which can be tested, is that viruses with the B allele might replicate poorly in primates. Tests of the appropriate reassortants confirmed that the NS B allele greatly attenuated the virus as determined by quantity and duration of virus shedding in squirrel monkey nasopharynx and trachea. The restriction of replication specified by the NS B allele was almost as great as that of the NP gene, which is generally the gene that specifies the most restriction. Reassortants with the NS A allele, as a control, replicated as expected.

POSSIBLE RESTRICTIONS ON HEMAGGLUTININ AND NEURAMINIDASE

There is also a very curious distribution of hemagglutinin (H) subtypes in the human population. Although there are 14 known hemagglutinin subtypes, only subtypes H1, H2, and H3 have been associated with influenza strains infecting humans. Subtypes H4 through H14 have never been isolated from humans, or detected serologically, despite the fact that these are widely distributed in avian species. Similarly, in humans there is evidence of infection only with three of the nine known neuraminidase (N) subtypes, namely N1, N2, and N8. There is very little information about why this distribution exists.

One obvious suggestion is that viruses possessing hemagglutinin subtypes H4 through H14 are restricted in humans or primates. Unfortunately, there is very little information on this subject, because of the concern that a new pandemic virus could be created by placing new surface glycoproteins, such as H4 and N5, into a human influenza strain. The hemagglutinin is of special importance, since neutralizing antibodies are directed against this protein, and it is variation in the hemagglutinin that allows new influenza strains to evade the immune system and infect. Because of these safety considerations, it is not permissible to study such recombinants in a normal laboratory. It could possibly be done under the highest levels of containment, called P4 or Biosafety Level 4 conditions, that are used for working with the deadliest viruses, but such facilities are rare.

As a substitute, we have tested in our monkey model a few naturally occurring avian isolates containing other H or N subtypes. Some can replicate efficiently in the respiratory tract of primates, for example one strain possessing hemagglutinin subtype H7. There is therefore no obvious indication that viruses with at least some non-H1, H2, or H3 hemagglutinin or neuraminidase subtypes are unable to infect humans. The possibility exists that such viruses might eventually be seen in the human population.

CONCLUSIONS

To summarize, NP genes from two different avian influenza viruses restricted replication of human influenza viruses in primates. Some varieties of avian M genes, but not others, can also restrict replication. For reasons that are not clear and may vary with different situations, specific combinations of genes from certain avian influenza can restrict replication. Finally, the NS B allele, but not the NS A allele, also severely restricts replication.

It is more difficult to make generalizations about hemagglutinin and neuraminidase subtypes, but it is possible that viruses with some subtypes, H4 or H14 or specific neuraminidases, might also be restricted in primates.

These results allow some answers to the questions originally posed about why pandemic influenza viruses do not appear more often. The presence of attenuating genes in the avian virus population is likely to be one reason for the relatively infrequent emergence of new pandemic influenza viruses. The vast majority of reassortants between avian and human (or mammalian) influenza viruses contain a gene, such as NP or the NS B allele, or gene constellation that prevents the virus from replicating efficiently in primates.

However, even if most of the avian NP genes and the NS B allele cause attenuation of the virus in primates, one can calculate that some 25 percent of the resulting recombinant viruses would still be potentially virulent for humans if one of the two parents is a human influenza virus. The fact that new human influenza reassortants do not appear with anything approaching this frequency suggests that there may be additional restrictions, such as limitations on hemagglutinin subtypes that can function efficiently in humans. The net result of all these constraints is that for any random reassortment between a human and avian influenza A viruses, the probability of emergence of a successful new virus that can readily infect humans is probably relatively small. On the other hand, there are avian influenza strains that can replicate in monkeys to levels equivalent to human viruses. Because many combinations of human and avian influenza genes can function efficiently in primates, new pandemic influenza viruses can emerge from time to time despite the numerous restraints imposed by the divergence of avian and human genes.

REFERENCE

Treanor, J., and B. Murphy (1990). Genes involved in the restriction of replication of avian influenza A viruses in primates. In *Applied Virology Research*, vol. 2 [*Virus Variability, Epidemiology and Control*] (E. Kurstak, R.G. Marusyk, F.A. Murphy, and M.H.V. van Regenmortel, eds.), pp. 150-176. New York: Plenum.

23

Recombination in the Evolution of RNA Viruses

JAMES H. STRAUSS

Recombination is a fundamental mechanism of genetic variation that results from the reshuffling of genetic material by processes including reassortment of chromosomes, breakage of a chromosome followed by rejoining to a chromosome from a second parent, or by a replicase enzyme switching strands during replication of the nucleic acid. Recombination in viruses is now known to arise from all of these mechanisms. The high frequency recombination characteristic of influenza virus and other viruses with segmented genomes has been well documented. This occurs by reassortment of the individual segments to make new combinations during mixed infection of cells with two virus strains. Within the past few years it has also become clear that recombination also plays a role in the evolution of viruses whose entire genome is a single piece of RNA. I will here discuss evidence for recombination in such viruses and the role of recombination in viral evolution.

RECOMBINATION IN THE ALPHAVIRUSES: WESTERN EQUINE ENCEPHALITIS VIRUS

We have studied RNA viral recombination in the alphaviruses, a genus in the family Togaviridae. Togaviruses are RNA viruses whose nucleocapsid core is surrounded by an envelope consisting of a lipid bilayer containing virally encoded integral membrane proteins (hence the name toga, like the Roman cloak). The alphavirus genus consists of about 25 members, with a wide geographic range (Calisher and Karabatsos, 1988). There are biological differences between the New World and Old World alphaviruses; New World alphaviruses often cause encephalitis, while Old World viruses cause arthritis and rash (Peters and Dalrymple, 1990).

The alphaviruses found in the United States include Eastern

equine encephalitis virus (EEE), present in the eastern United States
and extending into South America, and Western equine encephalitis
virus (WEE), which is present in the western United States, extending north to Canada and south to Argentina. Highlands J virus,
which is very closely related to WEE, and is thought by some to be
a subtype of it, is also found in the eastern United States.

Sindbis virus is an Old World alphavirus having a wide geographic distribution in Europe, Africa, Asia, and Australia, but it is
serologically most closely related to WEE. This has always been a
puzzle. Why should the closest relative of WEE, a New World virus,
be Sindbis, an Old World virus? The mystery is compounded by the
fact that the type of disease caused by WEE, a moderately severe
encephalitis, is more similar to the pathology of EEE than to Sindbis,
which is largely asymptomatic in man, although some strains of
Sindbis cause a typical Old World alphavirus disease characterized
by arthritis, rash, and fever. Furthermore, an evolutionary tree for
the members of the alphavirus genus can be constructed using the
amino acid sequences of the glycoproteins (Bell et al., 1984). On such
a tree, Sindbis and WEE are on the same branch, indicating that they
are very closely related. This agrees with the well-known antigenic
cross-reactivity between the two viruses, since the glycoproteins
carry the major antigenic determinants.

Nucleotide sequence analyses of Sindbis (Strauss et al., 1984),
WEE (Hahn et al., 1988), and EEE (Chang and Trent, 1987) have now
been completed throughout the region encoding the structural proteins, the adjacent upstream domain, and the 3′ noncoding region.
The data show clearly that WEE is, in fact, a recombinant virus, being
closely similar to EEE throughout most of its length, but the two
glycoproteins, E2 and E1, have been replaced by glycoproteins from
a Sindbis-like virus (Fig. 23.1). The virus that resulted from this
recombination event has been quite successful, since WEE is widely
distributed from Canada through South America. Biologically, the
disease symptoms of WEE mimic those of EEE, the parent from
which most of the virus genome is derived, but are somewhat less
severe, and WEE can be thought of as attenuated compared to EEE.
The recombination event also altered vector specificity, since WEE is
vectored primarily by *Culex* mosquitoes while EEE is vectored primarily by *Culiseta* mosquitoes.

The evidence for the recombination event is convincing (Hahn et
al., 1988). The capsid (coat) proteins of WEE and EEE show 85
percent amino acid sequence identity (Fig. 23.1), and the percent
identity is even higher (91 percent) in the C-terminal halves of the
proteins. On the other hand, the capsid proteins of WEE and Sindbis
show only 54 percent overall sequence identity, about the same as
the capsid protein similarities among other alphaviruses. Conversely,
the envelope glycoproteins show the opposite relationship, with 71

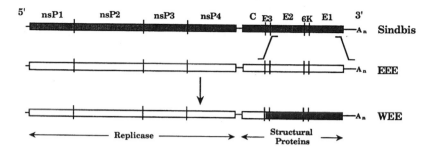

VIRUS	PROTEIN		
	nsP4	Capsid	Envelope
WEE/EEE	70	85	50
WEE/SIN	35	54	71
EEE/SIN	40	50	46

PERCENT SEQUENCE IDENTITY

Figure 23.1 WEE was produced by recombination between a Sindbis-like virus and EEE. In the top part of the figure are shown schematics of the Sindbis genome, the EEE genome, and the WEE genome. Shading is used to illustrate the part of the WEE genome that is derived from a Sindbis-like virus. The nonstructural proteins (nsP) are numbered 1, 2, 3, and 4, and together are required for RNA replication. The structural proteins are capsid (C), envelope (E) 1, 2, and 3, and a protein referred to as 6K. In the table below are shown the percent identities when proteins from different regions of the three viruses are compared. Note that the capsid protein and nsP4 of WEE are most closely related to EEE, whereas the envelope proteins of WEE are most closely related to Sindbis (SIN).

percent sequence identity between WEE and Sindbis, and only 50 percent between WEE and EEE. Although it seems clear that EEE was one of the two parents of WEE, Sindbis itself was probably not the actual second parent, event though Sindbis is the closest known relative to WEE. I suspect the true Sindbis-like parent is a New World alphavirus that has not yet been identified. Although it is very difficult to determine the exact time at which the recombination occurred, the high sequence similarity between WEE and EEE, in those portions that are common to both, indicates that this recombination event must have happened relatively recently. We originally estimated that WEE arose between 100 and 200 years ago, based upon the rates of sequence divergence commonly found in RNA viruses (Steinhauer and Holland, 1987; Strauss and Strauss, 1988). Recently, however, information on the rates of sequence divergence in alphaviruses has appeared (Burness et al., 1988; Shirako et al., 1991; Weaver et al., 1991), and it seems clear that these viruses diverge much more slowly than, say, poliovirus or influenza virus. Thus, WEE probably arose much earlier than we initially thought.

That a recombination event occurred to produce a virus is not surprising in itself. Recombination in various nonsegmented RNA viruses has been repeatedly demonstrated in the laboratory. But this is not the same as finding it in nature. Viruses are strongly selected for rapid growth and transmission. To be transmitted, an alphavirus infecting a vertebrate must achieve a sufficiently high viremia to infect a mosquito vector before host defenses are activated. Moreover, for efficient virus production, the envelope glycoproteins must interact specifically with the nucleocapsid core particle during budding of the virus from the infected host cell. A priori it would appear unlikely that the glycoproteins of Sindbis could interact with the capsid protein of EEE to give rise to virus that would replicate efficiently. And indeed it appears that the interaction of the capsid protein of EEE with the Sindbis glycoproteins was not optimal. The WEE capsid protein is a slight variant of the EEE capsid protein, in which a number of EEE amino acids have been replaced with their Sindbis counterparts. To be more precise, in the C-terminal half of the capsid protein there are only 7 differences between EEE and WEE, and of these six result in the replacement of the EEE amino acid with that found in Sindbis virus (Fig. 23.2). We believe that the capsid protein of WEE evolved after the initial recombination event, through selection, to a capsid protein that was better able to interact with its glycoproteins—that is, with the glycoproteins of Sindbis virus. The converse is also true. In the C terminus of the WEE E2 glycoprotein there are changes from the Sindbis sequence, such that the new protein now resembles the EEE sequence more closely (Fig. 23.2). This suggests that after the initial recombination event, continued selection resulted in further adaptation between the disparate elements derived from the two parental viruses.

PLASTICITY OF THE VIRAL GENOME

How is it possible to generate viable new combinations by recombination if critical functions such as the interaction between capsid and glycoproteins have already been optimized in extant viruses? This question can be approached by using the techniques of molecular genetics to make recombinants or to alter the genome in other ways. Alphaviruses contain several regions of sequence that are highly conserved at the nucleotide level among the alphaviruses examined (Strauss and Strauss, 1986). Even in these regions, many mutations can be tolerated and produce viable virus, illustrating

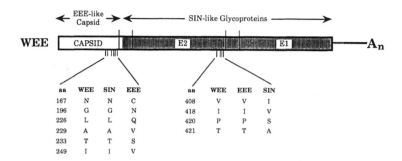

Figure 23.2 Evolution of the WEE capsid and E2 after the origin of WEE by recombination. In the capsid of WEE following residue 157, there are only seven differences from the EEE capsid. Of these, six residues are now the same as Sindbis, as shown in the figure. The tick marks shown the location of these differences, and the residue numbers and amino acids (in the single letter amino acid code) are shown below. In the C-terminal 16 residues of E2, there are six differences between WEE and Sindbis, and of these differences, four are now the same as EEE, as shown. We hypothesize that the WEE that arose by recombination between EEE and Sindbis evolved in these two regions so that the capsid and envelope protein 2 of the WEE recombinant could interact more efficiently during budding.

that the alphavirus genome possesses great plasticity. For example, deleting or altering many of the nucleotides in a conserved domain at the 3' end of the Sindbis viral genome had only modest effects on virus replication in chicken cells in culture (Kuhn et al., 1990). Although some residues were critical, most were not. Moreover, even very large deletions of the whole 3' nontranslated region, except for a few nucleotides at the absolute 3' end, had only modest effects on the ability of the virus to grow in tissue culture. Changes at the 5' end of the RNA also often yielded virus that replicated well (Niesters and Strauss, 1990a,b). The only major exception was that changes directly at the 5' end were lethal, and that deleting either the G or the C in a GC pair near the 5' end gave a temperature-sensitive mutant.

Although many of the resulting viruses appear to replicate well, none of these changes was truly neutral, in that these mutants are outcompeted by wild-type virus in mixed infections. In addition, the growth of many of the mutants in mosquito cells is much more dramatically impaired than in cells of mammalian and avian origin, and the mutants often grow much more slowly than wild type and yield a thousandfold fewer progeny. The failure to grow in mosquito cells is of great biological importance because alphaviruses are transmitted by mosquitoes and actively replicate in their arthropod vectors. Furthermore, we also found that some mutants grew well in mosquito cells but were severely impaired in chicken cells. These data lead to two conclusions. 1) The fact that the effect of any change

is different in mosquito cells than in chicken cells indicates that some
host cell components must interact with these mutagenized regions.
2) The requirement to alternate between a mosquito vector and a
vertebrate host imposes greater selective pressures than growth in a
single host, and may be one reason that all alphaviruses have re-
tained these highly conserved consensus sequences.

In the laboratory, we have also made various recombinants
between two alphaviruses, Sindbis and Ross River, and assessed
their ability to replicate in mammalian and insect cells (Kuhn et al.,
1991). As one would expect, the host range of the virus is usually
conferred by the structural proteins, the capsid protein and the
glycoproteins. Many of the recombinants were able to replicate
adequately in both mammalian and insect cell lines, but usually not
as well as the parents. The conclusion suggested by these experiments is that although recombination probably occurs with reasonable frequency in these viruses, often producing viable recombinants, most of the recombinants are at a selective disadvantage
compared to wild type, and do not spread. But the potential is
always there.

RELATIONSHIPS WITH PLANT VIRUSES

At this point, a little more detailed information about the structure
of the alphavirus genome is in order (Strauss and Strauss, 1986). The
alphavirus genome consists of one piece of single-stranded RNA
about 11,700 nucleotides in size that is divided into two regions (Fig.
23.3). The first region encodes the virus replicase, the RNA copying
enzyme made by the virus that is required in order for the virus to
make progeny RNA. The replicase is translated starting near the 5'
end of the incoming viral RNA as a long polyprotein. This product
is then cleaved into three individual proteins, designated simply
nonstructural protein (nsP) 1, 2, and 3, by a virally encoded protease
that is required for virus viability. There is a stop signal in the
genome after the information for protein 3, but the stop is sometimes
ignored (read through) to produce a fourth polypeptide, designated 4.

The second region of the genome consists of the 3' one-third of
the RNA. Here are located the genes for the structural proteins of the
virus, which are transcribed into a separate messenger RNA and
translated into another polyprotein; that polyprotein is cleaved to
yield the capsid protein and the glycoproteins, designated E1 and E2.

Studies of the Sindbis replicase and its processing by the protease led us to another remarkable example of apparent recombination in RNA virus evolution. Some time ago, we and others found
that there are three regions of protein sequence similarity shared by
Sindbis and a number of plant viruses (Ahlquist et al., 1985; Haseloff

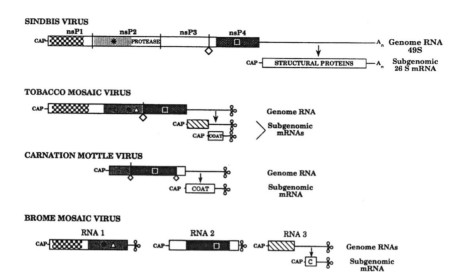

Figure 23.3 Sindbis, tobacco mosaic, carnation mottle, and brome mosaic viruses are related. Schematics of the genomes of these four viruses are shown. Three domains in the replicase genes that share amino acid similarity are indicated by the three different types of shading (checkerboard, stippling, and dark slanted shading, respectively). A helicase motif is indicated by the asterisk and an RNA polymerase motif by the solid square. Leaky termination codons that are readthrough are indicated by the open diamonds. All of these viruses transcribe subgenomic RNAs that are messengers for the structural proteins that form the virus particle. Note that brome mosaic virus has three genomic RNAs (it is tripartite), whereas the other viruses illustrated have a single RNA molecule as their genome.

et al., 1984), including tobacco mosaic virus (TMV), bromegrass mosaic virus (BMV), and carnation mottle virus (Fig. 23.3). These similarities involve large domains of 300 or 400 amino acids each and surely indicate that these protein domains are homologous. The genes are also organized a little differently in each of the plant viruses. BMV has the same regions of sequence homology, but unlike the other viruses, it has a segmented genome; two of the proteins are on the same segment, while the third is on a different segment. Carnation mottle virus has two of these three shared regions, but one of them is truncated. All of these viruses produce their capsid proteins by translation of subgenomic messenger RNAs derived from the 3′ ends of their genomes.

The genome organizations of these viruses and the homologies they share suggest that all of them arose from a common ancestor. During their evolution, the viruses not only underwent divergent evolution, but also recombinational events. The basis for this statement is the fact that despite the sequence similarities in their RNA replication enzymes, these viruses do not resemble each other morphologically. Sindbis is an enveloped virus with surface glycoproteins, while TMV is a helical rod without an envelope, and BMV is an icosahedron. Since the structural proteins that form the virion are responsible for these differences, this suggests that the structural proteins were derived from independent sources.

Furthermore, in addition to the regions that are more or less fully shared among all these viruses, there are other domains that are unique. The plant viruses, for example, contain genes that are required for such specialized functions such as transmission by aphid vectors and initiation of systemic infection. These genes have no counterparts in the alphavirus genome. However, some of the plant virus-specific genes resemble genes in other plant viruses that belong to other virus families, with different replicase genes. These partial relationships among viruses suggest that recombination events are continually occurring.

Conversely, Sindbis uses a specialized protease, present in nsP2, to carry out the cleavage of its nonstructural proteins to yield the individual proteins from the longer precursor (Hardy and Strauss, 1989). By contrast, in the plant viruses, the replicase proteins are produced as a unit that is never cleaved, and a protease is not present. Thus, in TMV, the two nonstructural domains always function together. The third domain, when present, simply adds to the polyprotein. The cleavage of the nonstructural proteins carried out by the alphaviruses therefore is interesting in view of the fact that the other viruses manage without it. One explanation may be that when proteins 1 and 2 are linked together in a domain, the polyprotein serves a different function than when the proteins are separated from each other. A second possibility is that separating the proteins allows for greater regulation of the virus life cycle (de Groot et al., 1990). This pattern might go back to the evolutionary roots of these viruses, when these domains presumably functioned together as a polyprotein, as they still do in the plant viruses. The alphaviruses have since evolved a mechanism to separate the two proteins, which may allow the virus to do things that its ancestor could not, such as adapting to new hosts.

Further support for the notion that the cleavage of proteins 1 and 2 was a later evolutionary development comes from studies of the Sindbis nonstructural protease gene itself (de Groot et al., 1990; Hardy and Strauss, 1989; Shirako and Strauss, 1990). As stated, the protease is in a region that is not shared with any of the plant viruses. There is a domain of 460 amino acids in the N terminus of nonstructural protein 2, which is homologous to a domain in the plant viruses and which presumably performs the same function in Sindbis RNA replication as the homologous TMV protein does in plant virus RNA replication (Ahlquist et al., 1985). Recent studies suggest that this domain functions as a helicase to unwind RNA during replication (Gorbalenya et al., 1988). Added on to the C terminus of the helicase of alphaviruses is a domain of about 300 amino acids that functions as a protease. These two domains are linked together by a sequence of approximately 15 amino acids, which are variable among alphaviruses, and that might function as a tether to link the two domains together. One can speculate that during evolution an ancestral virus acquired the protease gene by recombination with some other RNA, either cellular or viral, and in doing so gave rise to a virus with new capabilities.

CONCLUDING REMARKS

The comparisons of Sindbis and the plant viruses described above seem to represent a form of cassette or modular evolution, in which the different virus genes are evolving independently in different viruses (Strauss and Strauss, 1988; Zimmern, 1988). I suggest that modular evolution is going on all the time and is an important force in the evolution of RNA viruses. Through recombination and reassortment events, new combinations of virus can arise. Recombination can also lead to the insertion of new genes derived from host cells. Certain of these new combinations may expand the host range of the ancestral virus and lead to new replication strategies. Most of the RNA viruses of greatest medical interest today have relatively recent origins compared with the history of humans on the earth. Not only do RNA viruses diverge very rapidly by nucleotide substitution and point mutation, but it is clear that recombination can contribute significantly to the establishment of new virus families. These phenomena should not be considered merely a part of evolutionary history, but important elements of a process that is still ongoing today.

ACKNOWLEDGMENTS

I would like to thank Ellen Strauss for her many contributions to the development of this topic, and to thank many other members of my research group who have contributed to this story. The research from my group described herein has been supported by the National Science Foundation and the National Institutes of Health.

REFERENCES

Ahlquist, P., E.G. Strauss, C.M. Rice, J.H. Strauss, J. Haseloff, and D. Zimmern (1985). Sindbis virus proteins nsP1 and nsP2 contain homology to nonstructural proteins from several RNA plant viruses. J. Virol. 53:536-542.

Bell, J.R., R.M. Kinney, D.W. Trent, E.G. Strauss, and J.H. Strauss (1984). An evolutionary tree relating eight alphaviruses based on amino terminal sequences of their glycoproteins. Proc. Natl. Acad. Sci. USA 81:4702-4706.

Burness, A.T., I. Pardoe, S.G. Faragher, S. Vrati, and L. Dalgarno (1988). Genetic stability of Ross River virus during epidemic spread in nonimmune humans. Virology 167:639-43.

Calisher, C.H., and N. Karabatsos (1988). Arbovirus serogroups: Definition and geographic distribution. In The Arboviruses: Epidemiology and Ecology (T. P. Monath, ed.), vol. 1, pp. 19-57. Boca Raton, Fla.: CRC Press, Inc.

Chang, G.-J.J., and D.W. Trent (1987). Nucleotide sequence of the genome region encoding the 26S m RNA of Eastern equine encephalitis virus and the deduced amino acid sequence of the viral structural proteins. J. Gen. Virol. 68:2129-2142.

de Groot, R.J., W.R. Hardy, Y. Shirako, and J.H. Strauss (1990). Cleavage-site preferences of Sindbis virus polyproteins containing the nonstructural proteinase: Evidence for temporal regulation of polyprotein processing in vivo. EMBO J. 9:2631-2638.

Gorbalenya, A.E., E.V. Koonin, A.P. Donchenko, and V.M. Blinov (1988). A novel superfamily of nucleoside triphosphate-binding motif containing proteins which are probably involved in duplex unwinding in DNA and RNA replication and recombination. FEBS Lett. 235:16-24.

Hahn, C.S., S. Lustig, E.G. Strauss, and J.H. Strauss (1988). Western equine encephalitis virus is a recombinant virus. Proc. Natl. Acad Sci. USA 85:5997-6001.

Hardy, W.R., and J.H. Strauss (1989). Processing the nonstructural proteins of Sindbis virus: nonstructural proteinase is in the C-terminal half of nsP2 and functions both in cis and trans. J. Virol. 63:4653-4664.

Haseloff, J., P. Goelet, D. Zimmern, P. Ahlquist, R. Dasgupta, and P. Kaesberg (1984). Striking similarities in amino acid sequence among nonstructural proteins encoded by RNA viruses that have dissimilar genomic organization. Proc. Natl. Acad. Sci. USA 81:4358-4362.

Kuhn, R.J., Z. Hong, and J.H. Strauss (1990). Mutagenesis of the 3' nontranslated region of Sindbis virus RNA. J. Virol. 64:1465-1476.

Kuhn, R.J., H.G.M. Niesters, Z. Hong, and J.H. Strauss (1991). Infectious RNA transcripts from Ross River virus cDNA clones and the construction and characterization of defined chimeras with Sindbis virus. Virology 182:430-411.

Niesters, H.G.M., and J.H. Strauss (1990a). Defined mutations in the 5' nontranslated sequence of Sindbis virus RNA. J. Virol. 64:4162-4168.

Niesters, H.G.M., and J.H. Strauss (1990b). Mutagenesis of the conserved 51 nucleotide region of Sindbis virus. J. Virol. 64:1639-1647.

Peters, C.J., and J.M. Dalrymple (1990). Alphaviruses. In Virology (B.N. Fields, D.M. Knipe, et al., eds.), second ed., Chap. 26 (pp. 713-761). New York: Raven Press.

Shirako, Y., B. Niklasson, J.M. Dalrymple, E.G. Strauss, and J.H. Strauss (1991). Structure of the Ockelbo virus genome and its relationship to other Sindbis viruses. Virology 182:753-764.

Shirako, Y., and J.H. Strauss (1990). Cleavage between nsP1 and nsP2 initiates the processing pathway of Sindbis virus nonstructural polyprotein P123. Virology **177**:54-64.

Steinhauer, D.A., and J.J. Holland (1987). Rapid evolution of RNA viruses. Ann. Rev. Microbiol. **41**:409-433.

Strauss, E.G., C.M. Rice, and J.H. Strauss (1984). Complete nucleotide sequence of the genomic RNA of Sindbis virus. Virology **133**:92-110.

Strauss, E.G., and J.H. Strauss (1986). Structure and replication of the alphavirus genome. In *The Togaviridae and Flaviviridae* (S. Schlesinger and M. J. Schlesinger, eds.), pp. 35-90. New York: Plenum.

Strauss, J.H., and E.G. Strauss (1988). Evolution of RNA viruses. Ann. Rev. Microbiol. **42**:657-683.

Weaver, S.C., T.W. Scott, and R. Rico-Hesse (1991). Molecular evolution of eastern equine encephalomyelitis virus in North America. Virology **182**:774-784.

Zimmern, D. (1988). Evolution of RNA Viruses. In *RNA Genetics*, vol. 2 (E. Domingo, J.J. Holland, and P. Ahlquist, eds.), pp. 211-240. Boca Raton, Fla.: CRC Press, Inc.

24

Evolutionary Relationships of Vectors and Viruses

BRUCE F. ELDRIDGE

In a recent paper on the evolution of bunyaviruses, Calisher wrote that whereas creationism offers certainty without data, science offers data without certainty (Calisher, 1988). If this is true of the bunyaviruses, then what we can offer about the evolution of their mosquito vectors is very little data and very little certainty. Even so, we know more about the evolution of mosquitoes than we know about many other arthropod vector groups.

MOSQUITOES IN THE FOSSIL RECORD

Insects have a long evolutionary history, stretching back at least into the Carboniferous period, about 300 million years ago. We can say a few things with a fair degree of certainty about the antiquity of the Diptera, the flylike insects, and some authorities place the first Diptera as no later than the Triassic period, about 200 million years ago. There is no direct evidence in the fossil record to indicate when mosquitoes arose. There are specimens of what look like mosquitoes in amber, but the species cannot be identified with certainty, and most of the modern species are not represented at all in the fossil record. It is not until well into the Tertiary period, no more than about 50 million years ago, that the fossil record tells us anything about the origin of modern mosquitoes. *Aedes* and *Culex* are two major genera of mosquitoes. The first recognizable *Culex* dates to the Eocene epoch of the Tertiary period (roughly 40-50 million years ago). The first *Aedes* date to the middle Oligocene epoch, about 30 million years ago (Edwards, 1932).

Mosquitoes probably preceded the origin of warm-blooded animals, and most entomologists feel that the blood-sucking habits of mosquitoes were already established by the time birds and mammals arose. There is a small amount of circumstantial evidence for that. Most mosquitoes that feed on warm-blooded animals have receptors to help them locate their prey, but other mosquitoes completely lack these receptors.

VIRUSES AND THEIR VECTORS

From a medical point of view, arthropod vectors are arthropods that transmit pathogens causing human diseases. These include various species of insects and some ticks and mites. The present discussion will be confined to mosquitoes, most of them in the genus *Aedes*.

There are specific criteria for the incrimination of vectors that medical entomologists established many years ago (Barnett, 1962). Some people have suggested that mosquitoes may transmit the AIDS virus, but the presently understood relationship between HIV virus and mosquitoes satisfies none of these criteria. Modern concepts of vector-pathogen relationships involve more than just a physical transfer of pathogens to susceptible hosts. In nearly all instances of well-studied systems, there is a well-established biological association between vector and pathogen, so that the vector may also be considered a host for the pathogen. Such an association is lacking in the case of the AIDS virus. This is why mosquito transmission of AIDS seems implausible to most medical entomologists.

Mosquitoes transmit a variety of viruses to vertebrate animals. The best known of these are the arboviruses classified in the families Alphaviridae and Flaviviridae (examples are Western equine encephalomyelitis virus, an alphavirus; and yellow fever virus, a flavivirus). The California (CAL) serogroup viruses form a subgroup of the genus Bunyavirus in the family Bunyaviridae. They were discovered relatively recently and are thus less well known than alphaviruses and flaviviruses. The current classification of the CAL serogroup viruses is based on serologic relationships, determined by several methods, including the neutralization test (Calisher and Karabatsos, 1988). CAL serogroup viruses found in the United States are divided into three major subgroups, namely the Trivittatus, Melao, and California encephalitis virus serocomplexes. Melao is further subdivided into three major subtypes, Melao, Keystone, and Jamestown Canyon (JC), each with a single variety. The California encephalitis serocomplex includes the subtypes La Crosse, California encephalitis, and Tahyna (TAH). Finally, La Crosse subtype has two varieties, La Crosse and snowshoe hare (Calisher and Karabatsos, 1988).

CLASSIFICATION OF MOSQUITOES IN THE GENUS *AEDES*

The classification of mosquitoes is somewhat more controversial than that of bunyaviruses, possibly because quantifiable methods have rarely been used to classify mosquitoes. One of the most widely used classifications of the genus *Aedes* was published by Edwards in 1932, and is based primarily on male genitalia (Edwards 1932). Other systems of classification have used larval characters and other adult characters, but none has replaced the classification of Edwards.

The Edwards classification, as later modified, divided the North American *Aedes* vectors of CAL serogroup viruses into four subgenera, *Ochlerotatus, Protomacleaya, Aedimorphus*, and *Aedes*. Originally, the mosquito *Aedes triseriatus* was in the subgenus *Finlaya*, but subsequently other taxonomists stated that mosquito species in *Finlaya* occurred only in the Old World and placed all the New World species in *Protomacleaya* (Zavortink, 1972).

The subgenus *Ochlerotatus* dominates the North American *Aedes* fauna. The subgenus is defined on the basis of whether or not there is a basal lobe and an apical lobe on the largest structure of the male genitalia (the gonocoxite). The subgenus *Ochlerotatus* also contains most of the species that are vectors of the CAL serogroup viruses. Based on other characters of the male genitalia, the subgenus *Ochlerotatus* can be further divided into the species groups *scapularis, communis, stimulans*, and *dorsalis*. For example, *Aedes stimulans*, which is in the *stimulans* group, is an important vector of JC virus, in the Melao serocomplex (Boromisa and Grimstad, 1986).

ORIGINS OF NORTH AMERICAN *AEDES* MOSQUITOES

Another important consideration in the reconstruction of evolutionary histories is zoogeography. There is a classic paper by Ross in which he attempted to determine where the modern species of North American mosquitoes had originated (Ross, 1964). Ross's conclusion about the North American *Ochlerotatus*, which includes most of the species relevant to this discussion, was that three species groups were of tropical origin but had radiated into the Holoarctic region, then down into Europe and into North America across the Bering Strait. Two other collections of species, the *atlanticus* group and the *trivittatus* group, were also considered to be of tropical origin but were theorized to have entered North America directly from South America by crossing what is now Central America. These two groups are of interest because they are also vectors of certain CAL serogroup viruses.

Ross suggested that another subgenus, *Aedimorphus*, which includes *Aedes vexans*, an important vector of Tahyna (TAH) virus, came from central Asia and radiated into the tropics and, secondarily, into Europe and North America. The subgenus *Aedes*, which includes *Aedes cinereus*, another vector of a CAL serogroup virus, probably was also of tropical origin and radiated into North America (Ross, 1964).

For purposes of this discussion, it is important to note that most *Ochlerotatus* came to North America from Arctic regions, while species of other subgenera apparently arrived directly from the tropics. The hypothesis to be examined here is whether this knowledge can explain specific associations between vectors and individual viruses in the CAL serogroup group.

TECHNICAL DIFFICULTIES OF ASSOCIATING VECTOR AND VIRUS

Before discussing the information relating to this question, it is necessary to explain how the association of a mosquito species with a specific virus is identified. The traditional method involves collecting live mosquitoes, separating them by species and sex, placing them in pools of up to 50 individuals, and then testing them for virus by placing triturated suspensions of the pooled mosquitoes in vertebrate cell cultures. Any virus grown is then identified by serologic methods, such as a neutralization test, to classify the virus on the basis of its antigenic characteristics. Grimstad recently pointed out a number of problems with published data based on these procedures (Grimstad, 1988), to which a few more can be added. One problem is that data before 1970 often do not clearly identify the individual viruses within the CAL serogroup, usually describing them only as a California group virus. Often, the mosquito species were not identified below the generic level. Also, the mosquito species may have been misidentified, or the pools that were tested may have contained a mixture of species. Numerical data also were often lacking, so it is not now possible to calculate a minimum infection rate. Finally, name changes of mosquito species may have occurred. Ten or 15 years ago, it was not generally realized that many groups of mosquitoes do not represent single species but are actually groups of sibling species. The availability of modern molecular techniques has helped identify these groups, but it is not now possible to go back and reevaluate these earlier reports.

There are additional cautions. An isolation of virus from a blood engorged female mosquito may not represent an actual occurrence of an infected mosquito, but indicates only that the mosquito had ingested viremic blood. It is also difficult to interpret the many instances of low isolation rates, such as 1 in 500,000 mosquitoes, which represent rare natural occurrences.

REPORTS OF VIRUS-VECTOR ASSOCIATIONS

With these caveats in mind, all literature reports of isolations of CAL serogroup viruses from mosquitoes were reviewed, eliminating those that were equivocal based on the technical grounds mentioned above. There were more than 100 published papers where one could identify both the virus and the mosquito species involved, and where usable numerical data were available (Eldridge, 1990).

The question asked was whether there was a significant degree of vector selectivity observable and to what degree the classification of virus and vector correspond.

In the case of Trivittatus (TVT) virus, isolations came almost entirely from mosquitoes that were in the *scapularis* group. In fact, all were from two closely related species, *Aedes trivittatus* and *Aedes infirmatus*. The former species occurs in the southern United States; the latter is more common in the north.

In the Melao group (Melao, Keystone, and JC), Melao virus has been isolated only from *Aedes scapularis*, another member of the *scapularis* group. These isolations were made in the New World tropics.

Keystone virus has been isolated from the eastern United States, primarily from *Aedes atlanticus* and *Aedes infirmatus*. The latter species is also associated with TVT virus in the southern part of the United States. *Aedes atlanticus* is more common in the northern United States. Although these two species belong to different species groups, the two groups are closely related.

JC virus is still more interesting. The virus occurs all over North America, and has been isolated from a variety of mosquito species. Most of these represent snow pool *Aedes* of Arctic origin, such as *Aedes absseratus*, *Aedes communis*, and *Aedes stimulans*. Another species, *Aedes cantator*, is of Arctic origin but now occurs as far south as the Carolinas. One species that doesn't fit this pattern is *Aedes cinereus*, the only North American representative of the subgenus *Aedes*.

The members of the California encephalitis serocomplex include snowshoe hare (SSH), La Crosse (LAC), California encephalitis (CE) and TAH viruses. SSH itself is an Arctic virus, found mainly in Canada and Alaska. As one might expect, it is found mainly in mosquitoes belonging to three Arctic groups of the subgenus *Ochlerotatus*, although there have been reports of isolations from other species. LAC virus occurs in *Aedes dorsalis*, but far more commonly in *Aedes triseriatus*, which is a species supposedly of tropical origin. There is also evidence for transovarial transmission (from mother to offspring) in this species. In fact, the first instance demonstrated of transovarial transmission of an arbovirus by a mosquito involved LAC virus in *Aedes triseriatus*.

CE virus itself, the prototype strain, is almost completely restricted to two species, *Aedes melanimon* and *Aedes dorsalis*, both in the subgenus *Ochlerotatus* and therefore of Arctic origin.

The most complex relationships are found in the case of TAH virus, a California group virus that is not native to North America. TAH virus is distributed widely over Europe and Asia, including China. TAH virus has been isolated from a number of different mosquito species, involving more subgenera than any other virus in the CAL serogroup.

INTIMACY BETWEEN VIRUS AND VECTOR: TRANSOVARIAL TRANSMISSION

The natural occurrence of transovarial transmission, in which a virus infects the eggs of an infected female arthropod and in that way can be passed down to the next generation, has been documented many times. Transovarial transmission provides evidence of a long-standing, close relationship between a virus and an arthropod vector. Analyzing patterns of transovarial transmission can be helpful in sorting out relationships, because they can help differentiate biologically significant virus-vector relationships from apparent relationships based on rare occurrences or other factors discussed earlier.

Demonstrating transovarial transmission in nature is difficult, but isolation of virus from naturally collected eggs, larvae, or male mosquitoes represents much stronger evidence of the phenomenon than the artificial infection of female mosquitoes in the laboratory and the demonstration of virus in eggs or progeny.

PREDICTION OF UNIDENTIFIED VECTORS

Can one use knowledge of mosquito evolutionary relationships and viral origins to predict where new viruses can be found? Although this field is still in its infancy, a recent example offers encouragement that such knowledge could help direct future efforts.

A rather obscure mosquito, *Aedes squamiger*, occurs only on the coast of California. Although a salt marsh breeder, and therefore ecologically very different from the mosquitoes discussed so far, it is closely related to the snow pool *Aedes*. If there really is an evolutionary relationship between the CAL serogroup viruses and the *Aedes* mosquitoes of Arctic origin, one test of the hypothesis would be to obtain a CAL serogroup virus from a mosquito species that is a descendant of a snow pool *Aedes* species.

To test this hypothesis, collections of *Aedes squamiger* were made in 1988 and 1989 from a number of coastal areas in California. The first ten pools of *Aedes squamiger* tested (from San Luis Obispo County) yielded five isolations of a CE-like virus (Eldridge et al., 1991).

This type of analysis has never before been attempted with viruses and mosquitoes, and thus it is still a largely untried approach. It is based on a limited knowledge of evolutionary relationships among mosquito species and among viruses. The utility of this approach, and interpretation of the data, would be greatly improved by the development of more refined taxonomic systems based on modern techniques of molecular biology. However, this example does illustrate that, as a working hypothesis, correlating the evolutionary origins of viruses and vectors can be of predictive value and could serve to guide rational approaches for identifying virus-vector associations. If efforts in this area are ever to come to fruition, this work will require scientists trained for it. One concern is that the present critical shortage of vector biologists could well hinder future developments.

IMPLICATIONS FOR EVOLUTION OF ARTHROPOD-BORNE VIRUSES

Taken together, these data allow some tentative conclusions, albeit admittedly speculative, about the evolution of the CAL serogroup viruses. It would appear that the CAL serogroup viruses arose in association with the ancestors of the present day *Aedes* that are now in the subgenus *Ochlerotatus*. This is most likely to have occurred in the tropics before the Pleistocene, after which populations of snow pool *Aedes* were probably left on mountain tops in various places, including Canada, by retreating glaciers. The current varieties of the CAL serogroup viruses probably evolved in association with the present day descendants of the snow pool *Aedes* as they speciated after geographic isolation.

Some of the viruses may also have acquired secondary associations by horizontal transmission mechanisms (transmission between individuals of different species, or if the same species, transmission occurring simultaneously to different individuals), which may explain some of the apparent anomalies noted earlier. This may have happened with TAH virus, which shows transovarial transmission in *Culiseta*, a non-*Aedes* vector, as well as in *Aedes vexans*. A similar situation may have arisen with LAC virus, which is now associated with *Aedes triseriatus*, a mosquito of tropical origin. However, LAC virus is closely related to SSH virus, and LAC virus may have evolved from a SSH-like ancestor. SSH virus is associated with mosquito species of Arctic origin, as noted earlier.

In considering viral evolution occurring as a result of selection over time, one must also consider the selective pressures exerted by vertebrate hosts of these viruses. Possible physiological and ecological factors which may be involved in both vector and vertebrate host influences on viral evolution were discussed recently by Nuttall et al. (1991). However, in assessing the relative roles of invertebrate and vertebrate hosts on viral evolution, it is necessary to know the relative roles played by horizontal (both to and from vertebrate animals) and vertical transmission (invertebrate parent to offspring) in the total virus ecology. In the case of many CAL serogroup viruses, these roles are obscure. This is illustrated by a recent study by Heard et al. (1991), in which they found that *Aedes provocans*, a species frequently found infected in nature with JC virus, did not transmit the virus effectively to laboratory mice.

Much more research is needed on viruses and their mechanisms of infection of both vertebrate and invertebrate hosts at the molecular level. We also need to know much more about the systematics and evolution of viruses and their mosquito vectors. Until more detailed studies are completed in these areas, patterns of evolution will remain speculative. Such research would be scientifically rewarding and would have practical implications. They could increase our understanding of how these viruses evolve and how interactions with an arthropod could potentially affect the evolution of both virus and vector, and could also provide a rational foundation for future searches of presently unknown arthropod-borne viruses and their vectors.

REFERENCES

Barnett, H.C. (1962). The incrimination of arthropods as vectors of disease. Proceedings of the 11th International Congress of Entomology, pp. 341-345.

Boromisa, R.D., and P.R. Grimstad (1986). Virus-vector relationships of *Aedes stimulans* and Jamestown Canyon virus in a northern Indiana enzootic focus. Amer. J. Trop. Med. Hyg. 35:1285-1295.

Calisher, C.H. (1988). Evolutionary significance of the taxonomic data regarding bunyaviruses of the family Bunyaviridae. Intervirology 29:268-276.

Calisher, C.H., and N. Karabatsos (1988). Arbovirus serogroups: definition and geographic distribution. In *The Arboviruses: Epidemiology and Ecology* (T. P. Monath, ed.), vol. 1, pp. 19-57. Boca Raton, Fla.: CRC Press, Inc.

Edwards, F.W. (1932). Diptera, family Culicidae. Genera Insectorum, Fasc.

194. Brussels: Desmet Verteneuil.

Eldridge, B.F. (1990). Evolutionary relationships among California serogroup viruses (Bunyaviridae) and *Aedes* mosquitoes (Diptera: Culicidae). J. Med. Entomol. 27:738-749.

Eldridge, B.F., G.C. Lanzaro, G.L. Campbell, W.C. Reeves, and J.L. Hardy (1991). Occurrence and evolutionary significance of a California encephalitis-like virus in *Aedes squamiger* (Diptera: Culicidae). J. Med. Entomol. 28:645-651.

Grimstad, P.R. (1988). California group viruses. In *The Arboviruses: Epidemiology and Ecology* (T. P. Monath, ed.), vol. 2, pp. 99-136. Boca Raton, Fla.: CRC Press, Inc.

Heard, P.B., M. Zhang, and P.R. Grimstad (1991). Laboratory transmission of Jamestown Canyon and Snowshoe Hare viruses (Bunyaviridae: California serogroup) by several species of mosquitoes. J. Amer. Mosq. Contr. Assoc. 7:94-102.

Nuttall, P.A., L.D. Jones, and C.R. Davies (1991). The role of arthropod vectors in arbovirus evolution. Adv. Dis. Vect. Res. 8:15-45.

Ross, H.H. (1964). The colonization of temperate North America by mosquitoes and man. Mosq. News 24:103-118.

Zavortink, T.J. (1972). Mosquito studies (Diptera, Culicidae), XXVIII. The New World species formerly placed in *Aedes* (*Finlaya*). Contributions of the American Entomological Institute 8:1-206.

25

Global Change and Epidemiology: Nasty Synergies

THOMAS E. LOVEJOY

In the first 3 months of 1989, seven U.S. senators, in two groups, spent the night out in the Amazon jungle swinging in hammocks. One of the group, a certain distinguished senator from Pennsylvania slept very well indeed, judging from the noises he emitted during the night. The next morning, he explained to some of his companions, who did not sleep so well as a result, that he was not snoring but was communicating with the howler monkeys. Were he writing this chapter I am sure he would assert that he had been studying yellow fever in the sylvan cycle.

This is only one example of how environmental issues have now reached the national consciousness. As another example, a National Forum on Global Change, cosponsored by the Smithsonian Institution and the U.S. National Academy of Sciences, was held in May 1989 in the National Theater in Washington and drew over 1,500 people (DeFries and Malone, 1989), which indicates that indeed there is a great deal of appropriate concern throughout the country and around the world about major changes in the global environment. However rough the outlines of the future may be, it seems appropriate to consider how these problems may bear on emerging infectious diseases.

First, let me sketch in some of the aspects of global change that are worrying some of us very much indeed (DeFries and Malone, 1989; Committee on Global Change, 1990). The largest single element of it is a problem that has been building up for a very long time, namely the increased levels of carbon dioxide in the atmosphere and its relation to what is called the greenhouse effect. Although increased CO_2 in the atmosphere is not the only cause, it is certainly the largest part of the problem. Put very simply, the levels of CO_2 in the atmosphere are considerably higher than they have ever been in the history of our species, roughly 20 percent higher than in preindustrial times. Carbon is an element that absorbs radiant energy, trapping energy that otherwise would normally reflect off the surface of the earth, in fact, trapping that heat much as a greenhouse does.

For reasons I will discuss later, there is considerable imprecision in estimating exactly how far into a greenhouse warming we actually may be. The best estimates come from recent analyses of temperature data from seagoing vessels, going back into the last century; these data are free of confounding effects due to growth of cities around weather stations. Based on these data, I personally believe, as do many of my colleagues involved in the question, that the surface temperature of this planet is probably half a degree centigrade warmer, on average, than it was in preindustrial times.

That doesn't really sound like very much at all, but to give a sense of scale, I should point out that the average difference in global average temperature between the height of the glacial period and an interglacial period is only about 5°C. So if, in fact, global temperatures have already increased half a degree, this represents a step of 10 percent towards a magnitude of change that manifestly made huge differences in the ecology of the planet.

To give some numbers, the level of CO_2 in the atmosphere was estimated to be 200 parts per million (ppm) in glacial times. In the interglacial period, it had increased to 280 ppm. As far as we can tell, there is strong correlation between the temperature of the earth and levels of atmospheric CO_2; indeed, this correlation is borne out by general studies of planetary temperatures. The level of atmospheric carbon dioxide is now at 350 parts per million.

There are other gases as well. The chlorofluorocarbons, notably, have been implicated in thinning of the ozone layer, as well as serving simultaneously as greenhouse gases. This strengthens even further the argument that their use should be phased out as soon as possible. We should carefully monitor other gases as well, including methane, the natural cycling of which is really poorly understood. Atmospheric methane is in very small quantities, but the quantities are significant in terms of their ability to trap radiant heat. The dependence of our species on ruminant animals may be one of the major reasons for the increase in methane.

People try to project what increased CO_2, methane, and other greenhouse gases will do to average global temperature. It is clearly very difficult to project. A figure given at the National Forum in May 1989 was that a doubling of atmospheric CO_2 could produce a 3°C increase in average global temperature. There are enormous lags built into the system, because the heat trapped by the atmospheric CO_2 comes to thermal equilibrium slowly. In any case, this estimate of 3°C is based on a doubling of atmospheric CO_2 levels over a 50 year period, and doesn't even count the other greenhouse gases.

What is in store, to the best of our knowledge, in terms of global climate change? Most models show that most of the temperature increase will be towards the poles, as opposed to around the equator, so that 3°C **average** warming could easily mean increases on the order of 10°C in Canada. There will be also be concomitant changes in rainfall. It is very hard to predict, but most models seem to show a drying in the interior of continents during the summer months, which is why in certain senses, anyway, the recent dry summers in the United States can be considered a preview of the greenhouse effect. Not necessarily the first sign, but a preview of the kinds of alterations in physical climate that might be triggered.

What will happen in the tropics? That is even more vague, but it is perfectly possible that there will be major changes in the way moisture is distributed. Many of the other kinds of things we are doing to the face of our planet may also affect regional climatic processes. Conspicuous among these processes is the hydrological cycle of the Amazon basin. Three independent lines of evidence, in work done mostly by Brazilian scientists, demonstrate that up to about 60 percent of the rainfall in the Amazon basin is internally generated (Salati and Vose, 1984; Richey et al., 1989). The process also depends on the enormous insulating capacity of the Amazon forest vegetation, the way the vegetation breaks the fall of rain when it drums down on the forest and the ability of the forest soils to absorb a lot of that moisture so that it can return to the atmosphere as evaporation or transpiration.

Carlos Nobre, a Brazilian scientist who has been a visiting investigator at the University of Maryland, has been working on general climatic models, trying to determine what would happen if the Amazon forest were completely removed and replaced by pasture. His preliminary results show dramatic increases in temperature and decreases in rainfall in the Amazon basin. Since the Amazon basin is a source of rainfall and moisture throughout central Brazil and elsewhere in South America, these changes could alter fundamental physical conditions of that part of the world.

Is it ridiculous to think about the Amazon forest being replaced entirely by pasture? I think not. When I first met Robert Shope in Belém in 1965, I would guess that the amount of the Amazon forest that had been converted to such use was on the order of 2 to 3 percent. As of now, it appears that close to 15 percent of the Brazilian Amazon forest has been removed, and this process is continuing at the rate of about 3 percent a year. (Subsequent calculations show these to be overestimates but the numbers are still substantial.)

Brazil's National Institute for Space Research released figures estimating that 20 million hectares of Brazilian Amazonia went up in smoke in 1987, of which 8 million hectares had been primary forest. Even if those estimates were high by a factor of two, we are dealing with a massive rate of change. And to oversimplify it, I think that deforestation becomes an irreversible process long before. I suspect that when about 30 to 40 percent of the forest is removed, the hydrological cycle is undercut, and there is continual drying to the west. As it gets drier, the vegetation changes, and the amount of moisture returned to the atmosphere is reduced, so it becomes a runaway phenomenon.

And that, in fact, is one of the scary things about a lot of this climate change. Once the tundra is warmed, will there be a major input of methane into the atmosphere, which will create further warming? Authorities on the subject, speaking at conferences like the 1989 National Forum (DeFries and Malone, 1989), very frequently use words like "runaway effect", "feedback", and "surprise is lying out there for us".

One point should be clarified before I go on to discuss biological effects on epidemiology, the nasty synergies of my title. People often ask about our ability to predict specific effects of global change, sometimes arguing that the uncertainty of these predictions means that the threats are overstated. I feel that the general statements I am making in this essay are well substantiated by specific examples and data. But why do scientists argue about more specific predictions? One problem, which will come up again and again, is the complexity of world climatic and ecological systems. Another scientific limitation for trying to figure out what might happen in any particular place is that general circulation models, used to simulate climatic conditions on the computer, are extremely coarse. There are three major models, with numerous disagreements between models due to technical limitations. The best current model is so coarse that Panama, Japan, or the United Kingdom aren't big enough to show up. This model uses 25,920 grid points on a computer, representing a resolution to roughly five degrees latitude by five degrees longitude, or 300 nautical miles by 300 nautical miles. To get it down to one degree latitude by one degree longitude, you would have to advance to essentially 2.5 million grid points. This would drive up the cost of calculating the model by about five hundredfold. Advances in computer technology will eventually make this more feasible, but there are other severe technical limitations of climate data. Answers to the kinds of questions that a biologist or a specialist in infectious diseases would like to ask are always going to be ahead of the capacity of the models to provide.

On the other hand, many of the kinds of effects of environmental change are known because there are examples. All of the major environmental problems, population, deforestation, loss of biological diversity, global pollution, are really all part of one great interconnected problem and, in many senses, represent the greatest challenge that faces human society. That challenge is very near. What we are dealing with is a major change in the chemistry and physics of the planet, as represented by the processes in the atmosphere: how the atmosphere deals with energy and of what constituents it is composed. I personally feel that that is nothing to worry about, as long as biological systems are not affected. But with the kind of temperature changes and climatic changes that are in the offing, however imprecise we may be in predicting them, it is clear that biological systems will be affected.

Endless examples demonstrate how even relatively minor changes in ecology can cause epidemiologic effects. There is the classic example of tree cutting bringing woodsmen in contact with the *Haemagogus* mosquito and jungle yellow fever for which this mosquito is a vector. Thomas H.G. Aitken, of Yale University, brought to my attention the example of Lake Bayano in Panama (50 miles east-northeast of Panama City), which was created by a hydro-electric project. Quite rapidly, the water surface was covered by floating vegetation, particularly with "water lettuce", *Pistia stratiotes*. Certain mosquito species thrived on this vegetation, among them mosquitoes that are vectors for Venezuelan equine encephalomyelitis (VEE). The obvious consequence: cases of VEE appeared. Virus was recovered from three species of mosquitoes (*Culex erraticus*, *Culex ocossa*, and *Mansonia dyari*), as well as from sentinel hamsters and from humans around the lake (Adames et al., 1979).

In the Brazilian state of Rondônia, in the western Amazon, there are between 400,000 and 800,000 cases of malaria, all associated with the building of the infamous Brazil highway 364, and attributable to the clearing of 20 percent of the forest in Rondônia in only 5 years. Incidentally, never has so much forest been cleared or destroyed in such a short time.

Just the chance juxtaposition of a disease organism with an ecological situation can produce epidemics like the famous yellow fever epidemic that hit Memphis in 1878, and ran the population down to such a low number that the state insisted that it give back its city charter the following year.

Alterations in temperature and rainfall patterns induced by climatic change tie in a very coarse way to distribution of various kinds of organisms, which can include changes in vector populations. To speculate a little, the tsetse fly has a very defined distribution in Africa. How much that is tied to actual physical conditions I don't know, but, hypothetically, one could imagine that climatic change could widen the geographical range of its favored environmental conditions, thereby increasing the range of the tsetse fly.

Similarly, there would be changes in densities of host populations, alternate host populations, and vectors, which often make the difference between whether a disease organism can take off to cause an epizootic or not. There may be major changes in migration patterns. The ability of migratory organisms to move diseases around the globe has been a source of fascination for a very long time; it is quite clear that temperature changes might cause new migrations. There are also likely to be major changes in populations of migratory birds.

Eugene Morton and Russell Greenberg, of the National Zoo in Washington, D.C., have been following the populations of North American migratory passerine birds that hibernate in the tropical forest. It is suddenly becoming apparent that populations of many of those species have declined very dramatically in the last 10 years (Rappole et al., 1983; Robbins et al., 1989). This may occasionally upset the average bird watcher, but what does it mean to the rest of us? It turns out that most of those migratory passerines are very dependent on insect populations at the time they are raising young and are a major evolutionary influence on insect behavior and ecology. So even something as far fetched as conversion of Central American forest to cattle pasture could, in the end, have a major impact on the way viruses and other pathogens associated with birds or insects might behave in North America.

In considering effects of climate changes on the scale of interactions between species, it becomes impossible to really predict or even imagine what will happen. And on top of all of that, you have to throw in changes of seasonality, and entire changes in structure of ecological communities. Even if, for example, there were no global warming associated with increased carbon dioxide levels, there would still be changes in ecological communities, because higher atmospheric CO_2 levels have an enriching, or fertilizing, effect on plants. Different plant species will be affected differently. For example, plants used to growing under conditions of water limitation will benefit more from this effect because they can take in all the CO_2 they require during comparatively short periods of opening the stomata in their leaves during the day. All of these effects on relationships amongst the plant species in ecological communities, on top of effects caused by temperature and moisture changes, will be profoundly disturbing.

Historical and paleoecological data give us a little insight about this. If one charts, through pollen records, what happened to species like the American chestnut, or hemlock, as those species attempted to track their ideal climatic conditions, moving north and south with the advance and the retreat of the glaciers, one finds that they did not follow those changing conditions with the precision that one might expect. In fact, there were different communities composed of species that separated and moved at different rates, resulting in different kinds of communities. It is fairly well worked out now that tree species, moving in response to the advance or retreat of glaciers, could move up to 5 miles per century. The kinds of climatic changes we are discussing here are 40 times more rapid, which would require a movement rate of 200 miles per century. This may be well beyond the ability of many species.

All of this adds up to a great deal of turmoil in natural ecological communities. This is not to say that ecological communities are all highly structured entities, without any other random elements. But all these sudden changes probably add up to far greater chances of new epizootics and epidemics.

Agriculture will also be harmed by global change, especially in the poorer parts of the world, where gearing up an extension service to put in and distribute the newly appropriate crops to the small slash-and-burn farmer in the countryside is not really a viable option.

In addition, the changes in growing conditions elsewhere in the world will result in the transfer of the American agricultural focus, north into Canada into areas of poor soils. All of this suggests the possibility of nutritional problems in the future.

Another question, alluded to earlier, concerns the ozone layer and its depletion, which will allow more potentially dangerous ultraviolet light to reach us. I am not an expert on this problem, but I have been privy to some studies for the Environmental Protection Agency, which suggest that increased ultraviolet radiation can cause immune suppression. Another nasty synergy.

As I stated earlier, we are dealing with a series of interconnected environmental problems. In addition, the graph of human population growth from the beginning of history until today is flat until virtually the very end and then shoots up almost vertically. At the same time as these massive population increases, atmospheric pollution, greenhouse problems, and deforestation are shooting up also. The increase in population (essentially the pool of susceptibles for infections) together with nutritional problems and ecological destabilization make for some very frightening synergistic possibilities.

Lastly, in addition to these physical and ecological changes, there are tremendous consequences for biological diversity (Peters and Lovejoy, 1992). A workshop held in October 1988 on the consequences of the greenhouse effect for biological diversity concluded that, just about every way you looked at it, the problems were very severe. That becomes a matter of great concern because biological diversity is the great library of living systems that have come into existence and an important subset of what is biologically possible.

There is likely to be serendipitous discovery with practical application. One recent suggestive example (Fellows, 1989; Smith, 1983) involves a tropical day flying moth, *Urania*, which has episodic migrations. The migrations are triggered by changes in levels of specific compounds in leaves of the caterpillar food plant, *Omphalia*. These compounds affect sugar metabolism and also appear to have an effect on the polysaccharide coat of the AIDS virus, HIV (Fellows, 1989).

The loss of such serendipitous discoveries is, perhaps, the simplest demonstration of what global change will mean for our future. If it continues, its effects will be profound. It may well become a dominant force in epidemiology in the future.

REFERENCES

Adames, A.J., P.H. Peralta, R. Saenz, C.M. Johnson, and P. Galindo (1979). Brote de encefalomyelitis equina Venezolana (VEE) durante la formacion de Lago Bayano, en Panamá, 1977. Revista Médica de Panamá 4:246-257.

Committee on Global Change, National Academy of Sciences (1990). *Research Strategies for the U.S. Global Change Research Program.* Washington, D.C.: National Academy Press.

DeFries, R.S., and T.F. Malone (eds.) (1989). *Global Change and Our Common Future.* Washington, D.C.: National Academy Press.

Fellows, L. (1989). Botany breaks into the candy store. New Scientist, August 26, pp. 45-48.

Peters, R.L., and T.E. Lovejoy (eds.) (1992). *Global Warming and Biological Diversity.* New Haven: Yale University Press.

Rappole, J., E. Morton, T. Lovejoy, and J. Ruos (1983). *Nearctic Avian Migrants in the Neotropics.* Washington, D.C.: U.S. Department of the Interior, Fish and Wildlife Service.

Richey, J., C. Nobre, and C. Deser (1989). Amazon River discharge and climate variability: 1903 to 1985. Science 246:101-103.

Robbins, C., J. Sauer, R. Greenberg, and S. Droge (1989). Population declines in North American birds that migrate to the neo-tropics. Proc. Natl. Acad. Sci. USA 86:7658-7662.

Salati, E., and P. Vose (1984). The Amazon basin: a system in equilibrium. Science 223:129-138.

Smith, N.G. (1983). Host plant toxicity and migration in the dayflying moth *Urania.* Florida Entomologist 66:76-85.

26

Are We Prepared for a Viral Epidemic Emergency?

LLEWELLYN J. LEGTERS, LINDA H. BRINK, AND
ERNEST T. TAKAFUJI

News Report of the Future

I. PANDEMIC — New Virus?

Nybalo, Basangani,
December 6, 1994—
The impoverished na-
tion of Changa in Sub-
Saharan Africa is once
again a chaotic scene
of death and devasta-
tion. After a lull in the
long battle between
rebel factions in
Changa and the ruling
Marxist government,
tensions are again at a
high point. Terrorism
and destruction are
common, as rebels
battle for control of the
countryside surround-
ing the capital city.
Communities have
been plundered and de-
molished. Hundreds of
thousands of starving
Changans are fleeing
to the borders in search
of food and shelter. The
five-year civil war has

THIS SPECIAL REPORT, a "News Report
of the Future" in three parts, covers the "super-Ebola" Pandemic of 1994-95 and its aftermath. The articles are based on numerous in-
terviews, transcripts from the EIWG meetings,
and the top-secret Department of Health &
Human Services (DHHS) review.

Part I: PANDEMIC—New Virus? is the initial
report of the terrifying Ebola-like virus that
killed hundreds of Changan refugees before
spreading to every continent of the world during a two-month period in 1994-95.

Part II: "Dangerously Inadequate" covers the
DHHS review and the conclusions of the EIWG,
and defines the major deficiencies in United
States and global tropical medicine/infectious
disease capabilities.

Part III: EIWG Chair Speaks Out presents a
retrospective analysis of the pandemic, assesses
the increasing risks of infectious disease outbreaks, and outlines short- and long-term solutions. Legters proposes a system of "listening
posts" linked to the world's major research
institutions. Legters maintains that a global
surveillance/training network is feasible and
cost-effective using currently available telecommunications technologies.

killed an estimated 200,000 Changans and brought to a standstill the economy of this mineral-rich nation. The government has been unable to cope with the large number of malnourished displaced persons, forcing the refugees to seek asylum in the adjacent countries of Basangani and Lubawe.

A United Nations-sponsored peacekeeping force has been stationed in Basangani and Lubawe for 2 years, but because of recent medical events, the current status may be in question. The multinational unit, consisting of Australian, Kenyan, Swiss, British, Italian, French, American, and Malaysian soldiers, experienced an outbreak of hepatitis earlier this year, but has otherwise had few serious medical problems until now. The unexplained deaths in the last week of five soldiers who had returned to Fort Bragg after their tour of duty and the flu-like illness affecting other recent returnees have mystified health authorities.

In the border refugee camps housing the Changan refugees, sanitation is poor and the facilities are overcrowded. Heavy rains over the past month have made roads impassable, and supplies can only be airlifted into the camps when flying conditions are satisfactory. Strange illnesses and deaths have occurred in at least three Basangani camps. Three hundred refugees and four relief workers have died in the past month, and countless others are ill with a strange fever. Many volunteer workers have given up and returned to Europe and the Americas, partly dismayed at the futility of their limited effort, but mostly terrified with the disease and death that surrounded them in Basangani. Some of these workers have fallen ill at home and now worry about whom they might have exposed to the disease.

The governments of Basangani and Lubawe are concerned about the importation of this strange illness into their countries. The World Health Organization and other medical institutions, including the Pasteur Institute in Paris and the Centers for Disease Control in Atlanta, have been working around the clock to find the agent responsible for the deaths and illnesses. The disease agent is unlike anything ever seen before, different from Ebola, Marburg, and Lassa, and extremely difficult to isolate. The infection— probably a virus—seems to have a propensity to spread by both the blood-borne and respiratory routes, making it highly communicable. The hemorrhagic manifestations and multisystem involvement are similar to those seen with Marburg and Ebola virus infections.

The places and circumstances described in the "News Report of the Future" are fictitious; the substance of the article, however, is based on the presentations and discussion of participants in the Plenary Session of the Annual Meeting of the American Society of Tropical Medicine and Hygiene, Honolulu, HI, December 6, 1989, as they considered the hypothetical scenario. The opinions or assertions contained herein are the private ones of the authors and are not to be construed as official or reflecting the views of the Uniformed Services University of the Health Sciences, the Department of the Army, or the Department of Defense.

II. U.S. TROPICAL MEDICINE CAPABILITIES CALLED "DANGEROUSLY INADEQUATE"

Washington, D.C., February 10, 1995—A top-secret government evaluation of the nation's ability to respond to infectious disease epidemics has produced a sobering conclusion: the capabilities of United States tropical medicine are "dangerously inadequate." The report comes on the heels of the December 1994 "super-Ebola" epidemic that spread rapidly from the African country of Changa to every continent of the world. In the United States, the public has demanded to know how such a disease could reach American shores—and why United States health authorities were so unprepared to deal with it. Reliable sources say that the government's initial review has been expanded to focus on four major questions:

a. Why wasn't the disease discovered and confined within its region of origin (Central Africa)?

b. Why were our national surveillance and control efforts so ineffective and inefficient?

c. Why were our medical experts and facilities so ill-prepared to diagnose and respond clinically?

d. Was this situation unique, or could a similar outbreak occur with other diseases?

This reporter has just completed a 2-month, nine-country investigation into the consequences of this outbreak. Source material comes from informants within the administration; from portions of the top-secret review provided by a staffer who is dismayed by the limited resources and capabilities within the U.S. Department of Health and Human Services (DHHS) to deal with the outbreak; and from transcripts of the meetings of the 1994 Global Epidemic-Emergency Interagency Working Group (EIWG).*

It is clear that multiple factors permitted, and in some cases, actually encouraged, the spread of "super-Ebola" from continent to continent in a matter of days. EIWG representatives and other sources state that given the present deficiencies in our national and international surveillance systems, similar multicountry epidemics could occur with other viral, parasitic or bacterial diseases. The EIWG concluded that "The United States is not prepared to anticipate, identify or control the majority of the world's tropical diseases."

---

*The EIWG, an *ad hoc* committee convened by the United States Secretary of State during the second week of the epidemic, was composed of representatives from the Centers for Disease Control (CDC), National Institutes of Health (NIH), Department of Defense (DoD), and Department of State. Representatives from the World Health Organization (WHO), United Nations Disaster Relief, and various other international organizations participated in the almost daily EIWG meetings held during the first weeks of the epidemic.

A Decade of Warnings

More than a decade ago, Yale University virologist Robert Shope said, "It is not whether an epidemic will occur, but when!" Alarming reports of declining United States, and indeed worldwide, capabilities in the epidemiology, diagnosis, and treatment of tropical diseases had already appeared by 1980. During the last 10 years, concerned professional societies lobbied Congress, funded extensive public information campaigns, and in the spirit of Glasnost, invited the Soviet Union to join the United States in designing a worldwide surveillance system. In 1987, a report by the Board on Science and Technology for International Development (BOSTID) and the Institute of Medicine outlined the deficiencies in United States capability, agency-by-agency, and offered a detailed plan for recovery.** Yet despite repeated warnings, the succeeding administrations continued to cut relevant budgets. As one of our more outspoken senior senators admitted, "Much of the decline in preparedness and effectiveness of the nation's first-line medical defense systems can be traced to these ill-advised budget cuts, which forced the termination of essential research and training programs."

The question now must be, where are the deficiencies and just how bad are they? My investigation focused on five major areas:	1.	Organizational Response Procedures
	2.	Surveillance and Disease Assessment
	3.	Clinical Response and Management Resources Within the United States
	4.	Manpower Resource Pool
	5.	WHO and International Response

Organizational Response Procedures

Epidemics of the scope and severity of "super-Ebola" require immediate consultation and coordination of experts from many fields; rapid and continuous collection of the most accurate and up-to-date information; state-of-the-art means to communicate this information; and procedures for insuring that responsible actions are identified, implemented, and assessed. Overall, these requirements call for an established and proven procedure, not one that is "jury-rigged" as a response to an emergency. But the United States has no official, or even traditional, organizational procedure for responding to emergencies of this type, even at the highest government levels. In past incidents involving infectious diseases, the responses have varied widely. In

---

**Board on Science and Technology for International Development, Office of International Affairs, the National Research Council, and the Institute of Medicine, National Academy of Sciences (1987). *The US Capacity to Address Tropical Infectious Disease Problems*. Washington, D.C.: National Academy Press.

one case, the United States President personally approved emergency relief, and then assigned jurisdiction to various agencies (State, USAID, the Office of Foreign Disaster Assistance [OFDA], CDC, etc.). On another occasion, the Secretary of State responded directly to a request for help from a foreign government. In the latest case involving "super-Ebola," the United States Army became the first line of medical defense because of its presence in the International Peace-Keeping Forces.

Unfortunately, the blurred lines of overall responsibility continue into the actual implementation process. The relationships that should obtain between various government agencies and their responsibilities in responding to national and international causes of this sort are ill-defined, which results in underutilization of the full capacity of the government, including the military, to deal with the emergency. In situations where infectious disease agents pose a threat to the health of both humans and animals, the respective roles and responsibilities of DHHS and the Department of Agriculture remain ambiguous. This means that valuable time is lost as these organizations create a response system *de novo* for each emergency. More importantly, competition for immediate and long-term funding and duplication of efforts often surface at exactly the moment when a unified response is most crucially needed.

The EIWG found that:

a. There are no official definitions or classifications for disease-related emergencies.

b. Responses to emergency situations are on an *ad hoc* basis.

c. There is no official process for determining which organization(s) should assume administrative, technical, or financial responsibility, either within the United States or internationally.

d. The lack of a well-defined communications network connecting the various involved national and international organizations contributed significantly to the delays in effective response observed in this epidemic.

Surveillance and Disease Assessment

While the lack of a nationally organized response procedure contributed to the escalation and prolongation of the problem, it was the lack of a surveillance system, both in Africa where the disease began and at our own borders, that permitted entrance and spread of the disease within the United States

EIWG representatives suggested that the greatest deficiency is in the area of technical expertise for surveillance—the ability to rapidly test specimens and advise clinicians and state health departments of the threat. Within the United States, medical surveillance is based on data collection by public health personnel in the individual States. The forwarding of this information to the national database at the Centers for Disease Control (CDC) is for the most part on a voluntary state-by-state basis. Shortages of trained personnel in logistics and technical support were found in all areas of surveillance, from United States ports of entry to procedures for tracing contacts.

The report concluded that while there is a large cadre of United States epidemiologists who have been trained through CDC's Epidemic Intelligence Service (EIS) program (over 1,700 since 1951), there is no formal system for keeping track of these individuals or for mobilizing them when CDC's present capabilities are exceeded. Only under special cases are these epidemiologists available to conduct overseas epidemiology activities. Furthermore, overseas emergencies present unique problems and, as such, require that EIS personnel be trained and updated for each specific disease and in-country situation. Likewise, specific financial, logistic, and technical support must be provided. This leads to the question of who should finance CDC's emergency overseas activities. At present, there is no centralized long-term budget. Overseas activities are usually funded from within various related programs, and these programs would be depleted very quickly in an emergency.

Clinical Response & Management Resources Within the United States

The EIWG's review of medical and clinical responses to the "super-Ebola" outbreak concluded that the United States was unprepared to manage even small numbers of people with such a highly infectious and lethal disease. Almost all hospitals lack even the basic biocontainment equipment. Few, if any, personnel are trained in level-3 isolation techniques. And most hospitals, even when affiliated with a major medical school, lack the clinical expertise to diagnose and provide medical care for persons with unusual infectious diseases. For many of the world's major infectious diseases, there is a critical shortage or total lack of drugs for treatment, let alone drugs and vaccines for prevention. Even supplies of malaria chemoprophylactic drugs are dwindling as many drug companies stop production of these pharmaceuticals.

Other issues that surfaced but were left unresolved dealt with the procedures and facilities for medical evacuation and/or quarantine of patients and contacts. EIWG representatives noted that there are no special or separate treatment facilities available in the civilian community. All Public Health Service hospitals have been closed during the last decade, ostensibly for economic reasons.

Military representatives on the EIWG also noted that the

Armed Forces are organized for the defense of the country, not for civilian medical emergencies. They outlined the limited clinical expertise available in the military; the majority of the expertise is in the Research and Development (R&D) sector. The "super-Ebola" epidemic strained the military clinical capabilities to the breaking point. They were not optimistic about assisting the civilian community in the event of an outbreak in the future.

While the Army has deployable field hospitals that could be used for isolation purposes, these are configured mainly for surgical care. The capacity to provide for the isolation of patients is limited to routine nosocomial infections; it does not include the facilities and manpower to isolate patients with exotic, highly communicable diseases. The field hospitals would have to be reinforced with intensive care, pulmonary support, hemodialysis, and additional laboratory capa-bilities in order to diagnose and manage acute hemorrhagic diseases and illnesses such as malaria. There was a question of whether sufficient clinical expertise could be pulled from the Army, Navy, and one or two Air Force medical centers in the United States to staff these hospitals. Likewise, skilled serologists, virologists, and parasitologists, as well as preventive medicine support (entomologists, sanitary engineers, and environmental control specialists) would be needed, and these are in short supply within the military. Similarly, diagnostic equipment and supplies are limited and probably could not be shared with the civilian sector. Many military vaccines and drugs are under IND restrictions; while they can be released for military use by the Surgeons General of the military services in emergencies, their availability for use in civilian populations is problematic.

Manpower Resource Pool

As the BOSTID-IOM report warned in 1987, there is a paucity of expertise in the civilian sector in all areas of tropical medicine. Many people who gained their overseas experience during the war years are retiring or have died, and they are not being replaced by the present system. Few young people are being trained in the fundamentals of disease control; many medical students are not even offered a course in parasitology. An expert assessing the personnel response needed during the beginning of the "super-Ebola" outbreak said, "The four individuals sent to Africa represented nearly all of the professional capability within the USPHS for this type of disease. There was no one left to advise United States clinicians and local health authorities."

Military representatives question where they would find

sufficient expertise for *both* United States and overseas epidemiology and clinical care. Laboratory and preventive medicine manpower presently exists in the United States Army Medical Research Institute of Infectious Diseases, the Walter Reed Army Institute of Research and its overseas laboratories, and the Naval Medical Research Units. Of the two military labs in Africa, NAMRU-3 in Cairo has some virology capability and also biocontainment; Kenya has malaria expertise. Medical entomologists and virologists are available in other Army and Navy labs, but the requirements placed on the military during this epidemic considerably exceeded capabilities. As a military representative no longer with the Service put it, "The bottom line is that we have insufficient expert manpower to sustain the appropriate levels of health care and preventive medicine in several sites simultaneously. What we will wind up doing under these circumstances is to put very junior, inexperienced people in and hope they learn very, very fast."

WHO and International Response

During an infectious disease emergency, coordination among international organizations, including multinationals (WHO) and bilaterals (experts and institutions in other countries) would be essential. Additional academic, clinical, public health, laboratory and other personnel could be mustered in this manner, and extra logistical and financial resources identified and coordinated. An international group, such as WHO, would have to take the lead, and yet, as the EIWG representative from WHO observed, "WHO is always running on a shoestring—an annual budget of less than $250 million—not enough to run a decent-sized city hospital, and it is supposed to cope with the needs of 160+ member nations!"

III. EIWG Chair Speaks Out

To gain additional insights about the deficiencies that permitted this outbreak to get out of control, and the changes which might be made, we interviewed Dr. Llewellyn J. Legters, Chair of the Emergency Interagency Working Group. Dr. Legters was asked to propose ideal solutions and he emphasized cooperation, coordination, and communications without any massive additional funding.

Q: As Chair of the Emergency Interagency Working Group, or to use the acronym, the EIWG, Dr. Legters, are there any generalizations you could make now that the epidemic is over; any overall lessons learned from the experience?
Dr. Legters: Well, to put it succinctly, the outbreak has confirmed, in a very dramatic way, just how ill-prepared we are to detect global epidemic disease threats in a timely fashion, and, once detected, to respond appropriately.

Q: I suppose it's obvious why the U.S. Government should become involved in this kind of problem, since the epidemic did involve the United States directly; but surely, there have been outbreaks like this before that didn't spread to our borders. Why should Americans care?
Dr. Legters: You've implied by your question that the United States has self-interests that have to do with protecting the health of United States citizens from imported contagious diseases, and that's certainly true. Suppose, for example, that we had had an international surveillance system in place when AIDS first appeared, one that recognized the clinical presentation as being something different. And suppose we had had the capability then to isolate and characterize HIV? Almost certainly, we could have prevented a lot of cases, if only because we would have taken some actions earlier to protect our blood supply. Besides that, technologically speaking, we have world leadership responsibilities. The applicable medical technology should be exported. It's the humanitarian thing to do, and it's to our benefit, because it probably contributes to political stability. It certainly breeds good will on behalf of the United States.

Q: Does this outbreak mean that the world can expect more disasters like this in the future?
Dr. Legters: Well, certainly there are a number of factors operating that increase the risk. The human population is growing rapidly, and population pressures are resulting in overcrowding in the urban areas of most developing countries. The same pressures are causing human intrusions into areas that formerly represented exclusively animal habitats, increasing the potential for accidental transmission of zoonotic diseases to humans. Civil wars have produced massive dislocations of entire populations in many areas and the creation of refugee camps with crowded conditions. Add to this the factor of travel. Commercial jet aircraft move a lot of people around the world in a hurry these days. "We" go there; "they" come here, increasing the risk to United States citizens of exposure to tropical infectious diseases. All of these factors, taken together, increase the threat of widespread, even more devastating outbreaks than the one we've just seen.

Q: When you say we are ill-prepared to deal with this kind of emergency, what exactly do you mean?
Dr. Legters: Well, first of all, to respond quickly, we need to have a surveillance system that can identify unusual disease occurrences near their point of origin; a laboratory system that can quickly characterize the causative agents; a reporting system that alerts the world health community; and a way to institute controls. Of course, there are already national and international disease surveillance systems in many countries and regions. But, generally speaking, there are only *ad hoc* arrangements for communicating information about disease oc-

Chair Speaks Out (cont'd)_____

currences and for cooperation among agencies in epidemic disease diagnosis and control. Two sterling examples of international cooperation in disease control include the present system for global influenza surveillance and the smallpox eradication program. The latter program, in particular, was successful precisely because of the outstanding cooperation between First and Third World countries.

Q: Earlier, you implied that the U.S. didn't have sufficient trained professionals to manage this sort of problem. Would you elaborate?
Dr. Legters: It's true that there are not enough experts in tropical infectious diseases in the United States. The BOSTID-IOM report provides the most authoritative estimate. There are fewer than 2,500 Americans with research, clinical, or public health skills in tropical infectious diseases. Many of these got into the field by accident during World War II, and of course, their numbers are decreasing rapidly. We have a very limited training base to replace such professionals. There are only eight tropical medicine academic "centers" in the United States. The reason is the lack of incentives for people to undertake careers in the field. The dollars are simply not available to support any very large research and teaching programs in tropical infectious diseases. The question is, how many disasters like this will have to happen before enough dollars are appropriated?

Q: Let's talk about training. What's involved in training professionals in this field?
Dr. Legters: With some exceptions, medical schools in the United States include practically nothing in the basic science curriculum on tropical infectious diseases. This situation needs to be corrected, if only because the probabilities of seeing patients with tropical infectious diseases in the United States are increasing. Beyond that, I feel strongly that the most effective tropical medicine teaching programs are reciprocal. Third World students should have opportunities to come to U.S. institutions to learn technologies applicable to Third World problems; U.S. students should have opportunities to go to Third World countries for "hands-on" experience in the diagnosis and management of tropical diseases and doing field epidemiologic investigations. Without doubt, the fullest appreciation of the health and sanitation problems of Third World countries is best gotten by living and working there. Barring opportunities to actually work overseas, the new interactive videodisc (IVD) technology provides a means of offering realistic clinical and epidemiological training that's almost as good as being there. I've seen some IVD productions that are truly remarkable for the realism of the built-in clinical and epidemiological decision making.

Q: You mentioned the importance of training for Third World nationals in the United States. What sort of training?
Dr. Legters: The United States leads the world in the development of new medical technologies, in diagnostics, prophylactic and therapeutic drugs, immunizations, et cetera. The best way to transfer this technology is through appropriate training. I emphasize *appropriate*, not with equipment they will never see again after they leave the United

States, but, for example, in things like serodiagnostic tests using dipstick or conventional ELISA techniques. Such reciprocal programs are especially effective if there is continued collaboration after the formal training ends.

Q: That's fine, but this must be very expensive in terms of faculty time and energy, not to mention the cost of travel.

Dr. Legters: Well yes, it is. People who make careers of it surely have to have a genuine interest in Third World health problems and a fondness for working there. And, indeed, one has to travel some or a lot. But, I've already mentioned the potential for simulation training using IVD, and modern communications have vastly increased our capacity to maintain close contact with our overseas collaborators without actually being there. To get back to the specific problem of managing the global epidemic emergency, as I see it, modern telecommunications are a principal part of the solution to the problem of most efficient use of our currently scarce manpower. If you add the power of high definition television to capabilities for teleconferencing between widely separated locations around the world, you can bring the information to the experts, even if you can't send the experts to the field.

Q: Surely, this isn't the first time we've gotten concerned about the potential of a global epidemic emergency. Can you put the most recent outbreak in -perspective?

Dr. Legters: United States interest in tropical infectious diseases waxes and wanes with our political and military involvement overseas. As I said, many in the United States became experts while they were stationed in tropical countries in wartime. During the deepest cold of the "Cold War," the equivalent of my EIWG was formed under Centers for Disease Control (CDC) leadership to deal with the perceived threat of attack from biological warfare agents. So, in fact, there *are* organizational models to guide what we need to do, and there *are* significant capabilities to do it. Right this minute, however, these serve smaller organizational or regional purposes; they're not geared to participate as part of a global disease surveillance and control network. That's why I'm proposing use of telecommunications as a critical organizational link.

Q: Can you give me some examples?

Dr. Legters: The Department of Defense maintains medical research laboratories in a number of overseas locations. These are linked through the United States embassies by satellite communications with the Headquarters at Walter Reed Army Institute of Research. The CDC operates global EIS programs in eight countries. Various national systems in the Third World reflect a very high degree of competence in infectious disease epidemiology and control.

In the 1960s, the NIH sponsored a number of International Centers for Medical Research and Training, in which various United States academic institutions were affiliated with counterpart institutions in Third World countries. These served as foci for research in tropical infectious diseases and provided training opportunities for United States students. The NIH continues to sponsor a similar program on a somewhat smaller scale, called the

Chair Speaks Out (cont'd)

International Centers for Infectious Disease Research. In any case, to serve our immediate purposes, and to do this without massive additional budget outlays, I believe we have to organize what we already have in place a little better and supplement current capabilities by enlarging on organizational models that worked in the past, along the lines of the ICMRTs. I hasten to add that the ICMRT program did not provide the strengthening of the Third World clinical, laboratory, and epidemiological facilities that is needed to accomplish the purpose under discussion here. To do that, we need a specific program to support and foster a global disease surveillance and control network. An additional element, not available in the past, is a telecommunications systems necessary to link the various organizational entities into a well-coordinated network.

Q: Will your committee be making any recommendations in this regard and to whom will you make them?
Dr. Legters: In the aftermath of this particular epidemic, the climate seems to be right to initiate a set of national responses that would prepare us to cope with similar future episodes. We will, indeed, be making recommendations, and since the EIWG was the creation of the State Department, the recommendations will be made to the Secretary of State. First of all, we need to create an Interagency Working Group with representation from the several responsible federal departments (State, DHHS, DoD), but we also want to include private foundations and academia. The group will need to do more than simply prepare a "lessons learned" report of this particular outbreak. They will need to

function like a think-tank, modeling "worst case" scenarios and determining the resource requirements to deal with these. Of course, if our recommendations are to result in any improvements, the Government will have to act on them. The President himself should identify a lead agency within the Executive Branch, and that agency should translate the recommendations into proposed legislation and appropriations.

Q: Which agency should be given the lead?
Dr. Legters: The federal agency best suited to manage such a global surveillance system is the Department of Health and Human Services. The CDC would serve as a primary consultative resource and could respond appropriately to reports of epidemic disease.

Q: You've suggested that one of the things we will need to consider is strengthening our disease surveillance activities overseas. Could you be more specific?
Dr. Legters: The idea is not new with me. D.A. Henderson, former Dean of the Johns Hopkins School of Hygiene and Public Health, has suggested that for the modest sum of around 75 million dollars, we could create some 15 epidemiological research centers (ERCs) around the world that would serve as "listening posts" to identify the epidemiological events that might signal global epidemic disease threats. We on the EIWG agree with this proposal but would take it a few steps further. We should evaluate current overseas capabilities in this regard (e.g., the DoD overseas laboratories, CDC's global EIS program, national and international capabilities in various countries of interest, etc.) with a

view toward identifying geographical areas where there is no such capability and where, on theoretical grounds at least, there is the greatest potential for the emergence of human pathogenic viruses with global epidemic potential. We would not want to duplicate already-existing capabilities; rather, by agreement, these latter facilities could become formally incorporated into a global surveillance network. To be economical, the centers would have to serve other functions besides surveillance for emerging viruses. They should probably also become involved in field epidemiologic research activities directed at disease problems of major public health importance in the region (e.g., malaria). And these centers would be the logical loci for research directed at development of rapid diagnostic reagents, such as IgM and antigen capture systems, appropriate for the region.

Still another function of the ERCs would be training. There would be formal linkages of the ERCs with United States academic institutions, especially those with a track record in this arena. As I said, the BOSTID-IOM report identified eight United States academic institutions as tropical public health centers. However, there are certainly other United States institutions that have expertise and could be recruited if federal support were available. The affiliations should include arrangements for reciprocal training of foreign nationals.

As I've said, the key to an effective network is the telecommunication system. Among other things, it would make consultative expertise from the affiliated academic institutions and CDC readily available to the field and result in previously unimaginable teaching opportunities.

Q: How realistic is the idea of teleconferencing among a network of ERCs?

Dr. Legters: The experts say that if you can get the image (words, data or pictures) on a computer screen, you can transmit it via satellite anywhere in the world to someone else's desktop computer. I mentioned that the DoD overseas laboratories are already linked together with the Walter Reed Army Institute of Research via such a system. So it's real and doable with present affordable technology. There are still problems in synchronous transmission of full-motion video; it will be a few years before this can be done at an affordable cost. NASA did set up a "telemedicine spacebridge" in the aftermath of the Yerevan earthquake in 1989 that permitted Soviet doctors to present their patients in full-motion video to consultants at several United States institutions, but it was expensive.

Assuming teleconferencing among a network of ERCs in various locations, each affiliated with a United States teaching institution, imagine how exciting the daily or weekly clinical or epidemiological teaching rounds could become at both ends. In the event of an actual outbreak, the situation could be presented visually as well as verbally to the epidemiological consultants at CDC, the decisionmakers in the federal departments, and to Congress. Key people in the decision-making hierarchy could be kept updated through the telecommunications system. Students in the affiliated institutions could participate in the decision-making process while viewing "live" reports from the field, hospital, and laboratory.

Chair Speaks Out (cont'd) __

Q: As a closing comment, is there anything else that needs to be said about our preparedness, or lack of it, to deal with similar future emergencies?

Dr. Legters: The "quick fix" is to organize the assets that are already in place around the world to perform the surveillance function and to provide a "network coordinator" and a communications system that links them together for this purpose. Longer-term, this network of ERCs and the affiliated training programs should be expanded in number. I want to emphasize that the key to the effectiveness of the network is state-of-the-art telecommunications. Really, for a very modest outlay of money, epidemics of this sort can be contained closer to the original source. The American public can be protected from future disasters like this one.

27

Surveillance Systems and Intergovernmental Cooperation

DONALD A. HENDERSON

The recent emergence of AIDS and dengue hemorrhagic infections, among others, are serving usefully to disturb our ill-founded complacency about infectious diseases. Such complacency has prevailed in this country throughout much of my career. Indeed, it is a matter of record that in 1969 the Surgeon General, in a speech given at Hopkins, assured his audience that in this country we had effectively probed most frontiers of knowledge in the infectious disease field, that the remaining problems in this country were marginal, and that attention should now turn to the chronic diseases. It is evident now, as it should have been then, that mutation and change are facts of nature, that the world is increasingly interdependent, and that human health and survival will be challenged, ad infinitum, by new and mutant microbes, with unpredictable pathophysiological manifestations. Moreover, as we see with the Hantaviruses and others, their manifestations may be the chronic diseases. How are we to detect these at an early date so as to be able to devise appropriate preventive and therapeutic modalities? What do we look for? What types of surveillance and reporting systems can one devise?

Interestingly, some of these questions have been asked and responded to at least once before. One such time was 1950, soon after the onset of the Korean War. It was perceived then that a biological warfare attack on civilian populations in this country was a realistic possibility. A number of different microbial agents were candidates and several of them could be readily dispensed in crowded centers by a lone saboteur bearing no more than an innocuous appearing briefcase. To stop such an act was seen to be impossible. However, early detection was vital so that measures could be taken to prevent spread, to treat, and/or to decontaminate. Alex Langmuir, then head of epidemiology at CDC, the federal unit which is now the Centers for Disease Control, proposed that a special unit be created that would be on 24-hour call to investigate immediately any unusual disease outbreaks. Thus, the Epidemic Intelligence Service (EIS) came into being. Young medical officers were trained in field epidemiology and assigned to CDC, state health departments, and universities. Requests for help were responded to immediately on receipt of a request. The availability of resources that could be quickly mobilized increased the reporting of outbreaks. And, in due course, the states themselves strengthened their own capacity and capability to investigate outbreaks. CDC's role in defining and characterizing a wide range of new challenges is now well known, from AIDS to Legionnaire's disease to toxic shock syndrome to the problems of the 80/81 strain of *Staphylococcus*. What we don't know—and fortunately so—is how rapidly and effectively a biological warfare episode would have been detected and characterized had it occurred.

To detect the new or emerging viruses, the challenge we face bears some similarities to the challenge of 1950. We are uncertain as to what we should keep under surveillance, or even what we should look for. Moreover, the challenge differs in that the new or emerging viruses may not occur as outbreaks, as would be expected with biological warfare. Rather, new or emerging viruses may be manifested by scattered single cases, such as presumably has happened with AIDS and as now occurs with monkeypox. Secondly, and taking a global perspective, it seems to me most probable that new infectious entities of significance are more likely to occur first either in densely populated areas where crowding and poor sanitation are prevalent, or in tropical rain forests where man, monkeys and mammals live in close proximity. In sharp contrast to the 1950 challenge in the United States, such areas are minimally endowed with curative care facilities that might identify the unusual or unexpected illness and, moreover, they are all bereft of sophisticated, let alone competent, microbiological expertise and equipment.

Thus, the 1950 approach in the United States of creating a national Epidemic Intelligence Service, while providing a partial answer to detection of new entities, would not alone provide much assurance in other countries that newly emerging viruses would be detected in a timely manner. What therefore might be proposed?

A surveillance system to detect new and emerging viruses must inevitably consist of the same three components as any surveillance system. The first consists of units, customarily clinical, which are capable of detecting unusual cases or constellation of cases. In a tropical area this is an especially difficult task, given the background level of diverse conditions that present themselves. As was illustrated by Wilbur Downs with respect to Lyme disease, an effective unit must link clinical and epidemiological thinking. Such units are few and far between even in the industrialized world and I need only cite the prolonged delay in identifying the Thalidomide-phocomelia connection in Europe to further dramatize this point.

The second component: Having detected an unusual case or group of cases, there must be a defined channel for reporting the occurrence and a receptive, knowledgeable unit to receive it. This channel is the second component of the system. Health centers and hospitals throughout the world are customarily requested to provide no end of data and reports to some central unit of government. Our experience during the smallpox eradication program and more recently in the Expanded Program on Immunization (EPI) with respect to tetanus, poliomyelitis, and measles, indicates that most of these reports go to statistical offices that serve only an archival function. They are little concerned as to whether the reports are regularly received, only whether they have transcribed the correct numbers of reports of cases received. Rarely are analyses performed to assess whether there are unusual trends in incidence of any disease.

Finally, there must be some sort of capacity and responsibility at the national or regional or international level that is available to respond to unusual events or request for assistance. Indeed, the existence and responsiveness of such a unit itself serves to strengthen reporting from the network of clinical units. This has been the strength of CDC and its Epidemic Intelligence Service, but such a resource, charged with responsibility for the surveillance of a nation's health, is all but unique. Many illustrations could be offered, but let me cite experiences in European countries. The well-known typhoid epidemic in the Swiss ski resort of Zermatt was basically sorted out by an epidemiologist from Paris's Institut Pasteur, acting outside normal channels. And the origin of the 1965 epidemic of variola minor, mild smallpox, in the United Kingdom, a laboratory-originated outbreak, was worked out by a CDC epidemiologist sent to the United Kingdom as an observer. Admittedly, these events occurred some years ago but the situation today is little improved.

In summary, we are not today well-structured or staffed on a global level to detect either new or emerging viral diseases.

To identify the needs of a sensitive surveillance system that would detect new disease entities within a reasonable time frame, I found it helpful to consider different basic epidemiological characteristics of a new disease that need to be anticipated. One manifestation of a new entity might be an outbreak involving perhaps a hundred to several thousand clinical cases over a limited time frame and geographic area. If there were a number of associated deaths with rash or hemorrhagic manifestations, recent experience would suggest that even in some of the most remote areas these cases would soon come to notice, and assistance with dealing with them would be sought. I would cite the experience with Ebola and Marburg virus disease in illustration.

The likelihood of such outbreaks being properly investigated and characterized would depend on national governments utilizing appropriate expertise, but to do so they need assurance that competent assistance would be available to them and could respond in a timely fashion. The CDC has come to be recognized internationally as such a resource. Could or should the World Health Organization (WHO) be in a position to discharge such a role? In principle, the answer would appear to be in the affirmative. In fact, however, WHO has pathetically few resources of its own that are not specifically committed to specific diseases such as AIDS or other categorical programs. The Viral Diseases Unit at WHO headquarters in Geneva, however defined, consists of no more than five persons. Virus disease programs in most WHO regional offices are staffed by one or two persons only. Inevitably, those who staff such units are prized more for their administrative skills in bringing experts together rather than for their own professional expertise. Another problem for WHO is its basic character as an association of fairly independent regional offices, which generally are resistant to a coordinate responsibility discharged by a central office. I therefore see no option but to acknowledge CDC as an international resource, to fund it appropriately, and to acknowledge its mandate in legislation.

Another scenario for a new or emerging virus—less dramatic and less likely to be detected—would be represented by large outbreaks with few associated deaths and few of the dramatic manifestations of hemorrhage or rash. Small outbreaks with high case-fatality rates or hemorrhage and rash would similarly be more likely to escape detection. Illustrative of such events are perhaps the jungle-related yellow fever outbreaks of the 1920s and 1930s and the variety of outbreaks detected during the certification period of smallpox eradication. During the period of certification of smallpox eradication, we actively sought to obtain reports of possible smallpox cases. In such countries, hundreds of suspicious illnesses were reported annually by health service staff, news reporters, travelers, and private citizens. Most were outbreaks of measles with associated deaths, some were chickenpox involving adult populations, and some were typhus. In general, they were brought to notice within a matter of a few weeks to a few months. Had the national health services not been seeking to receive outbreak reports and to investigate them, most would probably never have come to official notice. The lesson I would derive from this is that national Epidemic Intelligence Service units, developed on the CDC model, would serve to encourage outbreak reports and would serve a valuable surveillance function. In part, these could be built in conjunction with the intensified polio surveillance systems now in place throughout the Americas, and which we hope will expand worldwide as the goal of global eradication is addressed. A few countries have already adopted the EIS model with encouragement and training support from CDC. It would seem logical and prudent to work with WHO in encouraging the expansion of such services, at least to the largest countries and those in the tropical rain forest.

A more difficult problem is posed by new or emerging viruses that cause only sporadic cases, or comparatively few severe cases over a limited time span. Such, presumably, was the scenario for the emergence of HIV. This poses the most difficult problem of all. Such cases might be identified and characterized at a reasonably early date if seen in an adequately staffed and equipped clinical center that was knowledgeable of tropical diseases and could identify the unusual and unexpected. Unfortunately, there are few such centers anywhere in the world, and, indeed, there are few persons now with real expertise in tropical medicine in either the industrialized or developing countries. In our own interest, let alone the interests of populations living in the tropics, it would seem prudent to foster the development of a network of units with expertise in tropical medicine. Cost alone would necessarily curtail the number that could be established, but with time and a mandate to provide training, it should be possible to expand national capacities. Here we have much to learn from the agricultural sector. Beginning with initiatives taken by the Ford and Rockefeller Foundations in the early 1960s, a network of international agricultural centers has developed, funded by many governments and agencies. In all, there are now more than 15 and these, in turn, have stimulated the creation of a complementary network of national centers. More than 50 United States academic institutions have received core support to permit them to relate to and participate in the international network. For health, there is exactly one comparably supported international center, and only a handful of United States academic centers that receive from NIAID (the National Institute of Allergy and Infectious Diseases of the National Institutes of Health) extremely modest support for a few specific programs in tropical medicine.

For purposes of improving a woefully inadequate surveillance system, I would argue for the development of a network of internationally supported health centers, which, in developing countries, I would recommend be based in periurban areas of major cities in the tropics. The periurban areas are customarily where migrants and travelers from rural areas are found. A clinical facility in such an area would thus serve to provide a window on events in surrounding areas. Preference, I believe, should be given to more densely populated areas and those near the tropical rain forest. I would propose that such centers have several components: (1) A clinical inpatient and outpatient service for infectious diseases. (2) supporting diagnostic laboratories, which, as needed, could serve as a locus for research studies. (3) an epidemiological unit that might serve as the national EIS resource and that would be engaged in a variety of ongoing studies in a population "laboratory" of perhaps two million to five million persons. By focusing research efforts within a defined area, rapport could be developed with local leaders and an invaluable data base would gradually accrue. In the course of various studies pertaining to disease epidemiology and the efficacy of interventions, observations of unusual events demanding special in vestigation would inevitably come to light. (4) An education-training unit for national as well as international staff. Finally, I would propose that such centers be formally identified as part of a network with designated counterparts in the United States (and other countries). The network should include such organizations as CDC, NIAID, and appropriate academic centers. It would be hoped that such a network might be sponsored jointly by WHO, as well as by other national governments, to assure the maximum of stability and legitimacy.

In brief, if we are to have a surveillance system with reasonable prospects for the timely detection of new or emerging viruses, an investment in manpower and capital will be required. Strengthening in mission, competence, and facilities is needed at three levels— internationally, nationally, and in selected cities. A beginning has been made or precedents established to address each of the components of such a system, but without a coherent vision of the whole. Thus, CDC serves now to respond to major or unusual epidemics in a number of countries. CDC has fostered the development of national EIS systems and has assisted in training of personnel. Finally, there are some centers in tropical medicine, although none wholly adequate for the purposes we are describing. These include the International Center for Diarrheal Diseases Research (ICDDR, B) in Dacca, Bangladesh, a number of military medical research units, and some national centers (e.g., Thailand). Thus, there is precedent for formally undertaking a broader program. In the best of all possible worlds, WHO would take a lead role but, as I have noted, most would have to conclude that WHO, on its own, would not do well in developing or managing a mixed research-service network such as this. A consortium of donors, a Consultative Group on Health (similar to the existing Consultative Group on International Agricultural Research), could be envisioned and indeed some discussions along this line are beginning to take place.

What might be this cost? Obviously, it would depend on the scope of activity, and this could be infinite. Let me sketch a modest core structure as an initial goal, which would begin to approach a counterpart agricultural network that is now being funded.

1. Fifteen broadly based tropical medicine centers of the type I have outlined, each to be funded at the level of $10 million per year, 50% of which is to be provided by the United States. *Net cost: $75 million.*

2. Expansion and funding of CDC epidemic response to training facilities. *Estimated cost: $10 million.*

3. Core funding for 10 United States centers to participate in the network of centers, at approximately $5 million per year. *Net cost: $50 million.*

4. A special grants program of $15 million to address special problems.

Adding all of this together, you derive a figure of $150 million. That figure was not decided by accident. In 1969, a study performed at CDC showed that the United States was spending $150 million annually in vaccination and quarantine activities to protect itself from smallpox. That was considered to be affordable. Today the United States spends $0 on these activities. And bear in mind that those were 1969 dollars, now worth more than $300 million.

Can we afford to invest in such a program? A better question is whether we can afford not to invest in a program that could be a determinant in our own survival as a species.

28

Afterword:
A Personal Summary Presented as a
Guide for Discussion

EDWIN D. KILBOURNE

I would like to do three things. The first is to present an anecdotal
report of an outbreak of influenza from personal experience. Then,
I would like to pluck out a few highlights and quotable quotes from
the contributions to this book. Finally, I would like to make a series
of arguable categorical assertions. These were written when I was, as
yet, unencumbered with the wisdom of this book's contents.

In 1976, I was sufficiently concerned about the emergence of two
pandemics of influenza within 2 decades that I brashly wrote an op-
ed article for the *New York Times*, in which I expressed this concern
and also made a prediction, that didn't seem too rash at the time, that
there would be another pandemic. Although we are still waiting, I
gather that many others share with me the concern that another
influenza pandemic is eventually going to happen.

What did happen was that 2 weeks after this piece appeared,
there was a flurry of excitement at Fort Dix because the swine
influenza virus suddenly appeared there among military recruits.
We believed that this swine influenza strain was related to the virus
responsible for the devastating pandemic of 1918-1919, and here the
virus appeared to be resurrecting itself. The specter of a new
pandemic was obvious, although illusory in this case. While I have
no wish to get into this somewhat emotionally charged arena again,
I think there are some instructive features about this example. Had
there not been good virologic surveillance going on at Fort Dix to
alert us to this influenza outbreak in the military, we would remain
ignorant, probably to this day, of the potential of the swine influenza
virus to come back, at least in partially resurrected form. The fact
was that there was a seasonal influenza epidemic that year, caused
by the A/Victoria strain (H3N2 subtype), and that buried under this
was a miniepidemic of the Fort Dix swine influenza strain, disguised

in the large number of A/Victoria infections and indistinguishable in the total epidemic curve. An analysis of this miniepidemic disclosed certain disturbing features. Of the 13 clinically well-documented cases, five progressed to lung involvement, an alarming sign with influenza, and there was one fatality in a previously healthy young male. Afterwards, it was possible to determine that about 230 people had been infected with this virus, based on serologic evidence.

Now the message here to me is not that one should not have surveillance, but rather that one should be aware of the consequences of surveillance and be prepared to take some action. I was delighted with Henderson's proposal, which ends up making a response, because we have been talking about detecting viruses and now, at last, we are talking about the probable necessity of doing something about it.

I would like to glean some of what I see as the important points raised in this book. One of the highlights is that many a rose is born to blush unseen, as Morse implied when he talked about viruses that may have emerged before, but have not emerged to our notice. The swine flu example is something we might easily have missed. Webster also reminds us that viruses not only emerge, they disappear. One variety of equine influenza virus (technically, the H7N8 subtype) has not been seen for 7 years, at least not in North America. Where has it gone? Possibly into ducks. But, in any case, we should be aware and count our blessings because occasionally things go away as well.

Joshua Lederberg said, "We have drastically tampered with human evolution." He also said that RNA and DNA, as units of evolution, are not always neatly packaged in viruses, but that there is an evolutionary continuum, which I suppose includes the mitochondria, among other things. Temin has pointed out the contrasting evolutionary rates of exogenous retroviruses (high, as in the case of HIV) versus endogenous retroviruses that have integrated themselves into the host germline (low). However, in general, viruses are ephemeral and changing entities. Holland elegantly reminds us that a particular virus, which we think of as homogeneous, is really a heterogeneous population. The RNA replicase, by which RNA viruses reproduce themselves, itself is subject to mutation, which confounds the issue and adds another dimension. The studies with monoclonal antibodies that, under the right laboratory conditions, drive a virus population to a very high rate of antigenic evolution, is a remarkable observation. He also referred to the nonpredictability of the direction of viral evolution. And, again, this is one of those things we are going to have to battle with because, truly, these events are extremely difficult if not impossible to predict. Temin sees new retroviruses emerging as a very rare event, despite high mutation rates, because of the multiple factors of genetic changes that may be necessary in evolving them. We have also learned from Temin that the mutation rate of a virus can depend on the cell in which it is propagated; Holland and Palese also have some information on this subject. As Strauss has so clearly demonstrated, true genetic recombination can occur in single-stranded RNA viruses. Some RNA viruses, at least, can recombine blocks, or cassettes, of information. For example, Western equine encephalomyelitis (WEE) virus originated by recombination of two "cassettes" from two other viruses, part of its genetic information—one cassette—coming from one virus and a larger cassette from eastern equine encephalitis (EEE) virus. To which I could add that we really haven't discussed at all the enormous potential gene pool that rapidly reassorting or recombining viruses have. Because they can reach into alien hosts, or seldom used hosts, and instantly recapture genetic material, tedious continuous mutation is not necessary for the very rapid evolution of these viruses. And, of course, this process of recombining is what we think classically happens with the introduction of pandemic influenza strains.

Many of McNeill's thoughts are highly quotable. First of all he reminds us that man is a tropical animal outside of his natural niche. I never quite thought of myself this way, but he is probably right. I think that the implications are clear: we have, over time, deadapted to a situation where, in the past, we were in daily intercourse with parasites; now, we so seldom meet them that they harm us when we encounter them again. I think this is one of the things Lederberg was referring to when he spoke of tampering with human evolution.

McNeill also pointed out, and his message here was the same as Fields's, that we cannot duplicate natural ecology, or natural ecologic circumstances in the laboratory. Therefore, our concern about high viral mutation rates has to be tempered by the realization that viruses have a critical necessity to adapt to their elegantly carved out niches, which imposes certain limitations.

He also had a phrase, "the conservation of catastrophe", which implied that man evolves from one state of vulnerability to another. Again, the message is, as Henderson has reminded us, that the infectious diseases are not dead and never will be. And we will always be substituting one set of diseases or reactions with viruses for another, depending on the changed ecologic circumstances.

Johnson pointed out the risk of the expanding, degenerating urban environment. Having recently been in Seoul, where highrise hotels border rice paddies, I know exactly what he means. Such places are highly appropriate, as Henderson also suggested, for establishing surveillance. In a similar vein, from both Johnson and LeDuc we have learned that we must also pick the rodent of our choice. We must also consider interactions between viruses. Some viruses, like the delta hepatitis agent, apparently cannot cause disease by themselves, but can cause serious disease in individuals infected with a helper virus. There has been some concern that this might happen in the Orient with the delta agent, which requires hepatitis B as a helper virus. Delta hepatitis agent is rare in the Orient, but hepatitis B virus is not.

Shenk pointed out the exquisite dependence of DNA virus replication on enhancer promoter regions in cells, a level of specificity

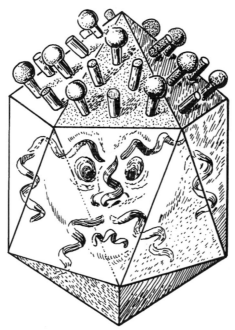

Figure 28.1 Hypothetical viral chimera. A maximally virulent virus would have the stability provided by icosahedral structure, a segmented genome for adaptability, surface spikes to optimize cellular attachment, pantropicity, and the capacity for persistence through chromosomal integration. Genetic and structural constraints operate to contain the emergence of an extremely virulent virus. [Reproduced with permission from Kilbourne, E.D. (1985). Epidemiology of viruses genetically altered by man - predictive principles. Banbury Report 22, *Genetically Altered Viruses and the Environment* (B. Fields, M. Martin and C.W. Potter, eds.), pp. 103-117. Cold Spring Harbor, N.Y.: Cold Spring Harbor Laboratory.]

in addition to surface receptors by which specific cells can be targeted by viruses.

Dear reader, I am sure you will have your own list of highlights, but that was mine. Forgive me for all the bright things that haven't been included.

As an intellectual exercise, I will try to construct a virus of maximal pathogenicity bearing in mind everything discussed here. I think we might try to make it icosahedral for stability, so that it can go through the gut and survive in vectors and so forth. We would certainly want to give it a segmented genome, like influenza, to allow easy reassortment of genes. I think we would like to give it some surface spikes to aid cellular attachment and to facilitate antigenic change. And, of course, we would endow it with a reverse transcriptase, which would enable it to integrate with the host cell genome. I have constructed such a virus (Fig. 28.1) and, as you can see, it has lethal potential, but it is not going to make it despite the frown. Anything this lethal is likely to put itself out of business in short order.

I would like to end with a few categorical assertions for future consideration. When I first wrote these down I was sure that they were surprisingly naive questions to ask after all this thinking, but in fact I think they are still relevant. First, how do we define what a new virus is? We haven't yet done so, particularly with the reminder of John Holland and others that a virus really is a statistical consensus of a genetically heterogeneous population, which, again, is in constant flux. The definition of what is really new becomes quite arbitrary and, I think, quite important. It must represent some change from the median phenotype. I asked Joshua Lederberg when a virus is new, and he answered, "When it matters". Perhaps that is the best answer for now.

My next assertion is one that Robert May might quarrel with, although I hope not. It is that viruses have evolved with a definitive host to a relatively steady state and balanced relationship. As a consequence, perturbation of virus-host balance in the individual host usually reflects impairment of host resistance, rather than any change in viral phenotype or intrinsic virulence. This is a very complicated way of saying that more often than not, if you are looking at individual patients, when one case is more severe than the other, these reflect differences in host reaction, due to immunosuppression, age, or other factors.

On the other hand, when we consider epidemic disease, if we recognize an epidemic as being more severe, then in that instance we *should* suspect that a viral mutant is operating or that some peculiar environmental changes have affected that virus host interaction.

My last assertion is that new viral diseases usually are caused by old viruses, either infecting under changed ecologic circumstances—for example poliomyelitis and perhaps AIDS—or crossing species barriers, as with Marburg disease. Conversely, new viruses can cause old diseases, which influenza virus is constantly doing; a disease with stable and characteristic manifestations for centuries is caused, again, by continuously mutating agents that preserve, apparently, enough of their structure to maintain their classical pathogenicity.

Therefore, early detection depends on the detection of both viral and disease changes, so both the virus and disease have to be under surveillance. And since part of the purpose of all the work that went into this book has to do with anticipating, if we are going to anticipate anything, which I hope we can do, we are going to have to look at total ecologic surveillance, of virus, host, and environmental change.

PREMISES

Facts, Reasonable Assumptions, and Historical Precedents as
a Guide to Surveillance and Control of Emerging Viruses

1) Any virus is the statistical consensus of a heterogeneous
   population in constant flux. A "new" virus, therefore,
   must represent change from a median phenotype.

2) Viruses have evolved with their (definitive) hosts to a
   relatively steady state and balanced relationship. If inter-
   specific transfer of viruses occurs, adaptive constraints
   on viral virulence are removed.

3) Increased disease severity *in the individual case* usually
   reflects impairment of host resistance rather than change
   in intrinsic viral virulence.

4) Change in the mean severity of disease *as manifest in
   epidemics* usually reflects viral mutation and/or environmental changes affecting virus-host interaction.

5) *New viruses* can cause old diseases. For example, influenza, a disease whose cardinal characteristics have not
   changed for centuries, is caused by a constantly changing
   virus.

6) *"New" viral diseases* usually are caused by old viruses
   a) infecting under changed ecologic circumstances, or
   b) infecting an unaccustomed species.

CONCLUSIONS

From the above premises,

1) **early detection** of new viral diseases demands both viral
   and disease surveillance;

2) **anticipation** demands ecological surveillance of potential changes in virus-host relationships;

3) **control** depends upon planned response to detection.

Index

Dowdle, W., 39
Downs, W.G., 111
Drug resistance, 212-14
Drugs, 214, 274, 276
    AZT, 215
    malaria chemoprophylactic, 274
    Ribavirin, 151
    thalidomide, 284
Dubos, R., 55
Ducks, 40, 234-37, 291
Duesberg, P., 124
"Duns", 47
Dura mater donation, 112
Duvenhage-like virus, 110

E. coli, 8, 206
E1A, 84-86
E1B gene, 85
E4 protein, 86
Earth
    first biosphere, 203
    surface temperature, 262
Earthquake, Yerevan (1989), 281
East Anglia, 184
Eastern equine encephalitis virus (EEE) , 19,
    147, 210, 242-43, 292
    geographic distribution, 242
    recombination in, 292
    relationship to WEE, 243
Eating customs, 182
Ebola virus, 25, 51, 113,115, 159-73, 270, 285
    antigen, 168
    causes for multiple introductions, 172
    disease, 285
    Ebola-like filoviruses, 164
    emergence of, 173
    identification of, 167
    impediments to research, 163
    infected animals dying, 168-70
    isolation and naming, 162
    monoclonal antibodies, 166
    morphology, 53
    strains, 165, 168, 172-73
Ecchymosis, 150
Ecology, 31, 46, 141, 265, 267, 292, 294-95
Ecosystem, 35, 55, 109-11, 267
Ecuador, 146
Edinburgh, 185
Education, health, 182
Edwards, F., 254
EEE. *See* Eastern equine encephalitis
Egypt, 32, 114, 143, 144
Eigen, M., 208, 212, 221
"EIWG", 276, 280
Electrolyte imbalance, 150
Electron microscopy, 91, 92ff., 165, 166, 169,
    208
Electrophoresis, denaturing gradient gel, 232

ELISA, 97, 100, 151, 154, 166-73, 188-89, 279
Emerging viruses, 10-20, 24-26
    definition, 10
    examples, 13-14, 113
Emergency situations,
    responses to, 273
Encephalitis, 73, 77, 110, 116-17, 141, 143
    in Brazil, 141
    by California group viruses, 253, 255-59
    Eastern equine encephalitis virus, 19,
        147, 210, 242-43, 292
    Japanese, 18
    LaCrosse, 11
    New World alphaviruses and, 241
    Rocio, 140
    St. Louis, 140, 142
    Venezuelan equine (VEE), 18, 146, 265
    western equine (WEE), 12, 138, 147, 241-
        43, 253, 292
    in Zimbabwe, 110
Encephalomyelitis. *See* Encephalitis
Endosymbiosis, 6
Endothelial cell, 162, 172
Enhancer sequences, 80-3, 292
Enteric infections, 34
Enterovirus, 209. *See also* Polio
Entry portals, 75
Envelope, 131-32, 242, 244
    HIV, 131-32
Environment
    altered conditions, 23, 142, 147, 264, 294-
        95
    environmental issues, 261
    factors affecting transmissibility, 138
    impacts on, 148
Environmental Protection Agency, 267
Enzootic cycles, 139
Enzyme
    activity, 91
    immunoassays. *See* ELISA
Eocene epoch, 252
Ependyma, 77
EPI, 20, 285
Epidemic. *See also* Epizootic
    curve, 60, 291
    e.-driven variation, 130
    Goddess of, 34
    model, 287
Epidemic Intelligence Service (EIS), 22, 274,
    284, 286
Epidemiological research centers (ERCs),
    280-82
Epidemiologists, 274, 285
Epidemiology, 25, 138, 274-88
    of hantaviruses, 156
    of primate filovirus epidemics, 171
Epifluorescence microscopy, 102
Epithelial cells, 75, 80-81

STD clinics, 122
Stenella, 184
Stomach, 74
Stomata, 266
Strauss, J. H., 12, 138, 291
Streptomycetes, 6
"Strong stop", 221
Suárez, Casa, 52
Subacute sclerosing panencephalopathy
    (SSPE), 73
Sudan, 53, 160, 163-64
    Ebola virus in, 163, 168, 171-72
    Rift Valley fever transported from, 113-4
Sumeria, 34
Superinfection, 145
Surface
    polysaccharides, 71
    receptors, 293
Surgeon General, 283
Surgeons General,
    of the military services, 275
Surgical care, 275
Surveillance, 21,118, 273-74, 285, 291-92, 294
    global disease, 21, 279-80, 295
    influenza, 21, 278
    monkeypox, 178, 181, 183
    polio, 286
    systems, 277, 283-85, 287-88
    technical expertise for, 273
SV40, 79-80, 130
"Swarm", 209, 221
Swelling, 141
"Swine flu". *See* Influenza
Swine vesicular exanthema, 16
Switzerland, typhoid, 285
Sylvan cycle, yellow fever, 48
Symbiosis, 3, 5
Symmetry, icosahedral, 198-99
Syncytia, 6
Synecology, 6
Synkaryosis, 6
Syphilis, 32
Syringes, unsterilized, 160, 162
Systemic lupus erythematosus, 115

T antigen, 81
T lymphocytes, 78, 81-82
T-cell epitopes, 78
Tahyna (TAH) virus, 253-54, 256-58
Talapoins, 128
Tandala (Zaire), 161
Tansmission, horizontal, 258
Tantalus, 125
"Target" sequence, 101
Tataguine, 111
Tautomeric forms of bases, 205
Taxonomic
    relatedness, 172

Taxonomic, *cont'd*
    systems for mosquitoes, 258
Taylor strain (influenza), 228
Telecommunications, 279, 282
"Telemedicine spacebridge", 281
Television, 279
Temin, H., 291
Temperature, 139, 262, 265
Temperature-sensitive (ts) mutants, 213
Tenochtitlan, 29-30
Teratocarcinoma cells, 82, 88
Ternstone, ruddy, 40
Tertiary period, 252
Tetanus, 285
Texas, 114
Thailand, 19, 131-32, 145, 171, 288
Thalidomide, 284
Thessaloniki (Greece), 152
Threshold phenomena, 60, 66
Thucydides, 32, 219
Ticks, 13, 139, 163, 253
    density, 141
Tiger mosquito, 14, 19, 146-47
Tires, 19, 112, 146-47
Tobacco mosaic virus (TMV), 247-48
Togaviridae, 13, 241
Toxins, 71
Traffic "signals", 23
Training, 278-79
Transcription, 80-83, 87, 105, 222. *See also*
    Reverse transcriptase; RNA polymerase
Transfer
    interspecies, 190-91
    passive, 163
Transformed cells, 104
Transmissibility, 67, 131, 138
Transmission
    aerosol, 171-72
    canine parvovirus, 196
    cycles, arbovirus, 138
    needle/syringe, 14, 73, 98, 112, 162
    transovarian, 139, 256-57
    vertical, 139, 143
Transport, 109, 187
    axonal, 76
    of infected vectors, 147
    to new ecosystem, 109
    to new geographic area, 109
Travel, 109-12,117, 220, 277, 287
Trees, 266
Triassic period, 252
Trinidad, 111, 142
Trivittatus (TVT) virus, 256
Tropics
    diseases, 117, 271, 278, 287
    dry seasons, 139
    New World, 256
    origins of N. Amer. mosquito, 254

CPSIA information can be obtained at www.ICGtesting.com
Printed in the USA
267539BV00001B/17/A